Hammertoes

Emily A. Cook • Jeremy J. Cook
Editors

Hammertoes

A Case-Based Approach

Springer

Editors
Emily A. Cook
Harvard Medical School
Mount Auburn Hospital
Cambridge, MA
USA

Jeremy J. Cook
Harvard Medical School
Mount Auburn Hospital
Cambridge, MA
USA

ISBN 978-3-319-16551-6 ISBN 978-3-319-16552-3 (eBook)
https://doi.org/10.1007/978-3-319-16552-3

Library of Congress Control Number: 2018967991

This Springer imprint is published by the registered company Springer Nature Switzerland AG
The registered company address is: Gewerbestrasse 11, 6330 Cham, Switzerland

Preface

As Aesop famously said, "familiarity breeds contempt," and the ubiquitous hammertoe deformity is proof to this statement as fact. We have attended many conferences, lectures, and workshops throughout our careers. At these meetings, we have often been surprised by the number of practitioners that ask for advice on the management of a complex digital deformity. Our ever-expanding expertise includes complicated multiplane limb deformity correction and ankle joint replacement, yet why should the statement "Nothing is as humbling as a hammertoe that has gone awry" still be true? The fact is that the biomechanics intrinsic to the toes are a marvel. The circumstances that disrupt that balance are equally complex which is why this book has been compiled.

The purpose of *Hammertoes: A Case-Based Approach* is to provide foot and ankle specialists with a comprehensive understanding of digital deformities of the foot and their management. An introductory chapter will establish the functional anatomy, while subsequent chapters provide a compilation of interesting cases and challenging pedal pathologies. The format is such that each case will present relevant clinical details that justify the subsequent decision-making and ultimately the final treatment option. The chapters are intended to be applicable for students and experts alike regardless of educational background.

In the initial stages of the process, it became apparent that to meet our lofty standards, we would need the expertise and most onerously, the time of our colleagues. We have assembled a virtual pantheon of experts and thought leaders to compile the information you now hold in your hands. It is with no small amount of pride that we can say that the contributing authors are drawn from diverse institutions, degrees, and far-flung locales. We cannot fully express our gratitude to them for their participation.

We recognize that surgery has a constantly evolving standard. Our objective is to provide a substantial foundation for the reader to draw from, with the understanding that time and knowledge march on. Although the details may change over time, we believe that principles expressed in these chapters may be applicable regardless of the technique or implant du jour. We encourage you to look at each chapter critically and see how it supplements your own current understanding. We hope that our efforts help you to continue to provide the exceptional care your patients deserve.

In the course of writing this book, one of the authors passed away. Bruce Richardson, PhD, served as the Dean for Preclinical Affairs at the California School of Podiatric Medicine at Samuel Merritt University. He masterfully taught human anatomy for decades with a kind spirit and a sharp wit. His list of accolades is a chapter unto themselves, but none greater than the living testament that his students, who improve the lives of patients everyday with the knowledge he provided. Several of the authors in this book owe their anatomic understanding to Dr. Richardson. We would like to dedicate this book to his memory and the spirit of education that was such an important part of his life.

Contents

Contributors

Gregory C. Berlet, MD, FRCS(C) Orthopedic Foot and Ankle Center, Westerville, OH, USA

Peter Blume, DPM Yale School of Medicine, New Haven, CT, USA

Melinda A. Bowlby, DPM Podiatric Section: Department of Orthopedics, Swedish Medical Center, Seattle, WA, USA

Michelle Butterworth, DPM, FACFAS Williamsburg Foot Center, Williamsburg Regional Hospital, Kingstree, SC, USA

Danielle N. Butto, DPM, AACFAS Trinity Health of New England Medical Group, Hartford, CT, USA

Saint Francis Hospital, Hartford, CT, USA

Thomas J. Chang, DPM Redwood Orthopedic Surgery Associates, Santa Rosa, CA, USA

Jeffrey C. Christensen, DPM Podiatric Section: Department of Orthopedics, Swedish Medical Center, Seattle, WA, USA

Ankle and Foot Clinics Northwest, Everett, WA, USA

Luke D. Cicchinelli, DPM Private Practice, Centro Clinico Quirurgico, Vigo, Spain

Emily A. Cook, DPM, MPH, FACFAS Harvard Medical School, Division of Podiatry, Department of Surgery, Mount Auburn Hospital, Cambridge, MA, USA

Jeremy J. Cook, DPM, MPH, FACFAS Harvard Medical School, Division of Podiatry, Department of Surgery, Mount Auburn Hospital, Cambridge, MA, USA

Robin Cook Harvard Medical School, Division of Podiatry, Department of Surgery, Mount Auburn Hospital, Cambridge, MA, USA

Drew Davidson, DPM McFarland Clinic, Ames, IA, USA

William T. DeCarbo, DPM, FACFAS St. Clair Orthopedic Associates, Pittsburgh, PA, USA

Lawrence A. DiDomenico, DPM, FACFAS Department of Surgery, St. Elizabeth Health Center, Youngstown, OH, USA

Northside Medical Center, Youngstown, OH, USA

Kris DiNucci, DPM, FACFAS Foot and Ankle Center of Arizona, Scottsdale, AZ, USA

Michael S. Downey, DPM, FACFAS Division of Podiatric Surgery, Penn Presbyterian Medical Center, Philadelphia, PA, USA

Department of Surgery, Temple University School of Podiatric Medicine, Philadelphia, PA, USA

The Podiatry Institute, Decatur, GA, USA

Private Practice, Philadelphia, PA/Southern NJ, USA

David Edwards, DPM Foot and Ankle Clinic, Logan, UT, USA

Mark Gilheany, B(Pod), G(Pod), FACPS Foot and Ankle Specialists, Traralgon, VIC, Australia

Kenneth Hegewald, DPM, AACFAS Cascade Orthopedics and Sports Medicine Center, Hood River, OR, USA

Christopher F. Hyer, DPM, MS, FACFAS Orthopedic Foot and Ankle Center, Westerville, OH, USA

Rene Hymel, DPM Baton Rouge General Hospital, Hammond, LA, USA

Robert Joseph, DPM, PhD, FACFAS Department of Podiatric Medicine and Radiology, Scholl College of Podiatric Medicine at Rosalind Franklin University of Medicine and Health Sciences, North Chicago, IL, USA

Rachel Baisch Kang, DPM The Foot and Ankle Center of Kirkland PLLC, Kirkland, WA, USA

Matthew Knabel Clinical Fellow in Surgery, Harvard Medical School, Department of Surgery, Mount Auburn Hospital, Cambridge, MA, USA

Adam Landsman, DPM, PhD Division of Podiatric Surgery, Cambridge Health Alliance, Cambridge, MA, USA

Harvard University, School of Medicine, Cambridge, MA, USA

Frank A. Luckino III, DPM, AACFAS Northeast Ohio Foot and Ankle Specialists, Canton, OH, USA

Mercy Medical Center, Canton, OH, USA

Elena Manning, DPM Department of Surgery, Division of Podiatry, Mount Auburn Hospital, Cambridge, MA, USA

Trevor S. Payne, DPM Private Practice, Augusta Foot & Ankle, PC, Evans, GA, USA

Eric G. Powell, DPM Podiatric Section: Department of Orthopedics, Swedish Medical Center, Seattle, WA, USA

Minor and James Surgical Specialists, Seattle, WA, USA

Christopher L. Reeves, DPM, FACFAS Florida Hospital, Winter Park, FL, USA

Bruce A. Richardson, PhD California School of Podiatric Medicine, Samuel Merritt University, Oakland, CA, USA

Douglas H. Richie Jr, DPM, FACFAS, FAAPSM Department of Biomechanics, California School of Podiatric Medicine at Samuel Merritt University, Oakland, CA, USA

Michael A. Rivera, DPM Memorial Hospital West, Pembroke Pines, FL, USA

Barry Rosenblum, DPM Beth Israel Deaconess Medical Center, Division of Podiatry, Department of Surgery, Harvard Medical School, Boston, MA, USA

Thomas S. Roukis, DPM, PhD, FACFAS Orthopaedic Center, Gundersen Health System, La Crosse, WI, USA

Nicholas D. Ryan, B.Pod (Hons) B. App Sci Footlab+, Ringwood, VIC, Australia

Ryan T. Scott, DPM, FACFAS The CORE Institute, Phoenix, AZ, USA

Michael L. Sganga, DPM, AACFAS Orthopedics New England, Natick, MA, USA

Amber M. Shane, DPM, FACFAS Orlando Foot and Ankle Clinic, Orlando, FL, USA

Simon E. Smith, B.Pod, M.Pod, FACPS Australasian College of Podiatric Surgeons, Melbourne, VIC, Australia

Mickey D. Stapp, DPM Private Practice, Augusta Foot & Ankle, PC, Evans, GA, USA

The Podiatry Institute, Decatur, GA, USA

Eric Swenson Clinical Fellow in Surgery, Harvard Medical School, Department of Surgery, Mount Auburn Hospital, Cambridge, MA, USA

Joshua D. Thun, DPM, AACFAS Western Orthopedics and Sports Medicine, Grand Junction, CO, USA

Christopher P. Tveter, MD, FRCS(C) Beth Israel Deaconess Medical Center, Division of Podiatry, Department of Surgery, Harvard Medical School, Boston, MA, USA

Beau Vesely, DPM Krohn Clinic, Black River Falls, WI, USA

Jacob Wynes, DPM, MS, FACFAS Department of Orthopaedics, University of Maryland School of Medicine, Baltimore, MD, USA

Francesca Zappasodi, DPM Foot and Ankle Associates, Mooresville, NC, USA

Chapter 1
Anatomy of the Intermetatarsal, Lesser Metatarsophalangeal, and Lesser Interphalangeal Joints

Bruce A. Richardson, Matthew Knabel, and Eric Swenson

Intermetatarsal Joints

Both the bases and the heads of the lateral four metatarsals are connected by ligaments forming the intermetatarsal joints (IMJ). The adjacent sides of the bases of the second, third, fourth, and fifth metatarsals articulate with one another via plane synovial joints. The synovial joint cavity of the second and third IMJ is continuous with the cavity of the great tarsal joint. The joint cavity of the third and fourth IMJ is occasionally continuous with the cavity of the general tarsal cavity and in other instances is continuous with the cavity of the lateral tarsometatarsal joint. The joint cavity of the fourth and fifth IMJ is continuous with the cavity of the lateral tarsometatarsal joint between the fourth and fifth metatarsal and the cuboid [1].

Articular surfaces do not exist between the metatarsal heads as they do not come close enough to one another to truly articulate. They are held together, however, by the deep transverse metatarsal ligament (Fig. 1.1a, b).

Components of the Intermetatarsal Joints

The bases of the four lateral metatarsals are connected by the dorsal intermetatarsal, plantar intermetatarsal, and interosseous intermetatarsal ligaments. The first metatarsal is connected with the second by interosseous fibers only; the fibers are weak and may be largely replaced by a bursa between indistinct facets on the two bones.

B. A. Richardson
California School of Podiatric Medicine Samuel Merritt University, Oakland, CA, USA

M. Knabel (✉) · E. Swenson (✉)
Clinical Fellow in Surgery, Harvard Medical School, Department of Surgery, Mount Auburn Hospital, Cambridge, MA, USA
e-mail: mknabel@mah.harvard.edu; eric.swenson@mah.harvard.edu

E. A. Cook, J. J. Cook (eds.), *Hammertoes*,
https://doi.org/10.1007/978-3-319-16552-3_1

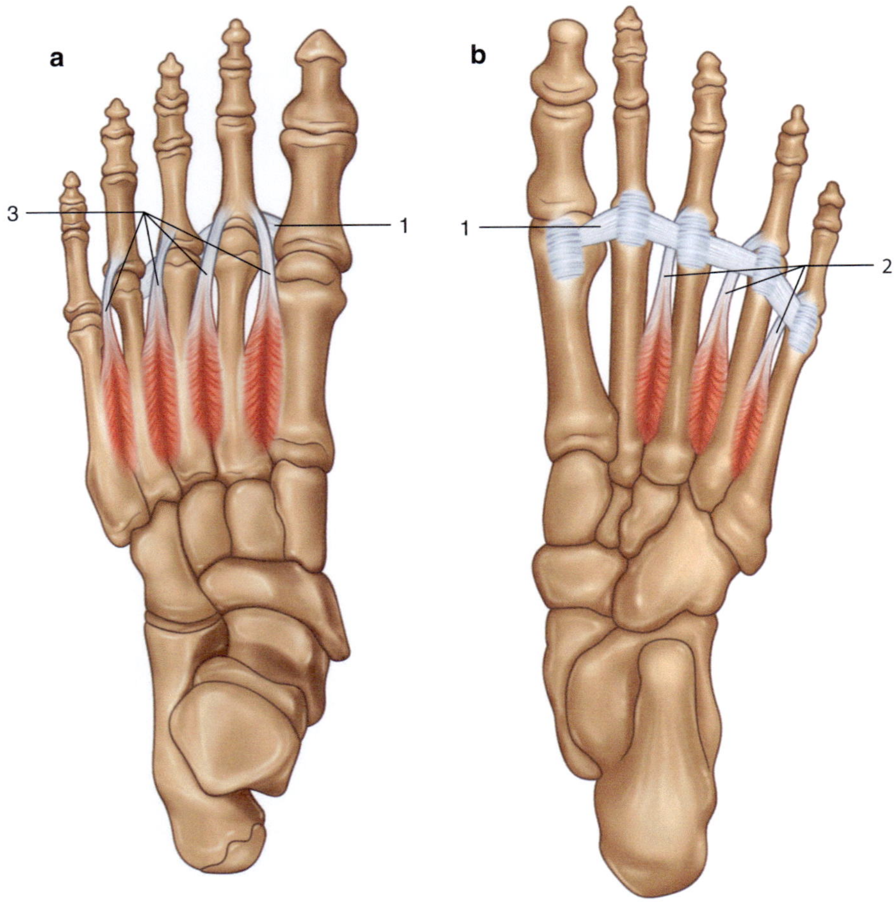

Fig. 1.1 (**a, b**) 1. The deep transverse metatarsal ligament connects the metatarsal heads. 2. Plantar interossei adduct toes 3–5 toward the midline of the foot. 3. Dorsal interossei abduct the toes away from the midline (second toe) of the foot. Both dorsal and plantar interossei lie dorsal to the deep transverse metatarsal ligament

The dorsal intermetatarsal ligaments pass transversely between the dorsal surfaces of the bases of the adjacent metatarsal bones. The plantar intermetatarsal ligaments extend transversely between the plantar surfaces of the bases of the adjacent metatarsal bones. The plantar ligaments are the stronger of the two sets being thicker than the dorsal ligaments. The strongest of the ligaments are the interosseous intermetatarsal ligaments. These ligaments attach to the non-articular areas of the adjacent metatarsal bases of the second, third, fourth, and fifth metatarsals.

The deep transverse metatarsal ligament extends medially as far as the lateral side of the head of the first metatarsal and laterally as far as the medial side of the head of the fifth metatarsal (Fig. 1.1). The fibers of the ligament are primarily connected to the plantar aspects of the metatarsophalangeal joints via the edges of the plantar plates.

Movements of the Intermetatarsal Joints

Gliding movements between the adjacent sides of the bases of the second, third, fourth, and fifth metatarsals occur at the IMJs. Although these movements are slight, they are important in that they contribute to movements of the forefoot relative to the midfoot and hindfoot, especially in forward propulsion and in excess weight-bearing, such as carrying a heavy object [2].

Innervation of the Intermetatarsal Joints

Innervation of the IMJs is provided by branches of the lateral plantar nerve and of the deep peroneal nerve [3].

Lesser Metatarsophalangeal Joints

The metatarsophalangeal joints (MTPJ) are of the condyloidal (ellipsoidal) synovial type. The MTPJs are both anatomical and functional joints in that they are true synovial joints, but each brings about significant movements or functions of the forefoot. They are formed by the reception of the rounded distal heads of the five metatarsal bones in the shallow cavities of the proximal bases of the five proximal phalanges. The lesser MTPJs are the articulations of metatarsals II through V with the corresponding proximal phalanges.

Components of the Lesser Metatarsophalangeal Joints

The joint surfaces of both the metatarsals and proximal phalanges are roughly oval in shape, with the head of the metatarsal contributing to the convex portion of the joint and the base of the proximal phalanx forming the concave portion. While the first MTPJ possesses sesamoid bones that are constant and contribute to the articular surfaces of this joint, the presence of sesamoids within the joint capsules of the lesser MTPJs is variable. The most common occurrence is at the second (1–1.6% of cases examined), fourth (2%), and fifth (11%) MTPJs. When present, typically there is one sesamoid of the second, one of the fourth, and two of the fifth MTPJ (Fig. 1.2). These sesamoids tend to be embedded within the joint capsules and the tendons of the short flexors of the toes [4, 5].

A loose fibrous joint capsule lined with a synovial membrane surrounds each MTPJ. The capsules are distinct dorsally and are attached further proximally on the plantar surfaces of the metatarsals than on the dorsal surfaces of the metatarsals. Dorsally, the capsule attaches very near the edge of the articular surface of each of the metatarsals and passes distally to attach near the dorsal edge of the articular surface of each of the proximal phalanges. The capsule in this region is very thin and is reinforced by the tendons of the long extensor muscles of the anterior leg. The tendons begin to expand into fibrous sheets at, or near, the MTPJs and are called extensor expansions. Occasionally situated between the tendons and the joint capsule dorsally are bursae [2]. On the plantar surface, the capsule attaches quite proximally on the metatarsal heads, approximately 5 mm posterior to the border of the

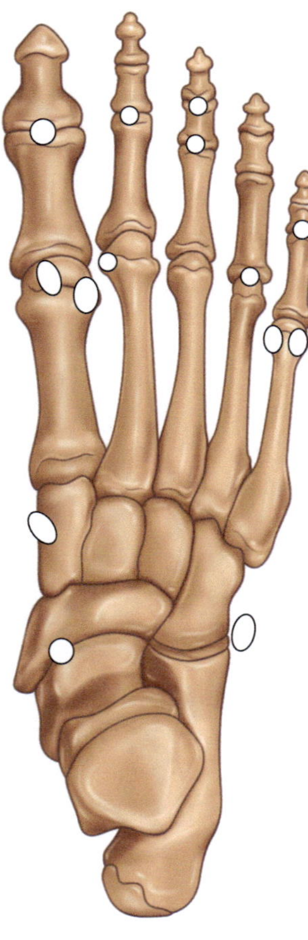

Fig. 1.2 The presence of lesser MPJ and IPJ sesamoids is variable

articular surface. Distally, the plantar portion of the capsule attaches near the plantar edge of the articular surface of the proximal phalanx.

Plantar metatarsophalangeal (MTPJ) ligaments (plantar plates, see below) reinforce the inferior aspect of the capsule and completely blend with it. The capsule is reinforced laterally and medially by strong metatarsophalangeal collateral ligaments as well as lateral and medial metatarsoglenoid suspensory ligaments [6]. The collateral ligaments also serve to restrict abduction and adduction as well as rotation at the joints (Fig. 1.3).

Plantar Plate and Collateral Ligaments

There are many different names for the plantar plates and collateral ligaments, and there is no standardized nomenclature. As described below, the plantar plate has also been called the plantar metatarsophalangeal ligament, plantar pad, and glenoid ligament. The medial and lateral proper collateral ligaments which run from the metatarsal to the phalanx are also simply called the metatarsophalangeal collateral ligaments. And finally, the medial and lateral accessory collateral ligaments which run from the metatarsal to the plantar plate are also called the metatarsoglenoid ligament or suspensory ligament (Figs. 1.3 and 1.4).

There are no dorsal ligaments per se, but the dorsal aspect of the capsules is reinforced by the extensor tendons and their expansions. The plantar metatarsophalangeal ligaments contribute to the overall strength of the plantar aspect of the capsule and are specialized in that they are partially fibrocartilaginous and form the

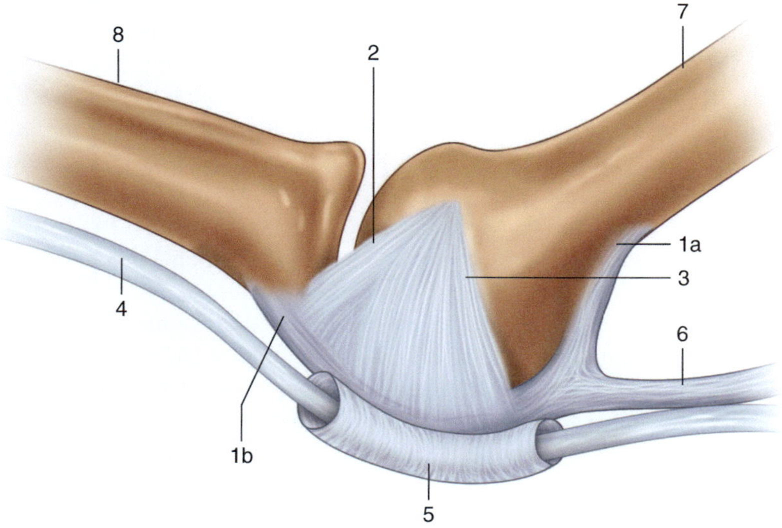

Fig. 1.3 Plantar plate and collateral ligaments. Labels: 1A = plantar plate origin (thinner), 1B = plantar plate insertion (thicker), 2 = proper collateral ligament, 3 = accessory collateral ligament, 4 = flexor tendons, 5 = flexor tendon sheath, 6 = plantar aponeurosis attaching into the plantar plate, 7 = metatarsal, 8 = proximal phalanx

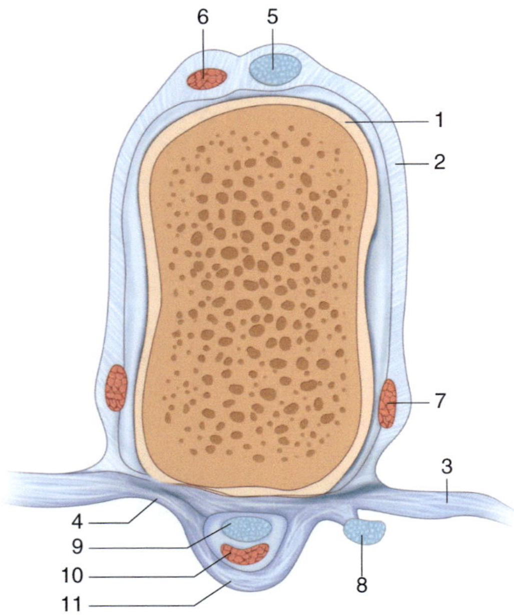

Fig. 1.4 Cross section of the metatarsophalangeal joint. Labels: 1 = joint capsule, 2 = extensor expansion with the sling and wing, 3 = deep transverse metatarsal ligament, 4 = plantar plate, 5 = EDL, 6 = EDB, 7 = interossei within the extensor sling, 8 = lumbrical with connections to the plantar plate, 9 = FDL, 10 = FDB, 11 = flexor tendon sheath

plantar plates, or plantar pads, of the MTPJs. The deep transverse metatarsal ligament attaches to the sides of the plantar plate between adjacent metatarsals (Fig. 1.4). The medial and lateral suspensory or metatarsoglenoid ligaments are also very strong and extend from the more dorsal aspects of the metatarsals to the sides of the plantar plate to which they attach [6] (Fig. 1.4). The plantar MTPJ ligaments, or glenoid ligaments, which form the plantar plate, reinforce the capsule inferiorly and blend with it such that the deep surfaces of these ligaments are lined with synovial membranes. The plantar plates are fibrocartilaginous thickenings within the plantar ligaments that average 18.8 mm in length (mean 20 mm for the second and third toes; mean 17 mm for the fourth and fifth toes) [7]. Most research related to the plantar plates has been carried out on the second MTPJ. The plantar plates are composed primarily of type I collagen and a minimal amount of elastin fibers [8].

In the lesser toes, the plantar plates are located deep to the metatarsal head and serve as the central attachment for ligamentous, tendinous, and capsular structures at the MTPJs (Fig. 1.4). Each plate is tightly bound to the proximal phalanx by a thick medial and lateral longitudinal bundles of fibers that attach directly adjacent to the articular surface of the proximal phalanx, thus forming a socket for the head of the metatarsus. Proximally the plantar plates are loosely bound to the head of the metatarsals but have strong fibrous proximal attachments consisting of the collateral ligaments and plantar fascia [2, 7] (Fig. 1.3). These attachments permit the plantar plates to move with the phalanges during flexion and extension of the MTPJs (e.g., during ambulation). The superior surface of the plate is smooth which glides along the metatarsal head during ambulation [9]. The edges of the plantar plates of the second, third, and fourth MTPJs are attached to the deep transverse intermetatarsal ligament (Fig. 1.4). The medial edge of the plantar plate of the fifth MTPJ is also attached to the deep transverse intermetatarsal ligament. The inferior surface of each plantar plate of the lesser digits is marked by a smooth groove formed by the flexor tendons as they cross the joint. The superior surface of the deep fibers of the central slip of the plantar aponeurosis of the foot also attaches to the inferior aspect of each of the plantar plates to form a sheath around the flexor tendons (Fig. 1.3).

The collateral ligaments of the lesser MTPJs are paired and triangular-shaped ligaments that extend from the tubercles on the dorsolateral and dorsomedial aspects of the metatarsals to tubercles on the lateral and medial plantar aspects of the bases of the proximal phalanges (Fig. 1.3). To distinguish the collateral ligaments from the adjacent paired metatarsoglenoid ligaments, Sarrafian refers to them as the metatarsophalangeal collateral ligaments [6]. Deland et al. refer to these ligaments as lateral and medial proper collateral ligaments [7]. Sarrafian describes the metatarsoglenoid ligaments as passing from the inferior aspects of the tubercles on the metatarsals to the medial and lateral sides of the plantar plates. The metatarsoglenoid ligaments are also referred to as suspensory ligaments as they assist in the suspension of the plantar plates [6]. Deland et al. call the suspensory ligaments accessory collateral ligaments [7]. The metatarsoglenoid ligaments fan out as they pass inferiorly to suspend the plantar plates and blend with the more anterior metatarsophalangeal collateral ligaments [6, 10]. Loretz and colleagues found in the dissection of 103 lesser MTPJs that the collateral and suspensory ligaments are distinct structures at proximal attachment to the metatarsal tubercles and blend distally with one another in 68% of the cases. In all dissections, the collateral ligaments attached to the tubercles of the proximal phalanges distally. In 32% of the joints dissected, the collateral and suspensory ligaments were fused together throughout their course and appeared as one triangular-shaped ligament [10] (Fig. 1.3).

The four lumbricals insert, in part, into the distal plantar aspect of tibial side of the plantar plate. Both plantar and dorsal interossei possess fibers that insert into the plantar plates as well [7]. Deland and colleagues also reported that fibers of the tendons of the transverse head of the adductor hallucis, flexor digiti minimi brevis, and abductor digiti minimi attach to the plantar plates of the lesser toes. Moreover, the flexor digitorum longus (FDL) and flexor digitorum brevis (FDB) tendons and the extensor hood and sling are also closely associated with the plantar plates of the lesser toes and contribute to the stability of the MTPJs [9]. Johnson et al. observed the flexor tendon sheath is situated centrally within the shallow groove on the superior surface of the plantar plate and is firmly anchored by a fibrous pulley. The FDB tendon, which splits to accommodate the FDL tendon at the proximal interphalangeal (PIP) joint, is inferior to the FDL tendon with the FDB inserting bilaterally onto the middle phalangeal base and the FDL inserting onto the inferior surface of the distal phalanges [8] (Fig. 1.5).

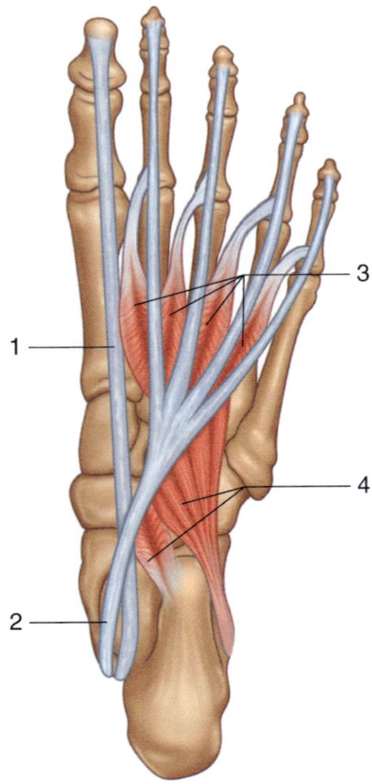

Fig. 1.5 Plantar foot containing the FDL, FHL, quadratus plantae, and lumbricals (not all four layers of the plantar muscles are shown). Labels: 1 = FHL, 2 = FDL, 3 = lumbricals (all four lumbricals lie plantar to the DTML, 4 = quadratus plantae

The extensor hood and sling is the fibroaponeurotic expansion of the extensor digitorum longus (EDL) tendon sheath and insert directly onto the plantar plate, the deep transverse intermetatarsal ligament, and the base of the proximal phalanx (Fig. 1.6a, b). The extensor mechanism, along with the lumbricals and interosseous tendons, contributes to the stability of the MTPJ in stance and during ambulation [11].

The anatomical unit consisting of the proximal phalanx, the plantar plate, the collateral ligaments (both proper and accessory), and the attachments of the above muscles, fibroaponeurotic dorsal expansion, and deep transverse intermetatarsal ligament is referred to by Sarrafian and colleagues as the phalangeal apparatus and represents the main articular unit of the ball of the foot [6].

Functionally, the plantar plates (phalangeal apparatus; see above) of the lesser metatarsophalangeal joints play a significant role in the stability of the lesser MTP joints as well as sustaining substantial tensile loads in the longitudinal direction making up an integral part of the windlass mechanism [7]. In addition, the fibrocartilaginous makeup of the plantar plates permits them to withstand compressive loads, thereby acting supportive articular surfaces for the metatarsal heads, similar to the menisci in the knee. Clinically, the plantar plates are also important in that pathological changes to the plates can lead to metatarsalgia, MTPJ instability, plantar plate rupture, and toe deformities such as hammertoe, claw toe, and medial crossover toe deformity [9].

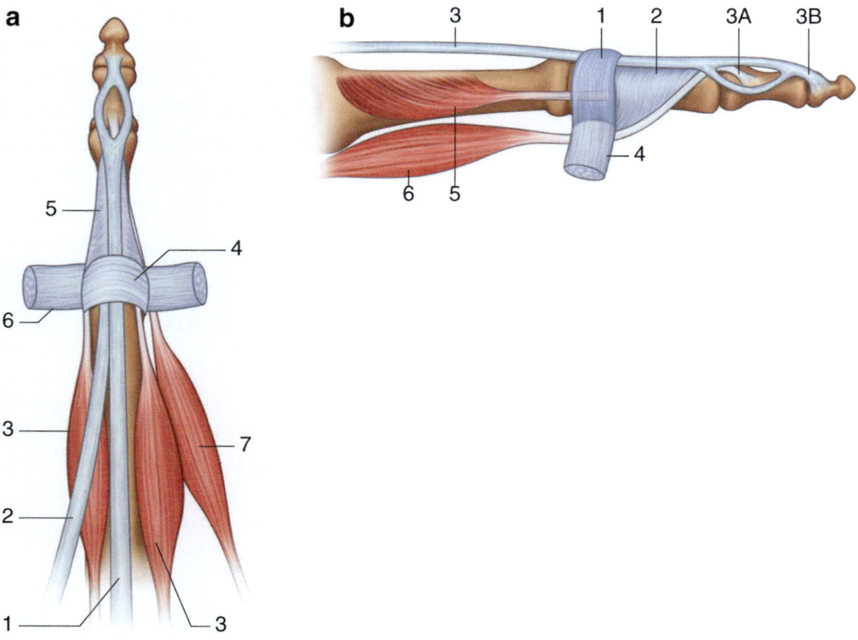

Fig. 1.6 (**a**, **b**) Top and side views. (**a**) top view labels: 1 = EDL, 2 = EDB, 3 = interossei (second MTPJ), 4 = extensor sling, 5 = extensor wing or hood, 6 = DTML, 7 = lumbrical. (**b**) side view labels: 1 = extensor sling, 2 = extensor wing or hood, 3 = EDL, 3A = central slip middle phalanx insertion of the EDL, 3B = terminal slip distal phalanx insertion of the EDL, 4 = DTML, 5 = interossei, 6 = lumbrical

Movements of the Lesser Metatarsophalangeal Joints

The lesser MTPJs are biaxial ellipsoidal joints; therefore movement is about two axes. One axis is in the transverse and frontal planes, perpendicular to the sagittal plane, permitting movements of plantar flexion and dorsiflexion or flexion and extension. The other axis is in the sagittal and frontal planes, perpendicular to the transverse plane, permitting the movements of abduction and adduction. The metatarsophalangeal collateral and suspensory ligaments function to restrict the degree of plantar flexion and dorsiflexion of these joints (Loretz et al. 1984). In addition, the suspensory ligaments, as a result of their attachment to the plantar plate, assist in the control of abduction and adduction. The glenoid ligament/plantar plate unit moves with the MTPJ through extension and flexion.

The range of extension at the MTPJs is much greater than that of flexion, while the range of abduction and adduction is quite small. The range of extension is 50–60°, while that of flexion is 30–40° [2]. When the foot is in the plantigrade position, the MTPJs are extended by about 25°, as the proximal phalanges are angled anterosuperiorly from the metatarsal heads which are in contact with the ground.

Some degree of abduction accompanies extension. Adduction and abduction also occur as independent movements, but their ranges are quite limited. As in the hand, the freest ranges of movement for abduction and adduction occur when the MTPJs are extended as this optimizes the line of pull of the interossei muscles which act to abduct and adduct most of the lesser digits. Even in this position, however, abduction and abduction of the toes is quite limited [12]. The abductor digiti minimi and the third plantar interosseous muscle act to abduct and adduct the fifth toe.

Innervation of the Lesser Metatarsophalangeal Joints

Innervation of the MTPJs is provided by the deep branch of the lateral plantar nerve and the medial plantar nerve to the second, third, and fourth MTPJs. The fifth MTPJ is supplied by the superficial branch of the lateral plantar nerve and the lateral dorsal cutaneous nerve. In addition, the lateral dorsal cutaneous nerve also assists in the innervation of the fourth MTPJ, and the deep peroneal assists in the innervation of the second MTPJ [3].

Blood Supply of the Lesser Metatarsophalangeal Joints

Nonunion, delayed union, and avascular osteonecrosis of the lesser metatarsal head are possible complications of distal osteotomies of the lesser metatarsal. These complications are a result of iatrogenic disruption of the blood supply [13]. Thus, knowledge of the vascular supply to the MTPJs is important when correcting various deformities such as claw toe deformities and metatarsalgia by distal osteotomies of the lesser metatarsals.

The metatarsal heads receive their blood supply from two main sources: the dorsal and plantar metatarsal arteries, both of which are branches of the posterior tibial artery. Petersen and colleagues also showed that the intraosseous arterial supply of the metatarsal head differs from that in the diaphysis. There are numerous arterial anastomoses between the vascular network of the bone and periosteum, whereas the arterial supply of the head consists of terminal end arteries. Thus, the metatarsal beads are more susceptible to osteonecrosis as a result of vascular injury than the diaphysis [13].

Interphalangeal Joints

The interphalangeal joints of the toes (IPJ) are the articulations between the proximal and middle and middle and distal phalanges of the lesser toes and between the proximal and distal phalanges of the hallux. They are all ginglymus or hinge joints that have their axes of movement in the frontal and transverse planes, perpendicular to the sagittal plane, permitting plantar flexion and dorsiflexion or flexion and extension of the toes. Typically, there are nine IPJs per foot, two for each of the lesser digits and one for the hallux. The two in each of the lesser toes are referred to as proximal and distal IPJs. In approximately 40% of the population, the middle and distal phalanges of the fifth toe are fused; consequently, no distal IPJ exists [1].

Components of the Interphalangeal Joints

The head of each proximal and middle phalanx resembles a pulley, and the base of the middle and distal phalanges possesses a reciprocally curved double concavity that fits into the pulley. The phalanges of the toes are smaller than those of the fingers, and often the joints between the middle and distal phalanges in the more lateral toes are ankylosed and nonfunctional (see paragraph above).

Each IPJ possesses a joint capsule that is thin dorsally and thickened by ligaments plantarly and bilaterally. Dorsally, the capsules reinforced dorsally by the long extensor tendons as they pass to their insertion on the dorsal aspects of the middle and distal phalanges. The capsules are strengthened medially and laterally by collateral ligaments. These ligaments for the proximal IPJ extend from the tubercles on the dorsomedial and dorsolateral aspects of the proximal phalanx to medial and lateral tubercles on the plantar aspect of the base of the middle phalanx. For each distal IPJ, the collateral ligaments extend from the dorsomedial and dorsolateral tubercles on the middle phalanx to the medial and lateral tubercles on the base of the distal phalanx.

On the plantar surfaces, the IPJs are reinforced by strong fibrous plantar ligaments, similar to the plantar ligaments of the MTPJs [2]. Moreover, the plantar ligaments of the IPJs may be thickened by cartilage (plantar plates), similar to those of the MTPJs [3]. Generally, the capsules and ligaments of the IPJs are tighter than those of the MTPJs.

Although inconsistent, sesamoid bones may be associated with the IPJs. When present, they are most commonly found in the IPJs of the hallux and the proximal IPJs of the second and third toes (Fig. 1.2).

Movements of the Interphalangeal Joints

As hinge joints, the only movements permitted at the IPJs are flexion and extension. The range of motion for flexion is greater than extension, with the latter being limited by the plantar and collateral ligaments. Flexion and extension are more extensive at the proximal IPJ than the distal IPJ [2].

Innervation of the Interphalangeal Joints

Innervation of the IPJs is provided by the proper plantar and proper dorsal digital nerves. The medial dorsal cutaneous nerve assists in the innervation of the IPJ of the hallux, while the superficial branch of the lateral plantar nerve is sole innervation of the IPJs of the fifth toe [3].

Muscular Involvement in Movement and Stability of the Lesser MTPJ and IPJS

Both intrinsic and extrinsic muscles act on the lesser metatarsophalangeal and interphalangeal joints. This section organizes these muscles into those that are located within the dorsal and ventral surfaces of the foot and those that are located within the plantar surface of the foot.

Dorsal Foot Extrinsic and Intrinsic Muscles

Extrinsic and intrinsic muscles acting on the lesser MTPJ and IPJs are found on both the dorsal and ventral surfaces of the foot. On the dorsum, the following muscles act on the lesser MTP and IP joints.

Extensor Digitorum Longus (EDL)
This pennate muscle is situated at the lateral part of the anterior leg, located laterally to tibialis anterior and superficially to extensor hallucis longus (Fig. 1.7). It takes origin from the lateral condyle of the tibia, the proximal two-thirds to three-fourths of the anterior surface of the body of the fibula, the proximal part of the interosseous membrane, the fascia cruris, and the intermuscular septa between it and the tibialis anterior medially and the fibularis (peroneus) laterally. As the muscle passes distally, it becomes tendinous in the inferior part of the leg and travels deep to the superior extensor retinaculum where it divides into two tendons. Deep to the superior retinaculum, it travels with the peroneus tertius or fibularis tertius. It splits into four tendons as it passes deep to the inferior extensor retinaculum through the lateral loop along with the tendon of the peroneus tertius or fibularis tertius where they are enclosed in a synovial sheath. The four tendons pass distally to each of the four lesser toes (Fig. 1.7). As the tendons approach the heads of the metatarsals, they spread out as membranous extension expansions. Joining the lateral side of the tendons to the second, third, and fourth digits are the tendons of the extensor digitorum brevis (see below). The four tendons split further to insert on both the distal and middle phalanges forming parts of the extensor expansion complex (Fig. 1.6a, b). Extensor digitorum longus extends the

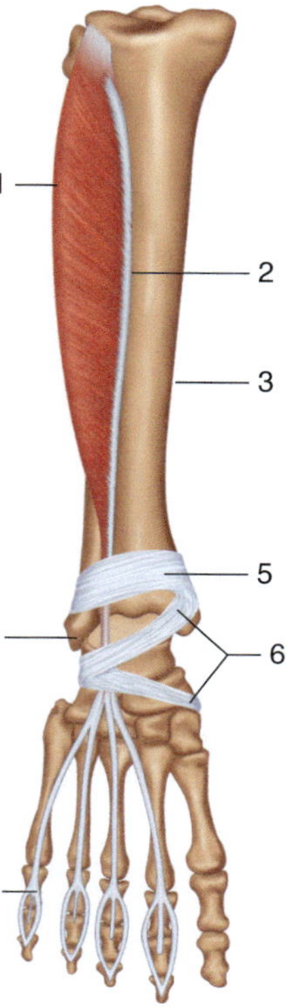

Fig. 1.7 Extensor digitorum longus. Labels: 1 = EDL, 2 = interosseous membrane, 3 = tibia, 4 = fibula, 5 = superior extensor retinaculum, 6 = inferior extensor retinaculum, 7 = EDL trifurcation with central slip insertion into the middle phalanx and terminal slip insertion into the distal phalanx

four lesser toes at the IP and MP joints. It also dorsiflexes the ankle and may al so be a minor evertor and/or pronator of the foot [12]. EDL is innervated by the deep fibular (peroneal) nerve and is provided with arterial blood from the anterior tibial artery.

Extensor Digitorum Brevis (EDB)

This muscle is broad and thin. It takes origin from a tubercle on the superolateral aspect of the calcaneus just anterior to the sinus tarsi. It also partially arises from the interosseous talocalcaneal ligament of the sinus tarsi and from the stem of the inferior extensor retinaculum. It passes diagonally across the dorsum of the foot medially and divides into four bellies and tendons which continue distally toward the first, second, third, and fourth digits. The most medial and largest tendon inserts onto the dorsal surface of the base of the first phalanx of the hallux and is called *extensor hallucis brevis*. The remaining slips insert into the lateral sides of the extensor digitorum longus tendons to the second, third, and fourth toes just distal to the MPJs of these digits and contribute to the extensor expansion (Fig. 1.6a, b).

EDB acts to assist the extension of the phalanges of the second, third, and fourth toes at the IPJs and MPJs. If EDL and EDB work alone without contribution of the plantar intrinsic muscles of the foot (e.g., lumbricals), they extend the MPJs by tightening the extensor sling and pulling the plantar pad up against the proximal phalanx and metatarsal. When in this position, they are unable to extend the IPJs because the wing of the extensor expansion is loose and the distal portions of the tendons are slack.

EDB is typically innervated by the lateral terminal branch of the deep fibular (peroneal) nerve (S1, S2). However, when an accessory fibular (peroneal) branch of the superficial fibular (peroneal) nerve is present, it may help to innervate EDB [14]. Blood is supplied by the lateral tarsal branch of the dorsalis pedis artery as well as the perforating fibular (peroneal) artery as it anastomoses with the lateral tarsal branch.

Plantar Foot Extrinsic and Intrinsic Muscles

The extrinsic and intrinsic muscles on the plantar surface of the foot that act on the IPJs and MPJs are as follows.

Flexor Digitorum Longus (FDL)
Found in the deep posterior compartment of the leg, this muscle is long and thin and takes origin from the posterior surface of the tibia, distal to the soleal line and medial to the vertical line, and from the fascia covering the muscles as well as the adjacent intermuscular septum. It is located medial to the tibialis posterior and flexor hallucis longus at its origin. As FDL narrows to a tendon distally, it passes superficial to the tendon of the tibialis posterior just superior to the medial malleolar sulcus. It then passes posterior to the medial malleolus in a groove along with tibialis posterior. At this point it is separated from the tibialis posterior tendon by a fibrous septum from the flexor retinaculum with each tendon being housed in its own synovial sheath. The FDL tendon continues distally into the foot to lie adjacent to the medial side of the sustentaculum tali, superficial to the calcaneotibial ligament. As it does so, it passes deep to the abductor hallucis and pierces the medial intermuscular septum of the plantar surface of the foot. At this point it also lies superficial to the tendon of flexor hallucis longus from which it frequently receives a tendinous slip (vinculum). It then expands, is joined by the quadratus plantae, and divides into four tendons which insert into the bases of the distal phalanges of the second, third, fourth, and fifth toes (Fig. 1.5). Each of these tendons passes through an opening in the corresponding tendon of the flexor digitorum brevis (see below) opposite the base of the proximal phalanx (Fig. 1.8).

FDL functions to flex the lesser four toes at the distal interphalangeal joints and, as it continues to contract, at the proximal interphalangeal joints and at the metatarsophalangeal joints, and, finally, it assists in plantar flexion of the ankle. FDL is innervated by the tibial nerve (S2, S3) and receives its blood supply via a muscular branch of the posterior tibial artery.

Flexor Digitorum Brevis (FDB)
The flexor digitorum brevis is situated deep to the central portion of the plantar aponeurosis from which it takes partial origin. It is also located between the medial

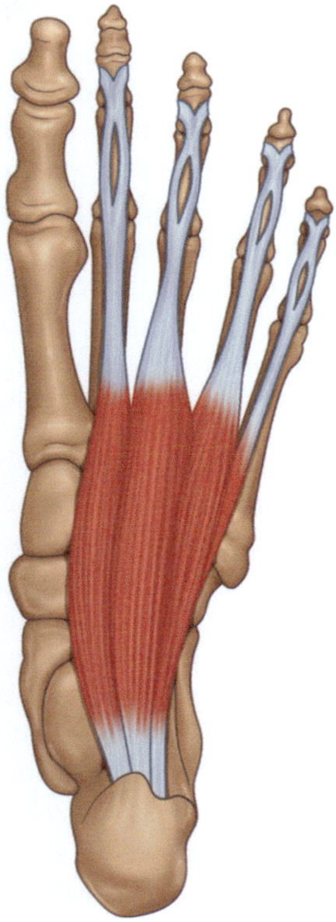

Fig. 1.8 The flexor digitorum brevis originates from the calcaneal tuberosity and plantar aponeurosis, divides into four tendon slips, and inserts into toes 2–5. Within each tendon slip, the FDB splits into two slips at the level of the proximal phalanx base, then reunites, and then splits again to insert onto the sides of the middle phalanges

and lateral intermuscular septa from which it also takes partial origin. Its deep surface is closely associated with the lateral plantar vessels and nerves by a thin fascial layer. It arises by a narrow tendon from the plantar aponeurosis, the medial and lateral intermuscular septa, and the medial process of the calcaneus tuberosity. The muscle runs distally in the center of the plantar aspect of the foot, and in approximately the middle of the sole of the foot, it divides into four tendons, one for each of the lateral four toes. Each of these tendons continues distally to run within the tendon sheaths of each of the corresponding tendons of FDL. At the bases of the proximal phalanges, each tendon splits into two slips. These slips diverge from one another to allow the passage of the tendons of FDL and then reunite distally, partially crossing over one another or decussating as they reunite and assist in forming a groove or channel for the tendon of FDL to which they now lie deep. The tendons of the FDB divide again and insert on the sides of the middle phalanges of the lesser toes (Fig. 1.8).

The FDB functions to flex the lateral four toes at the proximal interphalangeal joints. Continuing to contract, it will flex the proximal phalanges of the lesser four toes at the lesser MPJs. The FDB is innervated by the medial plantar nerve (L5, S1, S2). The medial plantar artery supplies the flexor digitorum brevis muscle.

Flexor Digiti Minimi (FDM)
Located in the lateral aspect of the third layer of muscles of the plantar foot, it arises from the base of the fifth metatarsal and from the sheath of the fibularis (peroneus) longus. It also takes origin from the plantar aponeurosis. The muscle travels distally parallel to the fifth metatarsal and inserts on the lateral side of the plantar aspect of the base of the proximal phalanx of the fifth digit along with the insertion of the abductor digiti minimi (see below). Deeper fibers often pass along the lateral aspect of the fifth metatarsal and may insert as part of the extensor expansion of the fifth digit or on the metatarsal shaft and head as a separate muscle sometimes referred to as *opponens digiti minimi*. The FDM flexes the proximal phalanx of the fifth digit at the MTPJ and helps to abduct the fifth digit.

Abductor Digiti Minimi (ADM)
The abductor digiti minimi lies along the lateral border of the foot with its medial margin adjacent to the lateral plantar vessels and nerves. It originates from the lateral process of the calcaneal tuberosity as well as, to some extent, from the medial process deep to the origin of the FDB. It also arises from the plantar surface of the calcaneus between the two processes, from the plantar aponeurosis as it passes to the fifth metatarsal, and from the lateral intermuscular septum. It then passes distally in the plantar surface of the foot along the lateral border and lateral longitudinal arch of the foot. Prior to its insertion, its tendon runs in a groove on the plantar surface of the fifth metatarsal. It inserts, along with FDM, into the lateral side of the plantar aspect of the base of the proximal phalanx of the fifth toe. The ADM, as its name implies, abducts the fifth toe and also helps to flex the fifth digit. ADM is innervated by the lateral plantar nerve (S 1, S2), the other terminal branch of the tibial nerve. Blood is supplied by lateral plantar artery (the other terminal branch of the posterior tibial artery).

Quadratus Plantae (Flexor Digitorum Accessories)
The quadratus plantae arises by two heads that are separated from each other by the calcaneal attachment of the long plantar ligament. The medial head is the larger and more muscular of the two heads and takes origin from the medial plantar surface of the calcaneus, inferior to the groove created by the tendon of flexor hallucis longus. The more tendinous and flatter lateral head arises from the lateral plantar surface of the calcaneus, just anterior to the lateral process of the calcaneal tuberosity and from the long plantar ligament. The two heads pass distally where they may join one another prior to inserting on the tendon of FDL just proximal to its point of dividing into four tendinous slips (Fig. 1.5). One variation is that the medial head joins the lateral head in part, while a medial tendinous slip extends to the FDL independently. In some cases, the medial head may fail to join the lateral head and, as a tendinous prolongation, may pass deep to the FDL and divide into slips to some of the digital tendons of the long flexor muscle.

Quadratus plantae acts to assist FDL in flexion of the distal phalanges of the lesser toes. It does so by helping to straighten the line of pull of the tendons of FDL so they have a more direct line of pull for flexion of the lesser toes [12]. Innervation is provided by the lateral plantar nerve (S2, S3). Blood is supplied by the lateral plantar artery.

Lumbricals

These are four small worm-shaped muscles that are accessory to the FDL, from which they arise, and are numbered one through four from the medial side of the foot. They tend to decrease in size from medial to lateral. As alluded to above, the lumbricals take origin from the tendons of FDL at the level of the separation of these tendons into four slips. Each lumbrical, except for the first (i.e., the most medial), originates from two adjacent tendons of FDL. The first lumbrical arises only from the medial aspect of the first tendinous slip of FDL. Each lumbrical then passes distally accompanying the tendon of FDL that lies lateral to the lumbrical. For example, the first lumbrical courses distally alongside the first slip of the FDL, while the second lumbrical passes alongside the second slip of the long flexor tendon and so forth. Each lumbrical crosses the medial side of its respective metatarsophalangeal joint and continues alongside the medial aspect of its respective digit (i.e., digits two through five) (Fig. 1.5).

The lumbricals all pass plantar to the deep transverse metatarsal ligament (Fig. 1.4). Each inserts into the medial aspect of the extensor expansion, somewhat more dorsally than plantarly. Thus, the first lumbrical inserts on the extensor expansion of the second toe, the second on that of the third toe, and so on. The lumbricals contribute to the wing portion of the extensor hood of each of these digits (Fig. 1.6b).

The actions of the lumbricals include flexion of the MPJ of digits two through five and extension of the IPJs of the same digits. The first lumbrical is innervated by the medial plantar nerve (L5, S 1), while two through four are innervated by the deep branch of the lateral plantar nerve (S1, S2). Blood supply is from the plantar metatarsal arteries, branches of the deep plantar arterial arch.

Plantar Interossei

Found in the fourth layer of the plantar aspect of the foot, there are three plantar interossei and four dorsal interossei (Fig. 1.1a, b). They are similar to the interossei of the hand, except that those of the hand are arranged relative to the third digit which is the midline of the hand, while those of the foot are arranged relative to the second digit which is the midline of the foot.

Lying inferior to the metatarsals, the plantar interossei take origin from the bases and medial sides of the shafts of the third, fourth, and fifth metatarsals. The second and third plantar interossei, in addition, may arise in part from the tendon sheath of peroneus longus. The plantar interossei insert on the medial sides of the bases of the proximal phalanges, the MPJ joint capsules, and the extensor expansions of the same digits from which they originate. All of the plantar interossei pass dorsal to or deep to the deep transverse metatarsal ligament (Fig. 1.1b).

The plantar interossei adduct (mnemonic, PAD) the third, fourth, and fifth toes toward the midline of the foot (i.e., second toe). They also assist in flexion of the proximal and extension of the distal phalanges of the third, fourth, and fifth toes. Innervation is provided by the superficial (third plantar interosseous) and deep branches of the lateral plantar nerve (S2, S3) (fourth and fifth plantar interossei).

Dorsal Interossei

Four in number, the dorsal interossei are situated more dorsal than the plantar interossei. Each of the four muscles is located in each of the interosseous spaces of the foot. Typically, they are bipennate and arise by two heads from the adjacent sides of adjacent metatarsals (Fig. 1.1a). For example, the first dorsal interosseous originates from the adjacent surfaces of the first and second metatarsals. The plantar interossei lie inferior to the lateral three dorsal interossei.

The posterior perforating arteries and the deep plantar artery pass along the posterior borders of each of the dorsal interossei as the two heads of origin of each muscle merge with one another. The two heads of each dorsal interosseous muscle converge on a central tendon that passes distally to insert on the base of the proximal phalanx and the extensor expansion of a certain digit (Fig. 1.1a). For example, the first dorsal interosseous inserts on the medial side of the proximal phalanx of the second digit, while the second dorsal interosseous inserts on the lateral side of the proximal phalanx of the second digit, the third dorsal interosseous inserts on the lateral side of the proximal phalanx of the third digit, and the fourth dorsal interosseous inserts on the lateral side of the proximal phalanx of the fourth digit. Like the plantar interossei, the dorsal interossei all pass dorsal to the deep transverse metatarsal ligament (Fig. 1.1a).

The dorsal interossei all function to abduct (mnemonic, DAB) the toes away from the midline of the foot (i.e., the second toes). Innervation to the dorsal interossei is provided by the deep branch of the lateral plantar nerve (S2, S3), except to the fourth dorsal interosseous which receives the superficial branch of the lateral plantar nerve. In addition, the first and second dorsal interossei each receive an extra nerve; the first dorsal interosseous receives a branch of the first interosseous nerve of the medial branch of the deep peroneal nerve, while the second interosseous receives a branch of the second interosseous nerve of the lateral branch of the deep peroneal nerve. There is some evidence that these additional twigs from the interosseous nerves are entirely sensory [12].

References

1. Draves DJ. Anatomy of the lower extremity. Baltimore: Williams & Wilkins; 1986.
2. Williams PL, Warwick R. Grey's anatomy. 36th ed. (British). Philadelphia: W. B. Saunders; 1980.
3. Gardner E, Gray DJ. The innervation of the joints of the foot. Anat Rec. 1948;161:141–8.
4. Bizarro AH. On sesamoid and supranumerary bones of the limbs. J Anat. 1921;55:256–67. Gardner E, Gray DJ, O'Rahilly R. Anatomy: a regional study of human structure. 4th ed. Philadelphia: W. B. Saunders; 1975.
5. Wood-Jones F. Structure and function as seen in the foot. London: Baillere, Tindall & Cox; 1949.
6. Kelikian AS. Sarrafian's anatomy of the foot and ankle. 3rd ed. Philadelphia: Wolters Kluwer/Lippincott Williams & Wilkins; 2011.
7. Deland JT, Lee KT, Sobel M, DiCarlo EF. Anatomy of the plantar plate and its attachments in the lesser metatarsal phalangeal joint. Foot Ankle Int. 1995;16(8):480–6.

8. Johnston RB 3rd, Smith DT. The plantar plate of the lesser toes: an anatomical study in human cadavers. Foot Ankle Int. 1994;15(5):276–82.
9. Umans HR, Eisinger E. The plantar plate of the lesser metatarsophalangeal joints: potential for injury and role of MR imaging. Magn Reson Imaging Clin N Am. 2001;9(3):659–69.
10. Loretz L, Gerbert J, Moss K. Significance of the suspensory and collateral ligaments in lesser metatarsal neck surgery. J Foot Surg. 1984;23:123–8.
11. Dalmau-Pastor M, Fargues B, Alcolea E, Martinez-Franco N, Ruiz-Escobar P, Vega J, Golano P. Extensor apparatus of the lesser toes: anatomy with clinical implications – topical review. Foot Ankle Int. 2014;35(10):957–69.
12. Hollinshead WH. Anatomy for surgeons: the back and limbs. Philadelphia: Harper & Row; 1982.
13. Petersen WJ, Lankes JM, Paulsen F, Hassenpflug J. The arterial supply of the lesser metatarsal heads: a vascular injection study in human cadavers. Foot Ankle Int. 2002;23(6):491–5.
14. Lambert EH. The accessory deep peroneal nerve. A common variation in innervation of extensor digitorum brevis. Neurology. 1969;19:1169–76.

Chapter 2
Biomechanics of Hammertoes

Jeffrey C. Christensen and Eric G. Powell

Overview

Hammertoe and related digital deformities are in most cases acquired digital conditions that appear to have genetic predisposition [1, 2]. While the occurrence of digital hammering is observed with other foot deformities such as cavus foot, flatfoot, and hallux valgus; it is not uncommon to see a normal-appearing foot to have isolated digital hammertoe deformities especially in a longer toe [3] (Fig. 2.1). Normal digital function involves a complex sequence of balanced events between powerful digital extensors and flexors and requires anatomic segmental alignment with functionally intact passive and dynamic stabilizers [4]. The development of hammertoes is an expression of compromised digital function; however, the precise etiological mechanism maybe unclear due to multifactorial influences over a variable time frame [5, 6]. Any functional deviation via muscle hyperactivity, motor weakness, anatomic malalignment, and/or structural compromise of stabilizing structures can lead to digital hammering, which can worsen over time. The basis of surgical treatment of digital deformities necessitates an understanding of the underlying biomechanical deficiency to ensure the best possible treatment outcome. A surgical plan without a rational mechanically based approach can potentially lead to overtreatment and unnecessary loss of function (Fig. 2.2a, b).

J. C. Christensen (✉)
Ankle and Foot Clinics Northwest, Everett, WA, USA

E. G. Powell
Minor and James Surgical Specialists, Seattle, WA, USA

E. A. Cook, J. J. Cook (eds.), *Hammertoes*,
https://doi.org/10.1007/978-3-319-16552-3_2

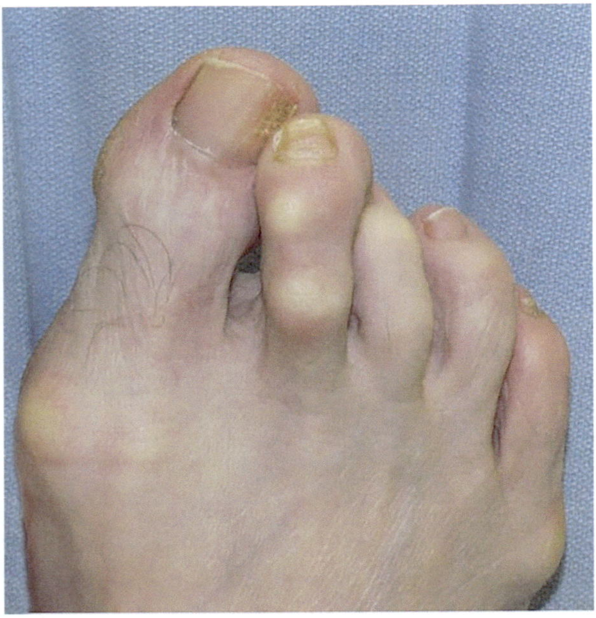

Fig. 2.1 Photograph of isolated second digital hammertoe associated with hallux valgus deformity. Second metatarsal overload from first-ray hypermobility or a long metatarsal segment can lead to mechanical compromise of the plantar plate and ultimately lead to digital hammering

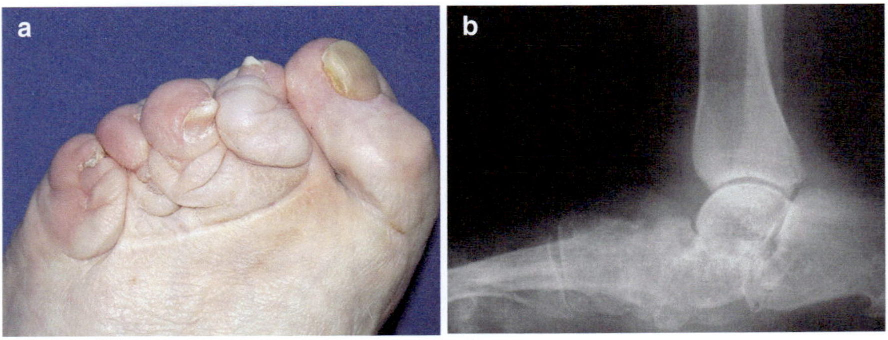

Fig. 2.2 (**a**) Photograph of a left foot deformity from an 80-year-old female with a history of pan digital base resections 40 years prior for moderate hammertoe deformities. Digital function including the windlass effect was fully lost, which further compromised foot function and arch integrity as the patient suffered a pure sagittal arch collapse. (**b**) Lateral radiographs from the same patient, illustrating sagittal collapse of arch with multi-segmental instability. The posterior tibial tendon was intact and had a normal appearance at the time of arch reconstruction, suggesting the loss of the windlass function contributed to arch collapse

Functional Role

It has been suggested that the role of digits in stance provides little benefit to foot function [7]. However, clinically in stance, as the foot is loaded, the plantar fascia tightens and the toes passively engage the ground maintaining a rectus segmental alignment with the proximal phalanx parallel to the ground. This action has been referred to as the reverse windlass and provides a preload to the arch segments creating stability in preparation for ambulation [8, 9]. While the first ray windlass function is clearly more powerful, the windlass effect of the lesser digits cannot be ignored [10]. When examining a normal lesser toe in stance, by action of the reverse windlass, individual toes will resist any effort to dorsiflex the proximal phalanx, at the metatarsophalangeal joint, while interphalangeal joint movements are supple. Dynamic motor influences are not active in this process. In gait, the role of normal lesser digital function becomes more evident. There is digital ground pressure for 75% of the gait cycle, and the digits collectively impart loads that are similar to the metatarsal heads [7]. While the toes are designed to purchase and remain stable on the ground, normal toe function provides a mechanism to stabilize the metatarsophalangeal articulations, which collectively is the primary fulcrum of the forefoot in gait mechanics [11]. Perhaps ever more important, the lesser toes as a byproduct of the windlass, significantly reduce dorsal stress to the metatarsal segments [12–14].

Anatomical Considerations

Stabilizing Structures

The plantar plate is the most important static stabilizer of the lesser digits [15–18]. It is a strong ligamentous structure on the plantar aspect of the metatarsophalangeal joint, that effectively extends the articular surface creating an acetabular-shaped socket for the metatarsal heads to rotate upon during propulsion (Fig. 2.3). There are several structures that attach to the plantar plate including the flexor sheath, the lumbrical, deep transverse intermetatarsal ligament, the plantar fascia, and the collateral ligaments. On the plantar plate of the fifth metatarsophalangeal joint, there is some minor insertion of the flexor digiti minimi brevis and abductor digiti minimi tendons to the fibular side of the fifth proximal phalanx base.

The anatomic layout is well described [17, 19, 20] and consists of the proximal plantar plate originating from the longitudinal septae and the associated vertical fibers extending from the superficial plantar aponeurosis [16] (Fig. 2.2). Distally, there is a lesser origination from the distal aspect of the metatarsal, just proximal to the articular cartilage plantarly with attachments to the periosteum in this area and a synovial recess for the proximal MPJ [19]. In the zone immediately plantar to the metatarsal head, the plantar plate is at its thickest ranging from 2 mm to 5 mm. As the plate progresses distally, it thins out and inserts onto the entire plantar base of the proximal phalanx directly into the bone. There is thickening of the plate at the margins both medially and laterally as it inserts onto the phalanx with central thinning noted. The shape of the plantar plate is trapezoidal to rectangular with the base oriented proximally. The plantar aspect of the plantar plate sees the flexor tendon sheath directly attached and forming the groove for the tendon sheath at this area. Medially and laterally, the deep transverse intermetatarsal ligament has direct attachments to the plantar plate. The medial and lateral collateral ligaments also attach to the plantar plate with a fanning out of the attachment to span onto the

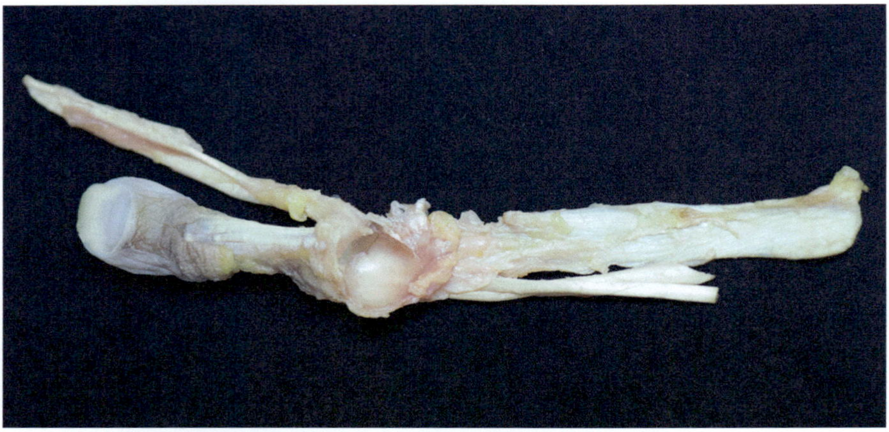

Fig. 2.3 Photograph of the dissected second toe with attached plantar plate and proximal slip of plantar fascia. Extensor tendons are reflected and the second metatarsal removed. Note acetabular shape of plate with fibrous tunnel for flexor tendons that are located superior to plantar fascia

medial and lateral phalangeal base as well. The mean width of the plantar plate averaged 11 mm proximally to 9 mm distally and the length averaged 19 mm [20].

In addition to the plantar plate, multidirectional stability is also achieved through a suspensory effect of the collateral ligaments, medial and lateral anchoring via deep transverse intermetatarsal ligament [16, 17]. This effectively creates a tie-bar system of ligaments to allow the forefoot to function as a unit [21]. A durable functional foot requires load sharing of digital supportive structures. Failure of these structures can occur with repetitive trauma, especially if individual joints are overloaded through various pathological mechanisms.

Extensor Tendon and Expansion

The extensor digitorum longus has dorsiflexory influence on the proximal phalanx through the action of the extensor sling apparatus [19]. This plays a contributory role in the progression of the hammertoe after plantar plate functional integrity is compromised. In situations where digital extensors are firing during forefoot loading, the extensors will have an antagonistic effect on the reverse windlass. If the reverse windlass is compromised, then extensor action will naturally contribute to a dorsiflexed alignment of the proximal phalanx in stance.

Deformity Progression

It is well described that digital deformities that include hammer or clawing of digits can be reducible (flexible), semi-reducible (semirigid), or non-reducible (rigid) in their presentation [6]. Clearly there is spectrum of deformity, which can be characterized by progressive dorsiflexion of the proximal phalanx and secondary interphalangeal contractures which individually progresses with time. It is generally accepted that long-standing deformities will undergo soft tissue contracture (including the skin) leading to a rigid deformity, which includes concomitant adaptive joint change [6, 22] (Fig. 2.4a). Dorsiflexion of the proximal phalanx combined with sagittal plane digital interphalangeal joint contracture induces an increase in retrograde forces plantarly onto the metatarsal heads. This plays a contributing role in the genesis of metatarsalgia, metatarsal stress fracture, and intractable plantar keratomas (Fig. 2.4b). While these are all common findings associated with prolonged hammertoe deformity, the true end stage of the disorder is total failure of the digital stabilizers, which results in digital dislocation at the metatarsophalangeal joint, which has a less frequent occurrence.

When a patient is examined in stance, irrespective of the etiological process involved, if the proximal phalanx remains dorsiflexed, it is certain that the natural length-tension relationship of the plantar plate/plantar fascia slip complex has been pathologically altered (Fig. 2.5). A hammer or claw toe deformity, with the foot plantigrade, cannot occur without compromise to this critical supportive unit. This is readily apparent when evaluating a patient with traumatic or iatrogenic shortening of a metatarsal resulting in floating toe [23–26]. Age-related deformity is however more difficult to appreciate because the rate of pathological change is more subtle. Simple but gradual thinning of the plantar plate centrally will allow the thicker portions of the plantar plate to migrate to the medial and lateral borders of the metatarsal head [21]. Therefore, the pulley effect of the metatarsal head is reduced (less arc of curvature), which effectively reduces the power of the windlass (as well as the

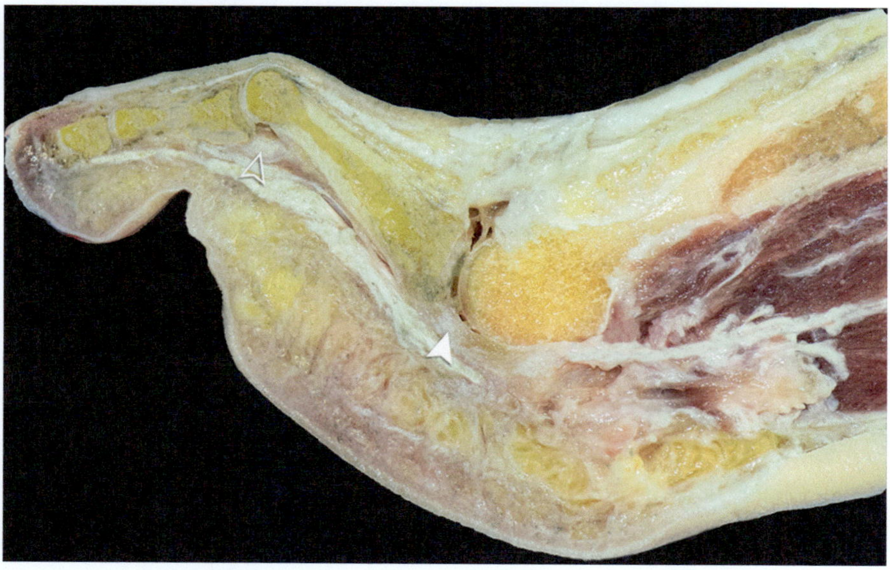

Fig. 2.4 Photograph of longitudinal section of a second ray with hammertoe deformity. The specimen age at death was 80 years. Note the plantar capsular thickening of the proximal interphalangeal joint and scarified appearance of plantar plate. This appearance is consistent with age-related attenuation of plantar plate (white arrowhead)

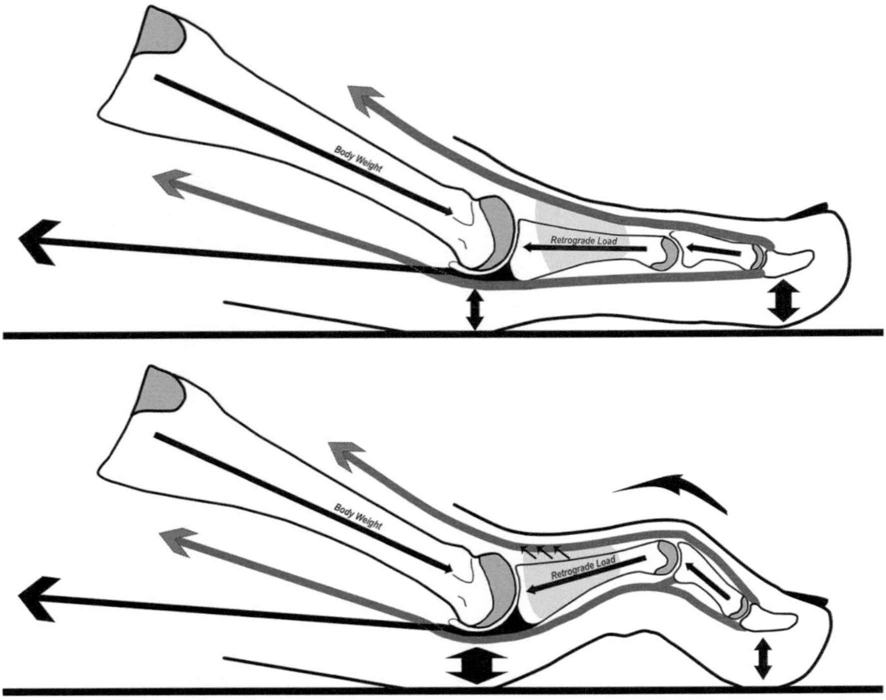

Fig. 2.5 Diagram of longitudinal section of a second ray. Note direction of force vector of hammertoe, where firing of digital musculature has capacity to generate plantarflexory retrograde pressure to the metatarsal head. Such retrograde pressure is associated with intractable plantar keratoma and plantar ulceration

reverse windlass). The plantar plate attenuation in these cases may require multiple decades before symptomatic hammertoe syndrome is clinically expressed. As the proximal phalanx migrates into a dorsiflexed position, any dynamic action of the digital flexors and extensors, whether normal or pathologic, can promote interphalangeal joint contracture, thus enhancing the deformity.

Etiological Factors

Hammertoe and related digital deformities have been thoroughly described in the past [6, 11, 22, 27, 28]. Various etiological mechanisms have been suggested when describing hammertoes, including shoe factors, structural variation, deformity, and trauma. Variability in deformity patterns can be observed between digits of the ipsilateral and contralateral foot. Multiple etiological factors can coexist and clinically cause confusing patterns of deformity.

Hallux Valgus and Hammertoes It is not uncommon to see the presence of a second toe hammering in conjunction with a hallux valgus deformity (Fig. 2.1). There are several plausible reasons for the occurrence. First with the formation of hallux valgus deformity, there is associated hypermobility of the first ray [29, 30]. With decreased ability to support ground load by the first metatarsal, there is greater than normal weight-bearing loads that are transferred over to the second ray [31]. This overload can gradually attenuate the plantar plate and allow the proximal phalanx to dorsiflex. If the overload is strictly absorbed by the second ray, the likely clinical expression will be an isolated hammering of the second digit. Additionally, as the hallux valgus progresses, the second toe position is encroached. Any loss or weakening of digital ground purchase can allow the hallux to underside the second toe and thus accelerate both deformities.

Metatarsal Parabola Abnormalities A relatively long metatarsal can lead to plantar plate attenuation and formation of an isolated hammertoe [32]. The long metatarsal head and periarticular structures are subjected to higher peak loads in propulsion and over time cause attenuation or frank tears to the plantar plate with repetitive microtrauma due to concentrated overload. Likewise, a short first metatarsal (Morton's foot) can also alter the load path to overload the lesser metatarsals [31, 33]. This also can cause mechanical overload of the second and third rays.

Shoe-Related Factors Digital deformity can be induced by restrictive shoes. The extreme of this effect is the use of shoe binding that inhibits foot growth and leads to foot as well as digital deformities [34]. As for modern shoe gear, women's dress shoes are believed to be significant contributors to the etiology of hammertoes [6, 35]. This perhaps occurs via digital crowding as a result of altered toe box volume that consists of nonanatomic shapes that focus on current fashion. Additionally, heeled shoes will clearly accentuate any aberrations of the metatarsal parabola.

Iatrogenic Effects Shortening of the first ray via amputation or surgical reconstruction can in some instance lead to formation of hammertoes. This occurs from a weakening or loss of the flexor hallucis longus tendon unit distal to the master knot of Henry. Flexor hallucis power can potentially be diverted through the master knot to the slips of flexor digitorum longus leading to hammertoe formation. Shortening of the first ray also can cause overload of the lesser rays especially second and third rays, which can also lead to attrition of the supportive mechanism digital tie-bar system. Furthermore, shortening of lesser metatarsals can induce floating toe. This is directly caused by loss of tension of the plantar plate and corresponding fascial slip and not from loss of structural integrity. In time a floating toe can progress to digital contracture with time.

Motor Imbalance Any pathological disorder that affects motor functional balance to intrinsic or extrinsic muscle function has the potential to develop hammertoes. Processes that result in altered or damaged motor function have a clear cause and effect relationship. However, processes that limit joint motion such as hallux rigidus or ankle equinus can create subtle motor imbalances between extrinsic digital musculature.

Equinus conditions have been reported to induce hammertoe deformity in neurologically intact extremities. While the exact mechanism for developing muscle

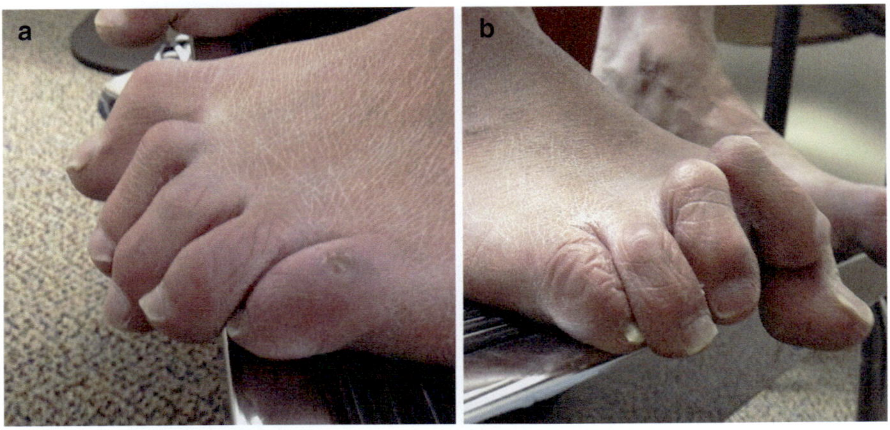

Fig. 2.6 Photograph of a patient standing on edge of a stool with digits overhanging. It is normal for toes to plantarflex with this maneuver. (**a**) Note in the asymptomatic left foot the proximal phalanges are in a rectus alignment parallel to the ground. (**b**) The symptomatic right foot there are hammertoe deformities 2/3, with dorsiflexed alignment of the proximal phalanx indicative to compromise of the reverse windlass mechanism. The second toe is end stage with dorsally dislocated at the metatarsophalangeal joint. The fourth and fifth toes are unaffected. Etiology of the hammertoes was osseous equinus from advanced ipsilateral post-traumatic ankle arthritis

imbalance is unknown, it is theorized that individuals recruit and overutilize EDL to assist tibialis anterior during functional activities during swing phase to assist with active ankle dorsiflexion to compensate for equinus contracture [27, 29] (Fig. 2.6).

Distal sensorimotor neuropathy like in diabetes affects the distal extremities particularly the lower extremity due to the longer neurons that are involved. This can create an intrinsic minus foot (progressively weakening foot instrinsics) [29]. While it is widely thought to lead to digital contracture, there are other mechanical factors that may be needed for this to occur [36].

Hereditary sensorimotor neuropathy or stroke-induced hemiparesis both have the tendency to develop a progressive cavus foot deformity [37]. Alteration in foot type architecture or muscle group spasticity can cause functional imbalance between flexors and extensor extrinsics leading to progressive digital contracture.

Trauma can lead to motor imbalance through direct nerve injury, muscle contracture seen in delayed treatment for compartment syndrome, or attritional loss of limb height (Fig. 2.7).

Load Path and Hammertoes

As a hammertoe becomes a rigid deformity the loss of its plantigrade orientation and dorsiflexed proximal phalanx, significant retrograde forces are generated with firing of digital toe motors. This results in increased plantar pressure at the level of the metatarsal head [10, 21, 38]. The severity of the hammertoe plays a predictive role in estimating elevated peak forefoot pressures in neuropathic feet [38].

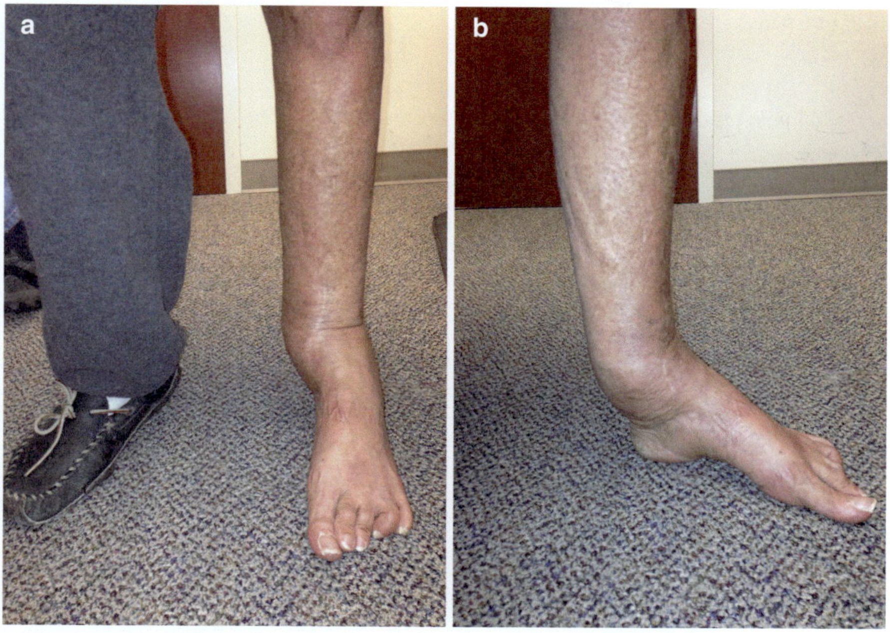

Fig. 2.7 Photographs (**a**, **b**) of a 65 year-old female that suffered a neglected tibial-fibular fracture 3 years prior. She had a complex tibial malunion/nonunion and limb shortening that lead to formation of hammertoes approximately 6–8 months after the injury. Lateralizing of the foot plus motor imbalance from the deformity are major contributing factors to her digital deformities

Digital Surgery Rationale

It could be argued that digital arthroplasty, which is the most common treatment for hammertoe, does not address deficiencies of the plantar plate tie bar or flexible hammertoes. In a clinical situation where there are acute post-traumatic changes or symptomatic changes with reducible digital deformity, a focused approach on compromised structures makes the most sense, as digital function can be normalized. However, with rigidly deformed toes, surgical efforts are best focused on reducing the magnitude of compensatory deformity with effort to reduce retrograde plantar pressure on the metatarsal heads.

Summary

The biomechanical basis of a progressive hammertoe deformity requires compromise of the length-tension relationship of the plantar plate tie-bar system. Contributory factors such as genetic predisposition, motor imbalance, metatarsal parabola discrepancies, iatrogenic surgical factors, floating toe, repetitive or overt trauma can accelerate the onset of hammertoe deformity.

References

1. Hannan MT, Menz HB, Jordan JM, et al. High heritability of hallux valgus and lesser toe deformities in adult men and women. Arthritis Care Res (Hoboken). 2013;65:1515–21.
2. Schnepp KH. Hammer-toe and claw foot. Am J Surg. 1937;36:351–9.
3. Smith BW, Coughlin MJ. Disorders of the lesser toes. Sports Med Arthrosc Rev. 2009;17:167–74.
4. Morris JL. Biomechanical implications of hammertoe deformities. Clin Podiatr Med Surg. 1986;3:339–46.
5. Shirzad K, Kiesau CD, DeOrio JK, Parekh SG. Lesser toe deformities. J Acad Orthop Surg. 2011;19:505–14.
6. Coughlin MJ. Lesser toe abnormalities. AAOS Instr Course Lect. 2003;52:421–44.
7. Hughs J, Clark P, Klenerman L. Importance of the toes in walking. J Bone Joint Surg. 1990;72-B:245–51.
8. Caravaggi P, Pataky T, Goulermas JY, et al. A dynamic model of the windlass mechanism of the foot: evidence for early stance phase preloading of the plantar apponeurosis. J Exp Biol. 2009;212:2491–9.
9. Song S, LaMontagna C, Collins SH, Geyer H. The effect of foot compliance encoded in the windlass mechanism on the energetics of human walking. 35th Annual Internaltiona Conference of the IEEE EMBS; 2013. p. 3179–3182.
10. Hicks JH. The mechanics of the foot II. The plantar aponeurosis and the arch. J Anat. 1954;88:25–31.
11. Lambrinudi C. Deformities of the toes. Clin J. 1935;64:57–61.
12. Gefen A. Stress analysis of the standing foot following surgical plantar fascia release. J Biomech. 2002;35:629–37.
13. Sharkey NA, Donahue SW, Ferris L. Biomechanical consequences of plantar fascia release or rupture during gait. Part II: alterations in forefoot loading. Foot Ankle Int. 1999;20:86–96.
14. Sharkey NA, Ferris L, Smith TS, Matthews DK. Strain and loading of the second metatarsal during heel lift. J Bone Joint Surg. 1995;77-A:1050–7.
15. Barca F, Acciaro AL. Surgical correction of crossover deformity of the second toe: A technique for tenodesis. Foot Ankle Int. 2004;25:620–4.
16. Bhatia D, Myerson MS, Curtis MJ, et al. Anatomical retraints to dislocation of the second metatarsophalangeal joint and assessment of a repair technique. J Bone Joint Surg. 1994;76-A:1371–5.
17. Deland JT, Lee KT, Sobel M, DiCarlo EF. Anatomy of the plantar plate and its attachments in the lesser metatarsal phalangeal joint. Foot Ankle Int. 1995;16:480–6.
18. Ford LA, Collins KB, Christensen JC. Stabilization of the subluxed second metatarsophalangeal joint: flexor tendon transfer versus primary repair of the plantar plate. J Foot Ankle Surg. 1998;37:217–22.
19. Sarafian SK. Anatomy of the foot and ankle: descriptive, topographic, functional. 2nd ed. Philadelphia: JB Lippincott Company; 1983.
20. Johnston RB III, Smith J, Daniels T. The plantar plate of the lesser toes: an anatomical study in human cadavers. Foot Ankle Int. 1997;15:276–82.
21. Stainsby GD. Pathological anatomy and dynamic effect of the displaced plantar plate and the importance of the inegrity of the plantar plate -deep transverse metatarsal ligament tie-bar. Ann R Coll Surg Engl. 1997;79:58–68.
22. Myerson MS, Shereff MJ. The pathological anatomy of claw and hammer toes. J Bone Joint Surg. 1989;71-A:45–9.
23. McGlamry ED. Floating toe syndrome. J Am Podiatry Assoc. 1982;72:561–8.
24. Migues A, Slullitel G, Bilbao F, Carrasco M, Solari G. Floating-toe deformity as a complication of the Weil osteotomy. Foot Ankle Int. 2004;25:609–13.
25. Perez HR, Reber LK, Christensen JC. The role of passive plantar flexion in floating toes following Weil osteotomy. J Foot Ankle Surg. 2008;47:520–6.

26. Brodsky JW, Passmore RN, Shabat S. Transection of the plantar plateand the flexor digitorum longus tendon of the fourth toe as a complication of endoscopic treatment of interdigital neuroma. A case report. J Bone Joint Surg. 2004;86:2299–301.
27. Boberg JS, Willis JJ. Lesser digital deformities: etiology, procedural selection, and arthroplasty. In: Southerland J, Boberg J, Downey M, Nakra A, Rabjohn L, editors. McGlamry's comprehensive textbook of foot & ankle surgery. 4th ed. Philadelphia: Wolters Kluer/ Lippincott Williams & Wilkins; 2013.
28. Kelikian H. Deformities of the lesser toes. In: Hallux valgus, allied deformities of the forefoot, and metatarsalgia. Philadelphia: W. B. Sanders; 1965.
29. Hansen STJ. Functional reconstruction of the foot and ankle. Philadephia: Lippincott Williams & Wilkins; 2000.
30. Rush SM, Christensen JC, Johnson CH. Biomechanics of the First Ray. Part II. Metatarsus primus varus as a case of hypermobility. A three-dimensional kinematic analysis in a cadaver model. J Foot Ankle Surg. 2000;39:68–77.
31. Morton DJ. The human foot: Its evolution, physiology and functional disorders. New York: Columbia University Press; 1935.
32. Klein EE, Weil L Jr, Weil LS Sr, Knight J. The underlying osseous deformity in plantar plate tears: a radiographic analysis. Foot Ankle Spec. 2012;6:108–18.
33. Christensen JC, Jennings MM. Normal and abnormal function of the first ray. Clin Podiatr Med Surg. 2009;26:355–71.
34. Blakeslee TJ, Chan RJ. Chinese bound foot. A literature review and case report. J Am Podiatr Med Assoc. 1986;76:502–5.
35. Thompson FM, Coughlin MJ. The high price of high-fashion footwear. J Bone Joint Surg. 1994;76-A:1586–93.
36. Bus SA, Maas M, Michels RP, Levi M. Role of intrinsic muscle atrophy in the etiology of claw toe deformity in diabetic neuropathy may not be as straightforward as widely believed. Diabetes Care. 2009;32:1063–7.
37. Perry J. Anatomy and biomechanics of the hindfoot. Clin Orthop. 1983;177:9–15.
38. Mueller MJ, Hastings M, Commean PK, et al. Forefoot structural predictors of plantar pressures during walking in people with diabetes and peripheral neuropathy. J Biomech. 2003;36:1009–17.

Chapter 3
First Ray Function, Metatarsalgia, and Hammertoes: How Are They Connected?

Douglas H. Richie Jr

Introduction

Digital deformities are commonly seen in patients with other foot pathologies such as hallux valgus and metatarsalgia. Many authorities have speculated about the cause-effect relationship between these three conditions. There are long-standing theories about the role of hypermobility of the first ray and the pathomechanics of a myriad of foot pathologies. Scrutiny of the medical literature reveals that many of these theories lack any foundation and many are simply untrue. Notwithstanding, several consistencies prevail which show an intriguing connection between first ray dysfunction, metatarsalgia, and digital deformities.

Metatarsalgia

The term metatarsalgia has been commonly used to describe a condition of pain in the plantar aspect of the forefoot [1, 2]. Often cited as a "garbage bag term," metatarsalgia does not describe a specific pathology, only a symptom. Despite the fact that the term metatarsalgia is commonly used in the medical literature, the condition has not been the focus of many quality scientific investigations.

Espinosa et al. have provided a comprehensive review and proposed a classification system of metatarsalgia [3]. Of note, this classification does not mention digital deformities a cause of metatarsalgia. Instead, hammertoes are listed with several factors which can cause a plantarflexed metatarsal, leading to metatarsalgia.

The Espinosa classification system proposes three categories of causative factors of metatarsalgia. Structural deformities within the foot, such as a long or plantarflexed

D. H. Richie Jr (✉)
Department of Biomechanics, California School of Podiatric Medicine at Samuel Merritt University, Oakland, CA, USA

E. A. Cook, J. J. Cook (eds.), *Hammertoes*,
https://doi.org/10.1007/978-3-319-16552-3_3

metatarsal, are classified as a *primary* cause of metatarsalgia. Also included in the structural category is the condition known as first ray insufficiency. Metabolic, systemic, and traumatic conditions are *secondary* causes of metatarsalgia. Finally, an *iatrogenic* category of metatarsalgia is proposed which can result from failed hallux valgus surgery or lesser metatarsal surgery.

In terms of relevance to hammertoe deformities, this chapter will focus on the structural or primary causes of metatarsalgia. In so doing, it becomes clear that there is lack of agreement about the role of each of the contributory factors for primary metatarsalgia which include first ray insufficiency, as well as abnormal length or abnormal position of the central metatarsals. We will begin with a review of current knowledge regarding the role of each of these three etiologies of metatarsalgia.

What Is the Role of an Elongated Metatarsal Causing Metatarsalgia?

Increased metatarsal length generally is believed to be a factor in the development of primary metatarsalgia [1, 3]. Morton suggested that a foot with a long second metatarsal was prone to develop metatarsalgia [4].

One of the most elaborate descriptions of variations in metatarsal parabola is provided by Maestro, who places great emphasis on metatarsal length for justification of metatarsal surgery to relieve metatarsalgia [5]. He speculates, like many others, that increased length of a metatarsal causes increased plantar pressure and metatarsalgia. In his paper, Maestro uses a standard AP radiograph and detailed measurements of metatarsal length to identify four different "morphotypes" of length patterns. Of these four, one morphotype is determined to be "harmonious" or "normal," yet this was only found in 31% of the feet they studied. Shortening osteotomies were recommended to restore the harmonious pattern of metatarsal lengths. Maestro used no other objective data such as plantar pressure measurements to verify the role of metatarsal length in creating metatarsalgia.

Elongated metatarsals have been attributed to be a cause of digital deformities [7, 12]. With little proof, many authors have speculated that elongated metatarsals will increase plantar pressure which leads to attrition and eventual rupture of the plantar plate. A review of the medical literature on this subject shows conflicting evidence linking elongated metatarsals to plantar plate injury.

Katz and Coughlin use the term "crossover toe" to essentially describe a plantar plate tear since the majority of patients in their study had a positive drawer test, consistent with this injury [11]. Many reports have theorized that a second crossover toe deformity is caused by a long second metatarsal [6–10]. However, Kaz and Coughlin challenged that notion when they found that less than half of the patients in their study (169 patients) with crossover toe deformity had an elongated second metatarsal [11]. The lower incidence of an elongated second metatarsal conflicted with Coughlin's previous study [7]. In that previous investigation, the second metatarsal was longer than the first metatarsal in 90% of cases with crossover toe. However, that earlier study used a simple measurement (i.e., "Coughlin measure") where a transverse line was drawn across the first to the third metatarsals and a long second metatarsal was determined if it crossed distal to that line. When Kaz and Coughlin used the metatarsal measurement technique of Hardy and Clapham [13] (i.e., drawing an arc with a compass rather than a line with a ruler), the prevalence of a long second metatarsal in patients with a crossover second toe dropped to 44%.

It appears that the detection of an elongated second metatarsal is dependent upon which method of measurement is utilized, and no specific technique has been verified as more accurate. For example, Bhutta and co-workers used the "Coughlin measure" of metatarsal length and found a positive correlation between increased second metatarsal length and incidence of crossover toe deformity [14]. This finding was published even though Coughlin had previously demonstrated that this measurement was misleading [11].

Fleisher et al. studied several radiographic measures of patients with documented tear of the plantar plate at the second metatarsophalangeal joint (MTPJ) [15]. Fleisher et al. utilized several methods of measuring forefoot metatarsal parabola including those described already by Couglin and Maestro, and another technique described by Nilsonne and Morton where a "metatarsal protrusion index" is determined by a simple direct measure of length between the first and second metatarsal [16, 17]. This "metatarsal protrusion index" was the only method of the four techniques used by Fleisher et al. which demonstrated a correlation with increased length of the second metatarsal and the prevalence of a plantar plate tear. It is important to note that the metatarsal protrusion distance will be negative (short first metatarsal) when there is a hallux valgus deformity causing increased medial rotation of the first metatarsal. Katz and Coughlin found that half of patients with a crossover second toe deformity also had accompanying hallux valgus deformity. This would be expected to greatly affect the metatarsal protrusion measurement in favor of demonstrating a "long" second metatarsal.

In summary, the only studies documenting a long second metatarsal correlating with increased risk of plantar plate tears used either the metatarsal protrusion distance or the Coughlin technique, both of which have shortcomings [18]. Coughlin himself demonstrated the shortcomings of his original measurement technique in his second study [11].

Do Long Metatarsals Can Elevate Plantar Pressures?

In their conclusion Fleisher et al. propagate a long-held notion about the role of elongated metatarsals, metatarsalgia, and digital deformity: "As the relative length of the second metatarsal increases with respect to the first metatarsal, the relative plantar loading beneath the second MTP joint can also be expected to increase, especially during the third rocker of gait. Repetitive, increased loading in this region of the foot is what we believe contributes to the initial attenuation of the plantar plate and eventual tearing" [15]. However, these authors provide no citations or evidence to support such a claim.

Kaz and Coughlin showed that only 7% of 169 patients with crossover second toe deformity showed evidence of callus under the second metatarsal head [11]. If length and subsequent pressure under the second metatarsal head were responsible for plantar plate injury, one would assume there would be a pressure-induced skin lesion at this location.

Setting aside plantar plate injuries, plantar pressure has been attributed to be the primary cause of metatarsalgia [19]. Furthermore, interventions which reduce plantar pressure under the metatarsals improve the symptoms of metatarsalgia [20, 21].

This amplifies the shortcomings of the term "metatarsalgia" as this condition embodies multiple pathologies which can have different etiologies and pathomechanics. Plantar plate tears may be the result of tensile strain rather than abnormal plantar pressure. To further complicate this issue is the possibility that shear stress may play a significant role in the pathomechanics of metatarsalgia [22, 23].

There is a long-held notion that elongated metatarsals cause metatarsalgia [1, 3, 5]. Plantar pressure studies reveal several myths and misconceptions about the role of elongated metatarsals and the development of metatarsalgia. The results of these studies are surprising. To summarize, elongated metatarsals do not cause increased plantar pressures and do not predictably cause metatarsalgia.

There are surprisingly few investigations of metatarsalgia, and most have focused on patients without hallux abductovalgus (HAV) deformity. Dreeben and co-workers studied radiographic and pedobarographic parameters in patients with primary metatarsalgia [24]. Thirty-seven patients (45 feet) with a diagnosis of primary metatarsalgia were followed preoperatively and postoperatively, and their contralateral symptom-free feet were used as healthy controls. The authors found no correlation between the length of the metatarsals and plantar-loading parameters (plantar pressures) or symptoms of metatarsalgia.

Kaipel and co-workers prospectively studied 46 patients with metatarsalgia compared to 45 asymptomatic patients and used radiographic and pedobarographic measures to determine the role of metatarsal length and plantar pressures in causing symptoms of metatarsalgia [25]. The relative lengths of the metatarsals did not correlate with the pressure or force under the respective metatarsal. Also, there was no difference in peak pressure under the central metatarsals comparing the group with metatarsalgia with the control group. There were no differences in metatarsal length patterns when comparing the groups with metatarsalgia to those without metatarsalgia. The only significant finding was a decrease in peak force under the first metatarsal in the metatarsalgia group. This validates a long-accepted notion that instability of the first ray is the primary cause of metatarsalgia.

This same finding of decreased peak force under the first metatarsal was also found in the study published by Dreeben et al. [24]. Other studies have shown a load transfer from the first ray to the symptomatic ray in patients with metatarsalgia [21, 26]. However, this is not always the case as Kaipel et al. did not see increased load under the central metatarsals despite decreased load under the first metatarsal [25]. Instead, the load appeared to increase in the fourth and fifth metatarsals, suggesting that patients may avoid painful plantar pressures by supinating their forefoot.

What Is the Role of Plantarflexed Metatarsals Causing Metatarsalgia?

Another cause of primary metatarsalgia is a plantarflexed metatarsal [3]. Global plantarflexion of metatarsals one to five, seen in cavus feet, will significantly elevate plantar pressures in the forefoot [27, 28]. Isolated plantarflexion of a single or multiple metatarsals can be the result of congenital deformity or can result from malunion after trauma or metatarsal surgery. The few limited studies of plantarflexed position of metatarsals verify that this parameter is more significant than metatarsal length in causing metatarsalgia.

A cadaver study was conducted by Jung et al. to determine the effect of dorsal elevation and shortening of the first metatarsal on plantar pressures [29]. Dorsal elevation had a greater effect on reducing pressure under the first metatarsal than shortening. Both dorsal elevation and shortening of the first metatarsal caused significant increased plantar pressure under the second metatarsal.

Dreeben studied 37 patients with primary metatarsalgia under the second metatarsal head [24]. Metatarsal length and height of the metatarsal head from the supportive surface were measured and then correlated with plantar pressure measurements obtained from a pedobarograph. In this study, plantar pressure did not correlate with metatarsal length but did closely correlate with metatarsal head position or height from the ground. When a second metatarsal osteotomy was performed, decrease in plantar pressure occurred when the metatarsal head was elevated, while shortening of the metatarsal had minimal effect on plantar pressure. In order to reduce plantar pressure and pain, the second metatarsal head required elevation by at least 3.5 mm; however, the reduction in plantar pressure was not predictable or linear with amount of elevation. The authors concluded that plantar pressure under the metatarsal heads is multifactorial and might be affected by the quality of the soft tissues and plantar fat pad.

To summarize, studies do not support the notion that elongated metatarsals increase plantar pressures or correlate with location of metatarsalgia. Instead, sagittal plane position of the metatarsal appears to play a more important role in plantar pressure. Finally, overall stability and position of the adjacent first metatarsal may be the most significant factor in central metatarsalgia.

What Is the Role of First Ray Instability and Metatarsalgia?

Instability or hypermobility of the first ray has been attributed to be the cause of a myriad of foot pathologies, most notably hallux abductovalgus (HAV), hallux rigidus, metatarsalgia, and hammertoes [30]. This critical skeletal segment of the human foot is comprised of the first metatarsal and the medial cuneiform. The first ray is the major load-bearing structure of the human foot [31].

The first ray of the human foot evolved from a grasping function in arboreal primates to become a stable beam of support to allow upright bipedal gait [32]. The grasping or "opposable" function of the first ray is demonstrated by its axis of motion which allows eversion with plantarflexion. This axis was originally defined by Hicks and later verified by other cadaver and kinematic studies [33–35].

Frontal plane rotation of the first ray into eversion with plantarflexion is critical to sagittal stability of this skeletal segment. The peroneus longus muscle plays a significant role in stabilizing the first ray in both of these planes. Johnson and co-workers verified that the first ray moves into eversion with plantarflexion [36]. They also demonstrated that the peroneus longus provides more frontal plane rotation than sagittal plane, moving the first metatarsal into eversion. Johnson and co-workers described a "locking" mechanism engaged by tensioning of the peroneus longus where the first ray was stabilized into a plantarflexed, abducted, and everted position.

Perez and co-workers subsequently verified the existence of a locking mechanism of the first ray [37]. This cadaver study measured significant reduction of sagittal plane motion when the first ray was moved from a position of inversion to a position of eversion. Perez et al. propose that, when the first metatarsal is positioned into plantarflexion and eversion.

The term "hypermobility" was first described by Dudley Morton, an anatomist who attributed forefoot pain to abnormal length or abnormal alignment of the first metatarsal resulting in excessive motion [38]. Since then, other terms such as "instability" and "insufficiency" have been used interchangeably with hypermobility when describing dysfunction of the first ray, contributing to many foot pathologies [30]. In reality all of these terms are misleading as they really should be describing the relative stiffness or load-bearing capacity of the first metatarsal during standing and walking. Without any norms for required stiffness of the first ray, clinicians still resort to more broad qualitative terms to describe poor performance of this skeletal segment. Furthermore, there is a large gap in reliability of static measures of first ray range of motion compared to actual stability of this segment during dynamic gait [39].

If the first ray has excessive motion in the sagittal plane, it is presumed to be hypermobile. One problem with assessing hypermobility is the fact that traditional clinical measures of mobility of the first ray are taken with the patient in a static, non-weight-bearing position [40]. Simple variations in positioning the foot and ankle can change these measures of mobility of the first ray [41]. The stiffness and performance of the first ray during dynamic gait are significantly dependent on the windlass mechanism which is not engaged during traditional static measurement [42].

Thus, clinicians should be wary when evaluating first ray range of motion and making conclusions about "hypermobility" which can lead to inappropriate decisions for surgical intervention. Allen and co-workers found that static measures of first ray mobility had very poor correlation with actual motion of this segment during ambulation [39]. The feet which demonstrated "hypermobility" of the first ray during the static exam did not show instability of this segment during dynamic gait.

Misconceptions about first ray range of motion can influence surgical decision-making. The primary joints of the first ray include the first metatarsocuneiform joint (first TMT joint) and the medial naviculocuneiform joint. Other articulations of the first ray include articulations between the first metatarsal and second metatarsal, the medial cuneiform articulation with the second metatarsal, as well as the articulation between the medial and intermediate cuneiform. A long-standing debate continues regarding which joint of the first ray contributes most to hypermobility. Lapidus proposed that the first TMT joint was responsible for first ray hypermobility [43]. This notion has become more popular over the past 30 years with many authorities advocating a Lapidus procedure to reduce first ray hypermobility [44, 45].

Yet, studies show that both joints of the first ray contribute equal amounts of motion. Fusion of either joint will give the same reduction in sagittal plane motion [46]. Other studies measuring motion at the two joints of the first ray have demonstrated that there is slightly more motion in the navicular-medial cuneiform joint than in the first TMT joint [47, 48]. Finally, no studies have been published showing any significant reduction of motion of the first ray when a single joint was fused.

In the healthy patient, the first ray bears 60% of the weight-bearing force in the foot [49]. With first ray insufficiency, load is shifted laterally to the lesser metatarsals, and this is the proposed underlying mechanism for second metatarsophalangeal joint synovitis, metatarsalgia, and stress fractures [50, 51]. While this theory is intuitive, the ability of the clinician to evaluate a patient and determine what parameters will predict first ray insufficiency remains challenging.

Pathologies of the First Ray

Hallux Abductovalgus and First Ray Hypermobility: Cause or Effect?

Hallux abductovalgus (HAV) deformity results from instability of the first ray when there is excessive mobility in both the transverse and sagittal plane [52]. As the first metatarsal rotates dorsally and medially, the axis of the first ray couples this motion with inversion of the ray in the frontal plane [33–36]. Reciprocally, the hallux moves laterally and into eversion [53]. This lateral shift of the hallux causes a lateral displacement of the soft tissues at the plantar aspect of the hallux including the flexor tendons as well as the distal extension of the plantar aponeurosis [54]. Inversion of the first metatarsal causes a plantar displacement of the abductor hallucis allowing further pronation of the hallux [55]. If the entire foot moves into excessive pronation, the first ray will appear pronated to the ground, while this segment is still dorsiflexed and inverted relative to the second metatarsal [56].

What is well established is a relationship between hallux abductovalgus deformity (HAV) and excessive mobility of the first ray [57, 58]. However, it is unknown if this is a cause-effect relationship. The degree of hypermobility of the first ray does not correlate with severity of hallux valgus [59].

In a systematic review of this subject, Shibuya found a significant increased range of motion in the first ray of patients with hallux valgus compared to those without hallux valgus deformity [60]. The authors make the astute observation that stabilization of the first ray does not necessarily require a Lapidus fusion of the first TMT joint as several studies have shown that simple correction of first ray alignment in the transverse plane will reduce hypermobility [61–65].

Rush and co-workers demonstrated that when the intermetatarsal angle in HAV deformity is corrected to normal alignment, a 26% increased stiffness and resistance to dorsiflexion will occur [42]. They attribute the hypermobility seen in HAV to a relative lateral shift of the sesamoids and distal slips of the plantar aponeurosis which appear critical to providing stability to the first ray, particularly during propulsion with engagement of the windlass mechanism.

Faber and co-workers conducted a cadaver study and demonstrated that the first TMT joint actually has more mobility in the transverse plane than the sagittal plane [66]. Furthermore, this joint is significantly stabilized by both the peroneus longus and flexor hallucis longus muscles. In particular, the flexor hallucis longus has effects to reduce medial displacement and dorsal displacement of first metatarsal.

It appears that hypermobility seen in HAV patients may be more the result of medial displacement of the first ray [58]. There is little evidence that sagittal plane hypermobility of the first ray is a primary cause of HAV but rather that this hypermobility is a result of the HAV deformity.

Hallux Rigidus and First Ray Hypermobility

Similarly, hallux rigidus also appears to have a paradoxical cause-effect relationship with first ray instability. Roukis and Scherer verified a well-accepted notion that elevation or dorsiflexion of the first ray will cause reduction in extension of the hallux. In their study, 8 mm of elevation of the first metatarsal reduced dorsiflexion of the first MTPJ by over 35% [67]. Lateral weight-bearing radiographs are commonly used to detect dorsal elevation of the first metatarsal, known as metatarsus primus elevatus (MPE).

However, studies of patients with hallux rigidus have provided conflicting results when looking at the role of first ray instability and MPE. In another study, Roukis showed that patients with hallux rigidus have greater degrees of metatarsus primus elevatus than patients with hallux valgus, neuroma, and plantar fasciitis [68]. But other studies of large groups of patients showed that as the grade or severity hallux rigidus increased, so did the amount of MPE [69, 70]. Significant MPE is only seen in late stages of hallux rigidus suggesting that this radiographic finding is a result, not the cause of hallux rigidus.

Metatarsus primus elevatus is not a valid measure of first ray hypermobility. Assessing a static radiograph and measuring alignment of the first metatarsal do not measure range of motion or stiffness of the first ray. As the hallux is progressively moved into plantarflexion with increasing severity of hallux rigidus, the first metatarsal is driven reciprocally into dorsiflexion or "elevatus."

Studies of mobility of the first ray in patients with hallux rigidus have refuted the notion that hypermobility is a causative factor of this condition. Coughlin and Shurnas studied 110 patients with hallux rigidus and used the Klaue device to measure first ray mobility [69]. These patients actually demonstrated decreased mobility of the first ray in the range of 6 mm, which is less than what is reported for healthy patients. Griesberg used another novel technique to measure first ray mobility and found no association between first ray hypermobility and hallux rigidus [71]. In fact, this study again documented decreased range of motion of the first ray in hallux rigidus patients. Griesberg et al. also found decreased range of motion of the first ray in patients with cavus feet, while patients with flat feet had greater range.

Does First Ray Hypermobility Cause Metatarsalgia?

While HAV has demonstrated a close association with first ray instability, few investigations have documented the true incidence of metatarsalgia in patients with this deformity. Coughlin and Jones have published the most comprehensive study of hallux valgus patients and did find a significant incidence of metatarsalgia which was found in 48% of patients with HAV deformity [72]. Yet, only 11% of all patients with HAV in this study demonstrated plantar callosities in the forefoot. Interestingly, metatarsalgia was the primary reason for seeking surgery for HAV deformity in 17% of the patients in the Coughlin study.

Hypermobility or instability of the first ray has been speculated to cause metatarsalgia due to a lateral shift of pressure away from the first metatarsal to adjacent metatarsals [73]. The specific conditions which result from lateralizing plantar pressures include synovitis of the lesser MTPs, plantar plate injury, neuroma, and metatarsal stress fracture [50, 74, 75].

Hypermobility of the first ray has been observed in patients without HAV deformity. Morton was among the first to speculate that a first ray which was abnormally short would be hypermobile [4]. However, a study of patients with metatarsalgia and HAV demonstrated that patients with a short first ray were actually less likely to have metatarsal pain [6].

Griesberg et al. measured first ray translation and elevation and correlated the findings in patients with various foot disorders [71]. The highest correlation of increased mobility of the first ray was found in patients with hallux valgus and patients with metatarsalgia. However, the authors did not separate the two patient groups, and the statistics suggest that most patients with metatarsalgia also had hallux valgus. There are no studies which show hypermobility of the first ray linked to metatarsalgia in any patient group other than those with hallux valgus.

Many clinicians attribute second metatarsal hypertrophy, seen on radiographic exam, as an adaptive change resulting from first ray instability. However, this sign may be misleading. Coughlin measured second metatarsal thickness on X-ray and then measured the mobility of the first metatarsal and found no correlation between the measurements [63]. In a retrospective case control study of women athletes with a history of lesser metatarsal stress fractures, Glasoe and co-workers found no correlation with increased first ray elevation and incidence of fracture [50].

In concluding this concept of first ray hypermobility, the existence of this condition in any foot disorder other than HAV has not been validated. Hypermobility of the first ray in the sagittal plane seems to occur only when there is medial shift of the first metatarsal and the stabilizing effects of the plantar aponeurosis and flexor hallucis longus are negated.

Pressure Studies of HAV Patients

Pressure studies have confirmed the critical role of the hallux in accepting load during gait. In fact, the hallux bears almost as much weight as any of the metatarsals and more than the third, fourth, and fifth metatarsals. Only the first and second metatarsals bear more weight than the hallux [76]. The lesser toes combined bear less than 50% the load of the hallux.

While it has been well established that patients with hallux valgus have excessive motion of the first ray in static exam and a significant number of these patients have metatarsalgia, few studies have documented increased pressure under the central metatarsal heads in these patients. It is assumed that there will be increased pressure under the second metatarsal resulting from simple load transfer from a hypermobile first ray. Not all studies show a significant load transfer to the second metatarsal in HAV patients. What is often overlooked is the effect of deviated alignment of the hallux in HAV deformity which significantly affects loading and plantar pressure across the forefoot.

This underscores two major obstacles when conducting pressure testing with human subjects. Plantar pressure can be altered by change in thickness of the integument and the plantar fat pad, a change often seen in HAV patients who have diminished fat pad under the first MTP [77]. Secondly, patients with metatarsalgia may compensate with an altered gait pattern to avoid pain. Commonly, this will show a lateral shift of loading across the forefoot as the patient supinates their foot during terminal stance [25].

Some studies have demonstrated the expected shift of pressure from the hallux to the central metatarsals in patients with HAV [58, 78, 79] (see Fig. 3.1). Other studies show that patients with HAV deformity will have increased plantar pressure under the hallux with lateral shift of pressure to the central metatarsals [80] (see Fig. 3.2). Other studies have shown no significant lateral shift of metatarsal pressure [81]. Finally, some studies show increased pressure under the first and second metatarsals in patients with moderate to severe HAV deformity [82, 83].

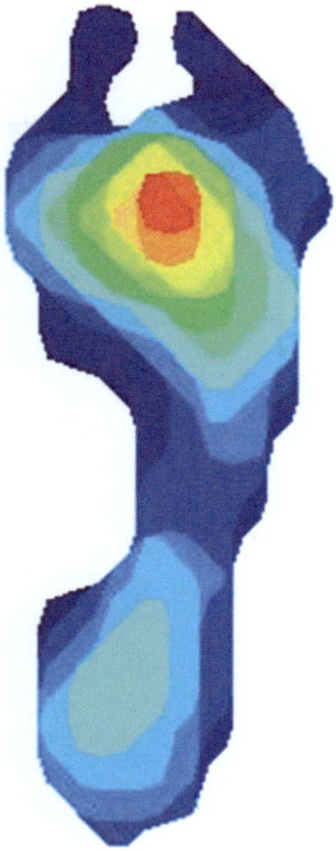

Fig. 3.1 Hallux valgus with transfer of load away from hallux to central metatarsals: the hallux has decreased pressure. (Study and images courtesy of Bruce Williams DPM)

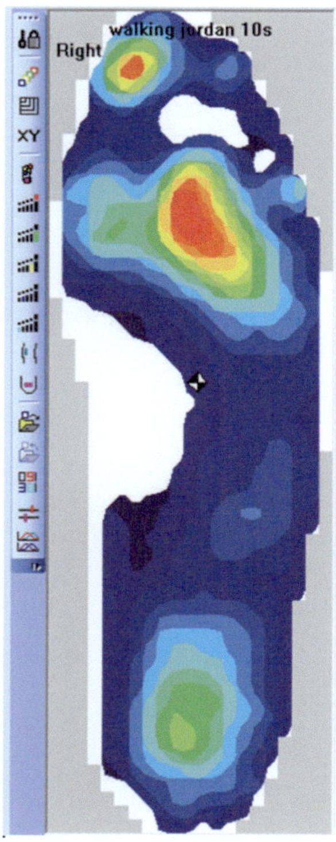

Fig. 3.2 Hallux valgus with load transfer to second MTPJ and increased pressure under the hallux. (Study and images courtesy of Bruce Williams DPM)

What is clear is that not all patients with HAV lose weight bearing under the hallux and first metatarsal and therefore do not transfer load to the lesser metatarsals. This was seen in the Kernozek study where patients with and without metatarsalgia were included [80]. Conversely, Waldecker studied HAV patients all of whom had metatarsalgia and documented a loss of weight bearing under the hallux resulting in a lateral shift of load to the central metatarsals [78]. Interesting, the major load transfer was from the hallux to the lateral forefoot, without unloading of the first metatarsal (see Fig. 3.3). Restoring load-bearing function under the hallux may be critical in the relief of symptoms of metatarsalgia in HAV patients.

Waldecker suggests a mechanism where loss of hallux purchase occurs in HAV deformity [78]. He noted that as the first metatarsal became more inverted with dorsiflexion, the hallux became more everted which distorts the orientation of the plantar fascia insertion and efficiency of the windlass mechanism. Cadaver studies have verified the enhanced functioning of the windlass mechanism and improved weight bearing of the first ray when hallux valgus deformity is corrected with first metatarsal realignment [42].

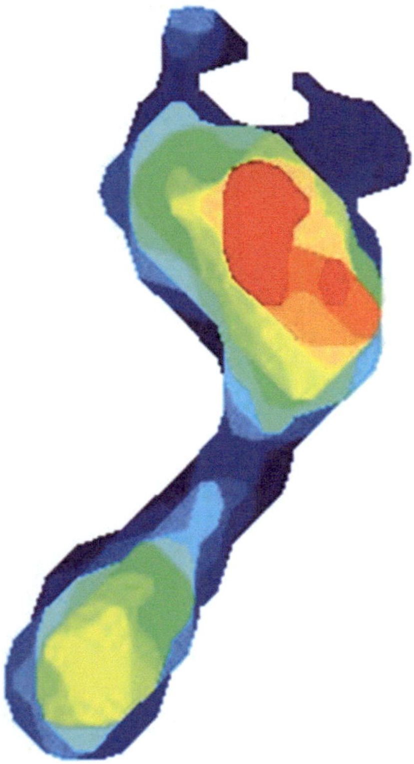

Fig. 3.3 Hallux valgus with transfer of load away from hallux to lateral metatarsals 3–5. (Study and images courtesy of Bruce Williams DPM)

First Ray Insufficiency and Digital Deformities

Many authors have linked a cause-effect mechanism for second digit hammertoe deformity developing from adjacent pressure of the hallux in HAV deformity [84–86]. Kaz and Coughlin found that 49% of patients with crossover second digit deformity had HAV deformity as well [11].

HAV has been linked to the development of hammertoes in other digits as well as the development of tarsometatarsal joint degenerative arthritis [87]. Gribbin and co-workers evaluated 163 patients who underwent surgery for HAV deformity [88]. A strong association was found between the severity of hallux valgus deformity and the presence of second digit hammertoe deformity as well as osteoarthritis of the second TMT joint. The authors point out that second digit deformity can precede or be the result of HAV deformity. As the second digit becomes elevated, lateral deviation of the hallux can accelerate in HAV deformity.

Pressure Studies on Hammertoes

Compared to HAV deformity, digital deformity can be expected to more predictably cause elevated plantar pressures under metatarsals 2 and 3 [82]. (see Fig. 3.4). It is interesting to note that there are very few plantar pressure studies of hammertoe deformities, and these mainly focus on patients with diabetes. Two of these studies showed that claw toes or hammertoes will cause lower hallux pressures but higher metatarsal pressures [83, 89].

High plantar pressures in diabetic patients are greatly exacerbated by digital deformities. Bus and co-workers showed that both peak plantar pressure and pressure-time integrals were significantly increased in diabetic patients with claw toe deformities compared to age and gender-matched diabetic patients without toe deformities [90]. Digital deformities are a significant risk factor for diabetic foot ulcerations [91]. In a study of 92 patients with diabetes, Holewski found that hammertoe deformities were present in 82% of patients with a history of ulceration and amputation, while these deformities were only found in 23% of patients who had no history of ulceration [92].

How Do Digital Deformities Elevate Plantar Pressures?

Mueller and co-workers studied 20 subjects with diabetes and neuropathy as well as 20 healthy control subjects [83]. The presence of hammertoe deformity as well as the magnitude of metatarsophalangeal joint extension had the most significant effect

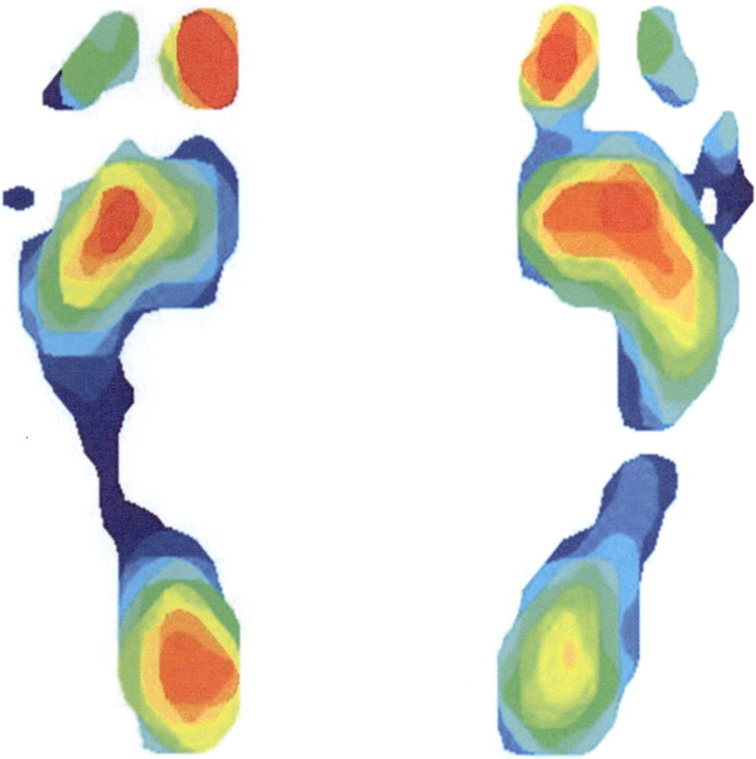

Fig. 3.4 Hammertoes with metatarsalgia. Decreased load on lesser digits, increased load under hallux, and diffuse increased load under central metatarsals. (Study and images courtesy of Bruce Williams DPM)

on peak pressure under the metatarsals compared to all other variables including ankle joint dorsiflexion. Mueller et al. concluded that loss of weight bearing by the hammertoe deformity caused a load transfer to the proximal metatarsal head. This would be plausible if the lesser digits bore significant load during standing and walking; however, pressure studies rule out this possibility [76]. Rozema studied 12 healthy adult subjects with in-shoe pressure measurements and determined that the lesser digits bear 50% less pressure during walking than the second metatarsal and 60% less pressure than the hallux [93]. This may explain why patients with hammertoes do not show significant loss of balance during ambulation or during static stance [82, 94].

A more logical reason that extension of the metatarsophalangeal joint would increase plantar pressure under the metatarsal head is the effect of retrograde force from the proximal phalanx causing plantar flexion moment at the tarsometatarsal joint. Multi-segment foot modeling has allowed insight into the motion of key skeletal segments of the human foot during dynamic gait [95]. Nester and co-workers found a significant amount of motion available at the tarsometatarsal joints [96].

Metatarsals 1–3 move an average of 6 degrees in the sagittal plane, while metatarsals 4–5 move 11 degrees. This dispels the myth that the tarsometatarsal joints are relatively rigid. It also allows understanding of how a metatarsal can plantarflex in response to extension of the proximal phalanx with a hammertoe deformity.

The Role of Plantar Fat Displacement and Digital Deformity

Another insight into the role of hammertoes creating increased plantar pressure is provided by Bus et al. [97]. This MRI study of diabetic patients with hammertoe or claw toe deformity revealed a significant anterior displacement of the plantar fat pad away from the weight-bearing surface of the metatarsal head [98]. This resulted in significant thinning of the submetatarsal fat pad which would explain increased plantar pressure in this location. In a follow-up study, Bus and co-workers found that claw toe deformity caused decreased fat pad thickness under the affected metatarsal, and this increased peak plantar pressure by almost twofold at that location [90]. These authors propose a "fat pad-plantar pressure exchange principle" whereby the fat pad migrates distally and plantar pressure increases proximally.

The Plantar Aponeurosis and Digital Deformity

Bojsen-Moller was the first to describe a mechanism whereby extension of the metatarsophalangeal joint, seen in hammertoe deformity, will cause the protective fat pad cushion to displace distally in the foot, exposing the head of the metatarsal to more focal and increased plantar pressure [98, 99]. He elegantly described and illustrated the key relationships between the plantar fat pad and the distal insertions of the plantar aponeurosis. Bojsen-Moller divides the "ball of the foot" into three transverse areas: (1) a proximal segment with subcutaneous transverse bands of the plantar fat pad interwoven with the deep sagittal septa of the plantar aponeurosis, (2) the area directly beneath the heads of the metatarsals which contain the submetatarsal fat cushions, and (3) the distal area which contains the insertions of the plantar aponeurosis into the skin. Just deep is the transverse interdigital ligament, also known as the superficial transverse metatarsal ligament. Bojsen-Moller describes the critical function of the plantar aponeurosis to restrain anterior migration of the integument during the third rocker or "push-off" phase of gait. He suggests that failure of the plantar fascia stability is critical to displacement of the metatarsal fat pad as well as overall digital stability.

Stainsby also attributes the development of plantar plate failure and digital deformity to malfunction of the windlass mechanism which relies upon stability of the plantar aponeurosis [100]. He also notes the common occurrence of claw toes in feet with HAV deformity and attributes the lesser digital deformity to failure of windlass mechanism when hallux valgus occurs. Stainsby describes a lateral overload of the plantar fascia shifting from the defective first MTPJ in HAV to the lesser toes which leads to rupture of the plantar plate.

The role of the plantar aponeurosis in the pathomechanics of digital deformity was elucidated by Hamel and co-workers [101]. They measured the contribution of the long toe flexors (FDL) and the plantar aponeurosis to stability of the lesser toes during gait. This important study reaffirmed the critical role that the plantar aponeurosis plays in providing flexion stability to the lesser digits with the same magnitude as the long flexor tendon (FDL). The plantar aponeurosis via the plantar plate has been identified to be the most important sagittal plane stabilizer of the lesser MTPs, preventing extension of the proximal phalanx [101].

Hamel et al. describe a windlass effect of the plantar aponeurosis at the lesser digits which applies flexion moment to the proximal phalanx [101]. This flexion moment develops during passive dorsiflexion of the digit during heel rise. Thus the plantar aponeurosis plays a critical role in stabilizing the toe and resisting dorsiflexion during toe off. Hamel et al. propose that a claw toe deformity can occur if the long flexor tendons are overloaded when the plantar fascia stabilizing mechanism is lost. Hamel et al. compromised the plantar fascia by performing a complete fasciotomy in cadaver specimens. They observed that loading shifted laterally to the lesser metatarsals during toe off and as they describe "a shift from the normal high-gear push-off to the less efficient low-gear push-off" [101].

Plantar Pressures, Push-Off, and Overall Foot Stability

The high-gear/low-gear push-off mechanism was first described by Bojsen-Moller [102]. Due to the shape of the metatarsal parabola, load can be transferred during terminal stance, i.e., the third rocker, to the first and second MTPs (the high-gear push-off) via a transverse axis or to the lateral MTPs 3–5 (the low-gear push-off) via an oblique axis. According to Bojsen-Moller, in the optimal functioning foot, the lateral column is stable due to anatomic locking of the calcaneal-cuboid joint [102]. Inversion of the calcaneus moves the calcaneal-cuboid joint into a close-packed position which allows anatomic locking, elevation of the joint from the supportive surface, and increased stiffness by loading of the long plantar ligament. This provides an optimal, stable fulcrum for the peroneus longus tendon which can now exert maximal force on the first ray. During terminal stance, the peroneus longus contracts to pronate the forefoot on the rearfoot as well as plantarflexing, abducting, and everting the first metatarsal. This facilitates load transfer to the first ray and engagement of the high-gear windlass mechanism through the hallux (see Fig. 3.5). The high-gear push-off optimizes tensioning of the plantar aponeurosis compared to the low-gear push-off. With a larger radius compared to the lesser metatarsals, the first metatarsal has a better mechanical advantage for increasing tension and "shortening" of the plantar aponeurosis as the hallux is driven into extension during toe off. The plantar aponeurosis invests the sesamoids, which, when properly situated beneath the head of the first metatarsal, greatly enhance the mechanical advantage of the hallux in engaging the windlass mechanism. The sesamoids provide a radius

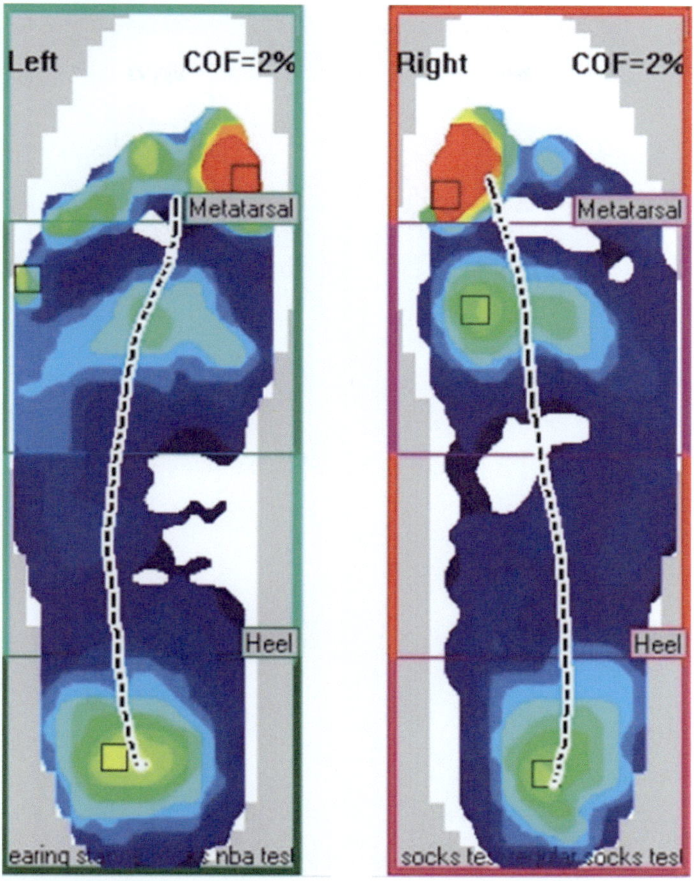

Fig. 3.5 High-gear push-off on the right foot through the first MTPJ and hallux. Low-gear push-off on the left foot, decreased loading of first MTPJ and increased loading of lesser digits. (Study and images courtesy of Bruce Williams DPM)

of curvature of the first MTP which is twice that of the third metatarsal [102]. When the sesamoids are shifted laterally in HAV deformity, this mechanical advantage of the windlass is compromised by shortening the radius of curvature of the first MTPJ.

Validation of this theory linking rearfoot position with loading of the hallux has been provided by the Framingham Foot Study [103]. This study of an extraordinary large group of human subjects allowed comparison of planar pressure and force among a group of patients with hallux valgus (1123 subjects), hallux valgus and other foot disorders (641 subjects), and people without hallux valgus (3707 subjects). This high-powered study evaluated foot posture, center of pressure excursion during gait, and distribution of peak pressure and force in eight regions of the foot. Subjects with hallux valgus demonstrated higher peak pressure under the medial rearfoot, as well as a smaller center of pressure excursion index and a lower arch profile than healthy subjects. All of these findings link hallux valgus to a pronated rearfoot alignment during gait. Furthermore, the subjects with hallux valgus demonstrated

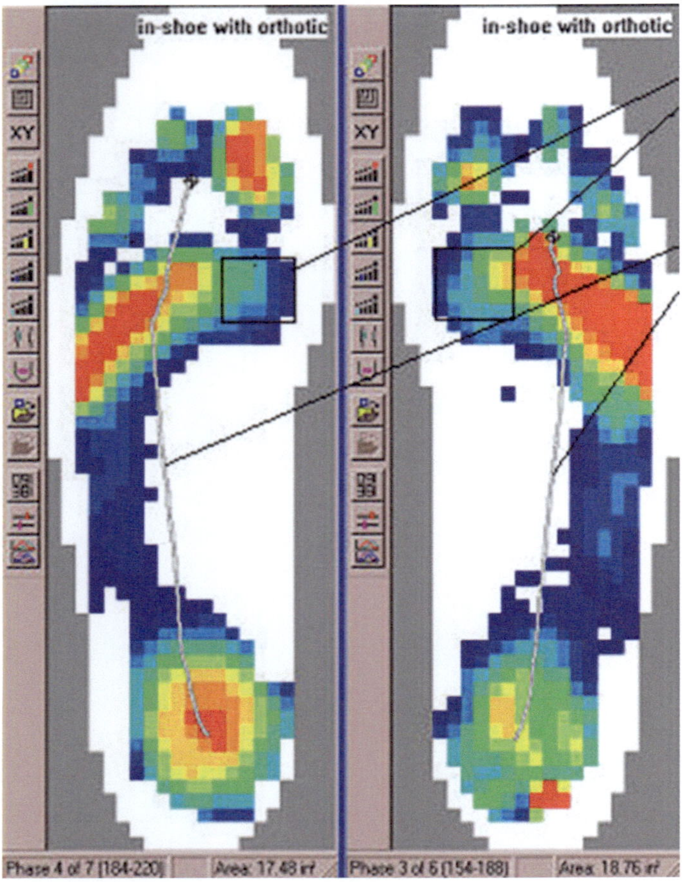

Fig. 3.6 Low-gear push-off through the central and lateral MTPJs and lesser digits. (Study and images courtesy of Bruce Williams DPM)

decreased loading of the hallux along with increased loading of the lesser digits. This shows a shift from a high-gear push-off to a low-gear push-off and lack of engagement of the windlass mechanism through the first MTPJ in hallux valgus patients (see Fig. 3.6). The pronated position of the rearfoot appears to be the predisposing factor for this low-gear push-off seen in HAV patients compared to healthy subjects.

Summary

Theories about function and stability of the first ray started with an anatomist, Dudley Morton, which have been propagated by clinicians and surgeons all over the world for nearly 100 years. Many of the concepts about the role of first ray dysfunction and the development of foot pathologies have been proven erroneous yet continue to be used as justification for certain surgical procedures. Simple structural variations of metatarsal alignment seen on plain radiographs do not explain metatarsalgia. Metatarsus primus elevatus does not predict first ray insufficiency. Shortened first metatarsals and elongated central metatarsals do not cause metatarsalgia.

Ironically, it was another anatomist, Finn Bojsen-Moller, who provided the best explanation for optimal foot function where the first ray and hallux accept the primary load during the critical phase of terminal stance during ambulation. The plantar aponeurosis and the peroneus longus muscle are the primary stabilizers of the first ray, and hypermobility occurs when the dynamic effects of one or both of these structures are compromised.

By looking back at the work of Bojsen-Moller and studying more recent research, we can now connect the dots and understand how the first ray function and lesser digital function are optimized. When first ray stability fails, digital deformity and metatarsalgia can result.

Optimal foot function starts with a stable hindfoot, which locks the calcaneal-cuboid joint, allowing efficient function of the peroneus longus muscle. This promotes pronation of the forefoot and locking of the first ray. With all of these positional changes, the windlass mechanism is optimized during terminal stance with a stiff, stable first ray enabling high-gear push-off through the hallux. When this mechanism fails, load is shifted laterally across the lesser MTPs which increases risk of digital deformity and metatarsalgia.

References

1. O'Kane C, Kilmartin TE. The surgical management of central metatarsalgia. Foot Ankle Int. 2002;23:415–9.
2. Coughlin MJ. Common causes of pain in the forefoot in adults. J Bone Joint Surg Br. 2000;82:781–90.
3. Espinosa N, Maceira E, Myerson MS. Current concept review. Metatarsalgia. Foot Ankle Int. 2008;29:871–9.
4. Morton D. Metatarsus atavicus: the identification of a distinctive type of foot disorder. J Bone Joint Surg. 1927;9:531–44.
5. Maestro M, Besse JL, Ragusa M, Berthonnaud E. Forefoot morphotype study and planning method for forefoot osteotomy. Foot Ankle Clin. 2003;8:695–710.
6. Slullitel G, Lopez V, Calvi JP, Seletti M, Bartolucci C, Pinton G. Effect of first ray insufficiency and metatarsal index on metatarsalgia in hallux valgus. Foot Ankle Int. 2016;37(3):300–6.
7. Coughlin MJ. Crossover second toe deformity. Foot Ankle Int. 1987;8:29–39.
8. Coughlin MJ. Subluxation and dislocation of the second metatarsophalangeal joint. Orthop Clin North Am. 1989;20:535–51.
9. Deland J, II-Hoon S. The medial crossover toe: a cadaveric dissection. Foot Ankle Int. 2000;21:375–8.
10. Thompson FM, Hamilton WG. Problems of the second metatarsophalangeal joint. Orthopedics. 1987;10:83–9.
11. Kaz AJ, Coughlin MJ. Crossover second toe: demographics, etiology, and radio- graphic assessment. Foot Ankle Int. 2007;28:1223–37.

12. Myerson MS, Shereff MJ. The pathological anatomy of claw and hammer toes. J Bone Joint Surg Am. 1989;71(1):45–9.
13. Hardy R, Clapham J. Observations on hallux valgus. J Bone Joint Surg. 1951;33-B:376–91.
14. Bhutta MA, Chauhan D, Zubairy AI, Barrie J. Second metatarsophalangeal joint instability and second metatarsal length association depends on the method of measurement. Foot Ankle Int. 2010;31(6):486–91.
15. Fleischer AE, Ahmad M, Shah S, Catena F, Weil LS Sr, Weil L Jr. Association of abnormal metatarsal parabola with second metatarsophalangeal joint plantar plate pathology. Foot Ankle Int. 2017;38(3):289–97.
16. Nilsonne H. Hallux rigidus and its treatment. Acta Orthop Scand. 1930;1:295–303.
17. Morton DJ. Structural factors in static disorders of the foot. Am J Surg. 1930;9(2):315–28.
18. Klein EE, Weil L Jr, Weil LS Sr, Bowen M, Fleischer AE. Positive drawer test combined with radiographic deviation of the third metatarsophalangeal joint suggests high grade tear of the second metatarsophalangeal joint plantar plate. Foot Ankle Spec. 2014;7(6):466–70.
19. Postema K, Burm PE, Zande ME, Limbeek J. Primary metatarsalgia: the influence of a custom moulded insole and a rocker bar on plantar pressure. Prosthetics Orthot Int. 1998;22:35–44.
20. Hsi WL, Kang JH, Lee XX. Optimum position of metatarsal pad in metatarsalgia for pressure relief. Am J Phys Med Rehabil. 2005;84:514–20.
21. Kang JH, Chen MD, Chen SC, Hsi WL. Correlations between subjective treatment responses and plantar pressure parameters of metatarsal pad treatment in metatarsalgia patients: a prospective study. BMC Musculoskelet Disord. 2006;7:95.
22. Yavuz M, Botek G, Davis BL. Plantar shear stress distributions: comparing actual and predicted frictional forces at the foot–ground interface. J Biomech. 2007;40(13):3045–9.
23. Yavuz M, Hetherington VJ, Botek G, Hirschman GB, et al. Forefoot plantar shear stress distribution in hallux valgus patients. Gait Posture. 2009;30:257–9.
24. Dreeben SM, Noble PC, Hammerman S, Bishop JO, Tullos HS. Metatarsal osteotomy for primary metatarsalgia: radiographic and pedobarographic study. Foot Ankle. 1989;9:214–8.
25. Kaipel M, Krapf D, Wyss C. Metatarsal length does not correlate with maximal peak pressure and maximal force. Clin Orthop Relat Res. 2011;469:1161–6.
26. Wanivenhaus A, Brettschneider W. Influence of metatarsal head displacement on metatarsal pressure distribution after hallux valgus surgery. Foot Ankle Int. 1993;14:85–9.
27. Ledoux WR, Shofer JB, Ahroni JH, Smith DG, Sangeorzan BJ, Boyko EJ. Biomechanical differences among pes cavus, neutrally aligned, and pes planus feet in subjects with diabetes. Foot Ankle Int. 2003;24:845–50.
28. Crosbie J, Burns J, Ouvrier RA. Pressure characteristics in painful pes cavus feet resulting from Charcot-Marie-Tooth disease. Gait Posture. 2008;28:545–51.
29. Jung HG, Zaret DI, Parks BG, Schon LC. Effect of first meta- tarsal shortening and dorsiflexion osteotomies on forefoot plantar pressure in a cadaver model. Foot Ankle Int. 2005;26: 748–53.
30. Van Beek C, Greisberg J. Mobility of the first ray: review article. Foot Ankle Int. 2011;32(9):917–22.
31. Saltzman CL, Nawoczenski DA. Complexities of foot architecture as a base of support. J Orthop Sports Phys Ther. 1995;21:354–60.
32. Olson T, Seidel MR. The evolutionary basis of some clinical disorders of the human foot: a comparative survey of the living primates. Foot Ankle Int. 1983;3(6):322–41.
33. Hicks JH. The mechanics of the foot. Part I: the joints. J Anat. 1953;87(4):345–57.
34. Cornwall MW, McPoil TG. Motion of the calcaneus, navicular and first metatarsal during the stance phase of gait. J Am Podiatr Med Assoc. 92:67, 2002–76.
35. Kelso SF, Richie DH Jr, Cohen IR, Weed JH, Root ML. Direction and range of motion of the first ray. J Am Podiatr Med Assoc. 1982;72(12):600–5.
36. Johnson C, Christensen JC. Biomechanics of the first ray part 1. The effects of the peroneus longus function. A three dimensional kinematic study on a cadaver model. J Foot Ankle Surg. 1999;38(5):313–21.

37. Perez HR, Leon KR, Jeffrey CC. The effect of frontal plane position on first ray motion: Forefoot locking mechanism. Foot Ankle Int. 2008;29(1):72–6.
38. Morton D. Hypermobility of the first metatarsal bone: the interlinking factor between metatarsalgia and longitudinal arch strains. J Bone Joint Surg. 1928;10:187–96.
39. Allen MK, Cuddeford TJ, Glasoe WM, DeKam LM, Lee PJ, Wagner KJ, Yack HJ. Relationship between static mobility of the first ray and first ray, midfoot, and hindfoot motion during gait. Foot Ankle Int. 2004;25:391–6.
40. Glasoe WM, Yack HJ, Saltzman CL. Measuring first ray mobility with a new device. Arch Phys Med Rehabil. 1999;80:122–4.
41. Grebing BR, Coughlin MJ. The effect of ankle position on the exam for first ray mobility. Foot Ankle Int. 2004;25:467–75.
42. Rush SM, Christensen JC, Johnson CH. Biomechanics of the first ray. Part 2: metatarsus primus varus as a cause of hypermobility. A three-dimensional kinematic analysis in a cadaver model. J Foot Ankle Surg. 2000;39(2):68–77.
43. Lapidus PW. Operative correction of the metatarsus varus primus in hallux valgus. Surg Gynecol Obstet. 1934;58:183–91.
44. Hansen ST. Hallux valgus surgery: Morton and Lapidus were right! Clin Podiatr Med Surg. 1996;13(3):347–354, 1996.
45. Hofbauer MH, Grossman JP. The Lapidus procedure. Clin Podiatr Med Surg. 1996;13(3):485–96.
46. Gellman H, Lenihan M, Halikis N, Botte MJ, Giordani M, Perry J. Selective tarsal arthrodesis: an in vitro analysis of the effect on foot motion. Foot Ankle Int. 1987;8(3):127–33.
47. Ouzounian TJ, Shereff MJ. In vitro determination of midfoot function. Foot Ankle Int. 1989;10(3):140–6.
48. Roling BA, Christensen JC, Johnson CH. Biomechanics of the first ray. Part IV: the effect of selected medial column arthrodeses. A three- dimensional kinematic analysis in a cadaver model. J Foot Ankle Surg. 2002;41:278–85.
49. Feibel JB, Tisdel CL, Donley BG. Lesser metatarsal osteotomies. A biomechanical approach to metatarsalgia. Foot Ankle Clin. 2001;6:473–89.
50. Glasoe WM, Allen MK, Kepros T, Stonewall L, Ludewig PM. Dorsal first ray mobility in women athletes with a history of stress fracture of the second or third metatarsal. J Orthop Sports Phys Ther. 2001;32:560–5.
51. Weinfeld SB, Haddad SL, Myerson MS. Metatarsal stress fractures. Clin Sports Med. 1997;16:319–38.
52. Coughlin MJ. Hallux valgus. J Bone Joint Surg Am. 1996;78:932–66.
53. Helal B, Rowley DI, Cracchiolo A, Myerson MS. Hallux valgus and rigidus. In: Surgery of disorders of the foot and ankle. 1st ed. London: Lippincott-Raven; 1996. p. 303–26.
54. Thomas S, Barrington R. Hallux valgus. Curr Orthop. 2003;17:299–307.
55. Saltzman CL, Aper RL, Brown TD. Anatomic determinants of first metatarsophalangeal flexion moments in hallux valgus. Clin Orthop Relat Res. 1997;339:261–9.
56. Root ML, Orien WP, Weed JH. Normal and abnormal function of the foot. In: Clinical biomechanics. 1st ed. Los Angeles: Clinical Biomechanics Corporation. p. 1977.
57. Klaue K, Hansen ST, Masquelet AC. Clinical, quantitative assessment of first tarsometatarsal mobility in the sagittal plane and its relation to hallux valgus deformity. Foot Ankle Int. 1994;15(1):9–13.
58. Dietze A, Bahlke U, Martin H, Mittlmeier T. First ray instability in hallux valgus deformity: a radiokinematic and pedobarographic analysis. Foot Ankle Int. 2013;34:124–30.
59. Glasoe WM, Allen MK, Saltzman CL. First ray dorsal mobility in relation to hallux valgus deformity and first intermetatarsal angle. Foot Ankle Int. 2001;22:98–101.
60. Shibuya N, Roukis TS, Jupiter DC. Mobility of the first ray in patients with or without hallux valgus deformity: systematic review and meta-analysis. J Foot Ankle Surg. 2017;56:1070–5.
61. Coughlin MJ, Jones CP, Viladot R, Golano P, Grebing BR, Kennedy MJ, Shurnas PS, Alvarez F. Hallux valgus and first ray mobility: a cadaveric study. Foot Ankle Int. 2004;25:537–44.

62. Faber FW, Mulder PG, Verhaar JA. Role of first ray hypermobility in the outcome of the Hohmann and the Lapidus procedure: a prospective, randomized trial involving one hundred and one feet. J Bone Joint Surg Am. 2004;86-A:486–95.
63. Coughlin MJ, Jones CP. Hallux valgus and first ray mobility: a prospective study. J Bone Joint Surg Am. 2007;89:1887–98.
64. Kim JY, Park JS, Hwang SK, Young KW, Sung IH. Mobility changes of the first ray after hallux valgus surgery: clinical results after proximal metatarsal chevronosteotomy and distal soft tissue procedure. Foot Ankle Int. 2008;29:468–79.
65. Faber FW, van Kampen PM, Bloembergen MW. Long-term results of the Hohmann and Lapidus procedure for the correction of hallux valgus: a prospective, randomised trial with eight- to 11-year follow-up involving 101 feet. Bone Joint J. 2013;95-B:1222–6.
66. Faber FW, Kleinrensink GJ, Verhoog MW, Vijn AH, Snijders CJ, Mulder PG, Verhaar JA. Mobility of the first tarsometatarsal joint in relation to hallux valgus deformity: anatomical and biomechanical aspects. Foot Ankle Int. 1999;20:651–6.
67. Roukis TS, Scherer PR, Anderson CF. Position of the first ray and motion of the first metatarsophalangeal joint. J Am Podiatr Med Assoc. 1996;86:538–46.
68. Roukis TS. Metatarsus primus elevatus in hallux rigidus: fact or fiction? J Am Podiatr Med Assoc. 2005;95:221–8.
69. Coughlin MJ, Shurnas PS. Hallux rigidus: demographics, etiology, and radiographic assessment. Foot Ankle Int. 2003;24:731–43.
70. Horton GA, Park YW, Myerson MS. Role of metatarsus primus elevatus in the pathogenesis of hallux rigidus. Foot Ankle Int. 1999;20:777–80.
71. Greisberg J, Sperber L, Prince DE. Mobility of the first ray in various foot disorders. Foot Ankle Int. 2012;33:44–9.
72. Coughlin M, Jones C. Hallux Valgus; demographics, etiology and radiographic assessment. Foot Ankle Int. 2007;28:759–77.
73. Meyer JM, Tomeno B, Burdet A. Metatarsalgia due to insufficient support by the first ray. Int Orthop. 1981;5:193–201.
74. Grebing BR, Coughlin MJ. Evaluation of Morton's theory of second metatarsal hypertrophy. J Bone Joint Surg Am. 2004;86-A(7):1375–84.
75. Cooper AJ, Clifford PD, Parikh VK, Steinmetz ND, Mizel MS. Instability of the first metatarsal-cuneiform joint: diagnosis and discussion of an independent pain generator in the foot. Foot Ankle Int. 2009;30(10):928–32.
76. Mueller MJ, Strube MJ. Generalizability of in-shoe peak pressure measures using the f-scan system. Clin Biomech. 1996;11:159–64.
77. Abouaesha F, van Schie C, Griffths G, Young R, Boulton A. Plantar tissue thickness is related to peak plantar pressure in the high-risk diabetic foot. Diabetes Care. 2001;24:1270–4.
78. Waldecker U. Pedographicanalysis of hallux valgus deformity. Foot Ankle Surg. 2004;10: 121–4.
79. Nyska M, Liberson A, McCabe C, Linge K, Klenerman L. Plantar foot pressure distribution in patients with hallux valgus treated by distal soft tissue procedure and proximal metatarsal osteotomy. Foot Ankle Surg. 1998;4:35–41.
80. Kernozek TW, Elfessi A, Sterriker S. Clinical and biomechanical risk factors of patients diagnosed with hallux valgus. J Am Podiatr Med Assoc. 2003;93:97–103.
81. Bryant A, Tinley P, Singer K. Plantar pressure distribution in normal, hallux valgus and hallux limitus feet. Foot. 1999;9:115–9.
82. Mickle KJ, Munro BJ, Lord SR, Menz HB, Steele JR. Gait, balance and plantar pressures in older people with toe deformities. Gait Posture. 2011;34:347–51.
83. Mueller MJ, et al. Forefoot structural predictors of plantar pressures during walking in people with diabetes and peripheral neuropathy. J Biomech. 2003;36:1009–17.
84. Branch HE. Pathologic dislocation of the second toe. J Bone Joint Surg. 1937;19:978–84.
85. Coughlin MJ. Lesser toe deformities. Orthopaedics. 1987;10(1):63–75.

86. Yu GV, Judge MS, Hudson JR, Seidelmann FE. Predislocationsyndrome:progressive subluxation/dislocation of the lesser metatarsophalangeal joint. J Am Podiatr Med Assoc. 2002;92:182–99.
87. Shirzad K, Kiesau CD, DeOrio JK, Parekh SG. Lesser toe deformities. J Am Acad Orthop Surg. 2011;19:505–14.
88. Gribbin CK, Ellis SJ, Nguyen J, Williamson E, Cody EA. Relationship of radiographic and clinical parameters with hallux valgus and second ray pathology. Foot Ankle Int. 2017;38(1):14–9.
89. Ahroni JH, Boyko EJ, Forsberg RC. Clinical correlates of plantar pressure among diabetic veterans. Diabetes Care. 1999;22:965–72.
90. Bus S, Maas M, de Lange A, Michels R, Levi M. Elevated plantar pressures in neuropathic diabetic patients with claw/hammer toe deformity. J Biomech. 2005;38:1918–25.
91. Lavery LA, Armstrong DG, Vela SA, Quebedeaux TL, Fleischli JG. Practical criteria for screening patients at high risk for diabetic foot ulceration. Arch Intern Med. 1998;158:157–62.
92. Holewski JJ, Moss KM, Stess RM, Graf PM, Grunfeld C. Prevalence of foot pathology and lower extremity complications in a diabetic outpatient clinic. J Rehabil Res Dev. 1989;26:35–44.
93. Rozema A, Ulbrecht JS, Pammer SE, Cavanagh PR. In-shoe plantar pressures during activities of daily living: implications for therapeutic footwear design. Foot Ankle Int. 1996;17(6):352–9.
94. Menz HB, Lord SR. Foot pain impairs balance and functional ability in com- munity-dwelling older people. J Am Podiatr Med Assoc. 2001;91:222–9.
95. Leardini A, Benedetti MG, Catani F, Simoncini L, Giannini S. An atomically based protocol for the description of foot segment kinematics during gait. Clin Biomech. 1999;14:528–36.
96. Nester CJ, Liu AM, Ward E, Howard D, Cocheba J, Derrick T, Patterson P. In vitro study of foot kinematics using **a** dynamic walking cadaver model. J Biomech. 2007;40:1927–37.
97. Bus SA, Maas M, Cavanagh PR, Michels RP, Levi M. Plantar fat-pad displacement in neuropathic diabetic patients with toe deformity: a magnetic resonance imaging study. Diabetes Care. 2004;27(10):2376–81.
98. Bojsen-Moller F. Anatomy of the forefoot, normal and pathologic. Clin Orthop Relat Res. 1979;142:10–8.
99. Bojsen-Moller F, Flagstad KE. Plantar aponeurosis and internal architecture of the ball of the foot. J Anat. 1976;121:599–611.
100. Stainsby GD. Pathological anatomy and dynamic effect of the displaced plantar plate and the importance of the integrity of the plantar plate- deep transverse metatarsal ligament tie-bar. Ann R Coll Surg Engl. 1997;79(1):58–68.
101. Hamel AJ, Donahue SW, Sharkey NA. Contributions of active and passive toe flexion to forefoot loading. Clin Orthop Relat Res. 2001;(393):326–34.
102. Bojsen-Møller F. Calcaneocuboid joint and stability of the longitudinal arch of the foot at the high gear and low gear push off. J Anat. 1979;129:165–76.
103. Galica A, Hagedorn TJ, Dufour AB, Riskowski JL, Hillstrom HJ, Casey VA, Hannan MT. Hallux valgus and plantar pressure loading: the Framingham foot study. J Foot Ankle Res. 2013;6:1–18.

Chapter 4
PIPJ Arthroplasty Without Fixation

David Edwards

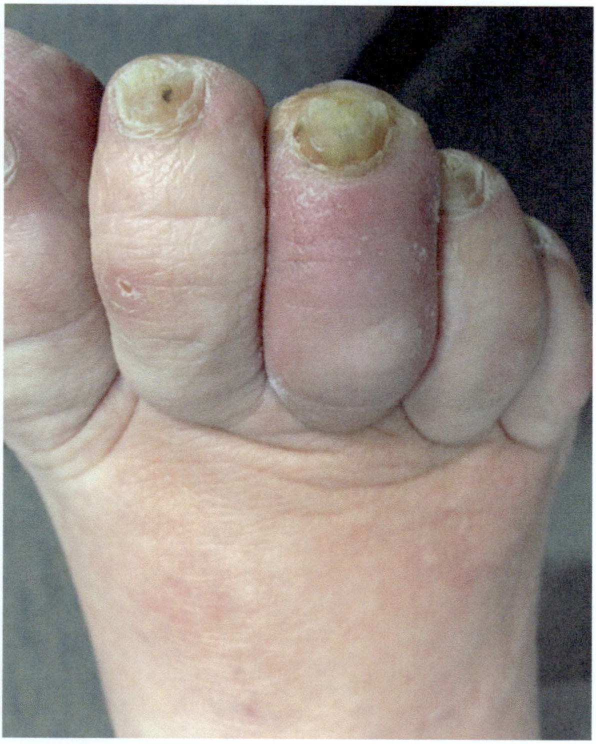

D. Edwards (✉)
Foot and Ankle Clinic, Logan, UT, USA
e-mail: DGEdwards@apma.org

E. A. Cook, J. J. Cook (eds.), *Hammertoes*,
https://doi.org/10.1007/978-3-319-16552-3_4

History

The patient is a 77-year-old female who had been in my practice for at-risk diabetic care for 6 years. After missing an appointment and failing to follow up in a timely manor, she presented with cellulitis and an open lesion on the distal third toe of the right foot. Her diabetes was stable and no other medical concerns were noted. Standard conservative care was followed, and improvement in cellulitis was noted, but the distal lesion showed little improvement. After 3 weeks of failed resolution via conservative care, we decided to proceed with surgical intervention.

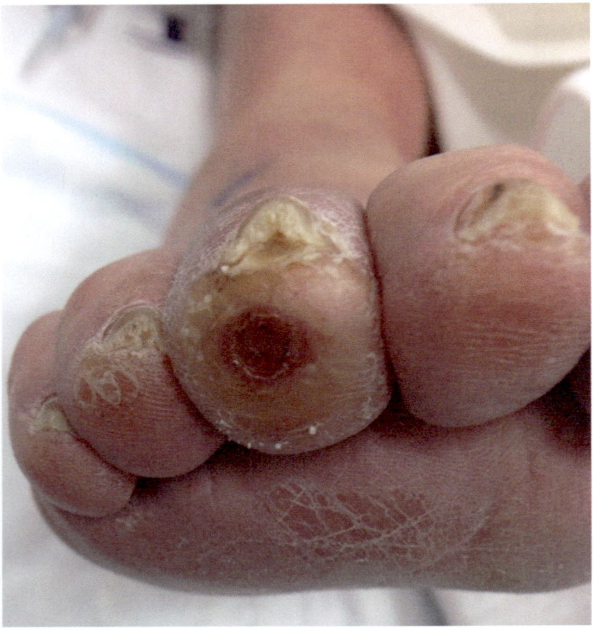

Treatment Plan

The goal of surgery was to relieve the plantar pressure off the distal third toe. This was necessary to allow for healing of the distal lesion. Because of the open lesion distally and some remaining mild cellulitis, the decision was to perform a non-fixated PIPJ arthroplasty to minimize any postoperative complications. Although other deformities existed, they were relatively non-symptomatic and had responded well to her ongoing at-risk care. The decision was to do no other procedures at this time.

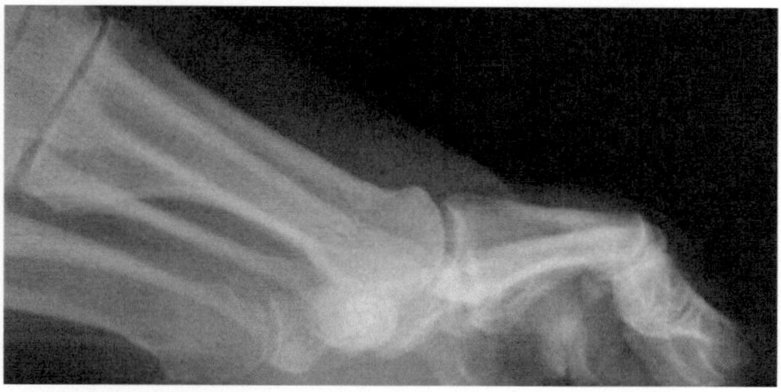

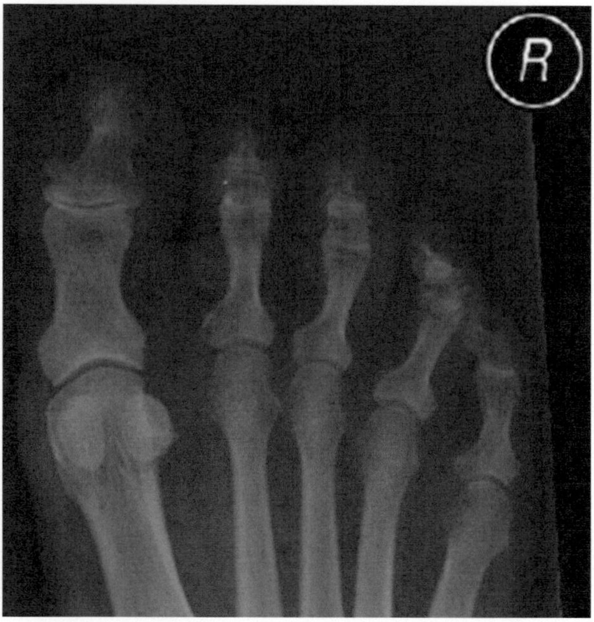

Surgical Technique

The surgical technique will be described in a stepwise photographic sequence on the pages that follow.

- Dorsal transverse elliptical incision at the PIPJ level
- Skin wedge resection to assist dorsiflexion of the digit at the closure

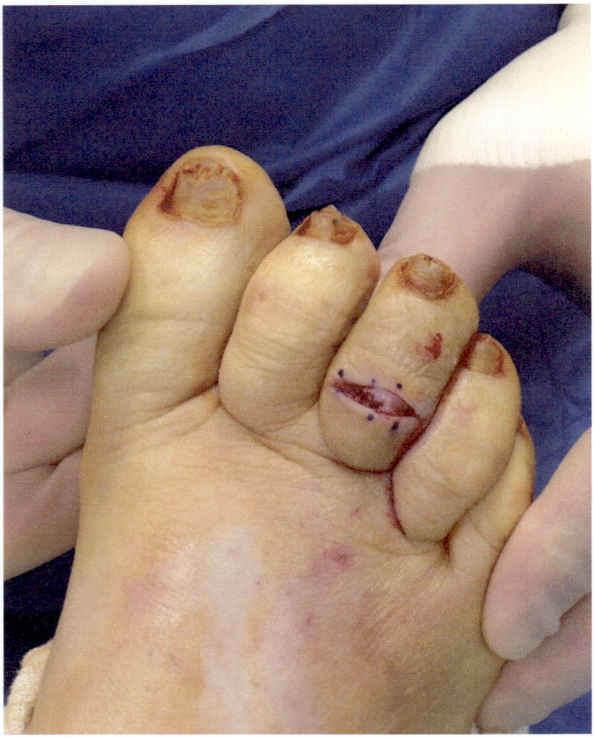

- Identify and isolate the extensor digitorum longus tendon.

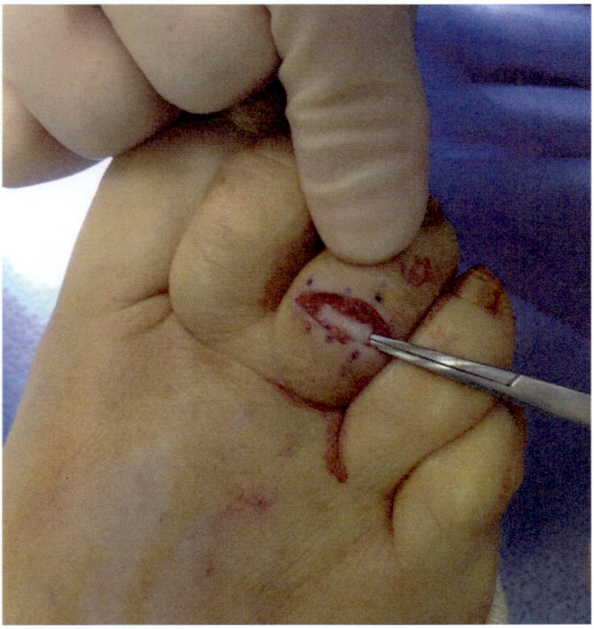

- Perform EDL tenotomy at the joint level.
- Reflect the proximal and distal ends of the tendon for later re-approximation.

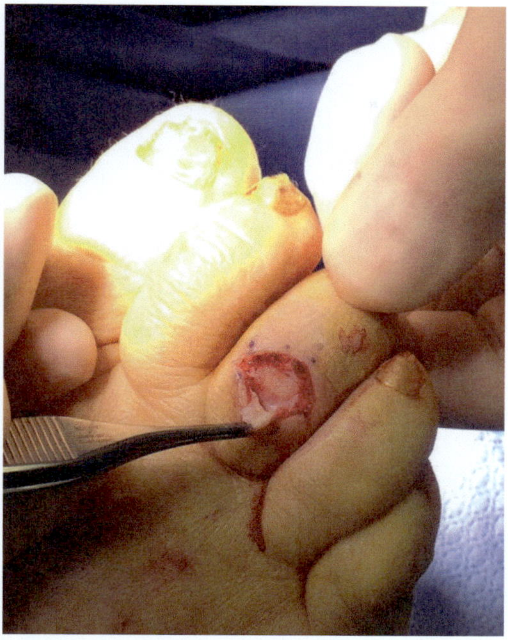

- Isolate and free the head of the proximal phalanx.

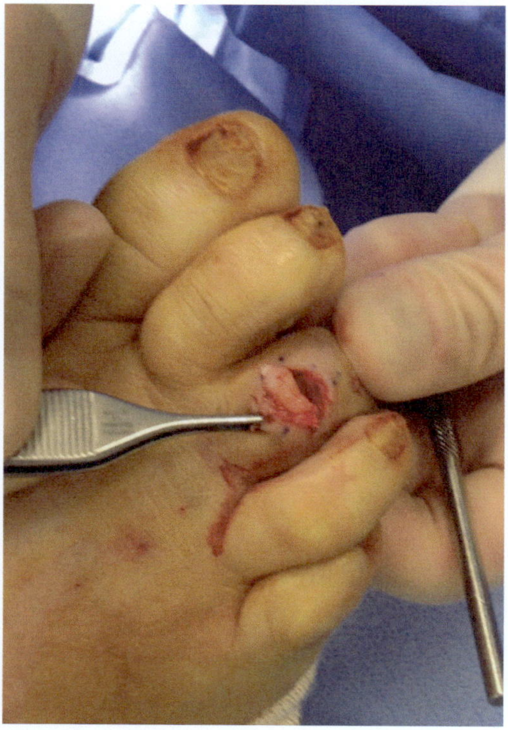

- Remove the necessary amount of the bone for the needed correction.

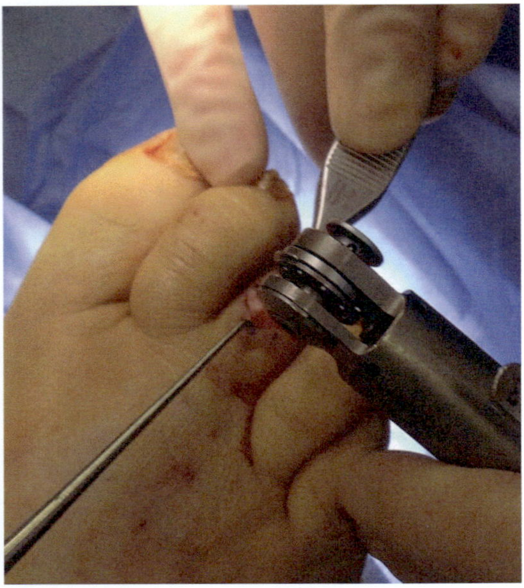

- Remove the cartilage surface off the base of the intermediate phalanx.

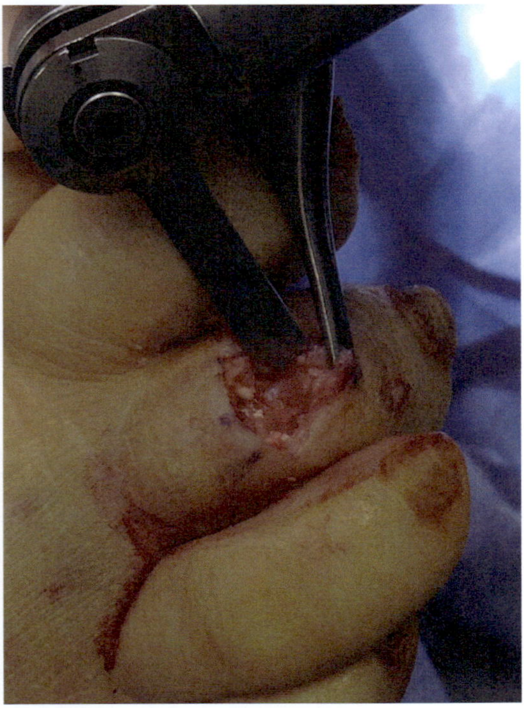

- Shorten the tendon for appropriate correction and dorsiflexion.
- Re-approximate the EDL using a horizontal mattress with 4–0 absorbable suture.

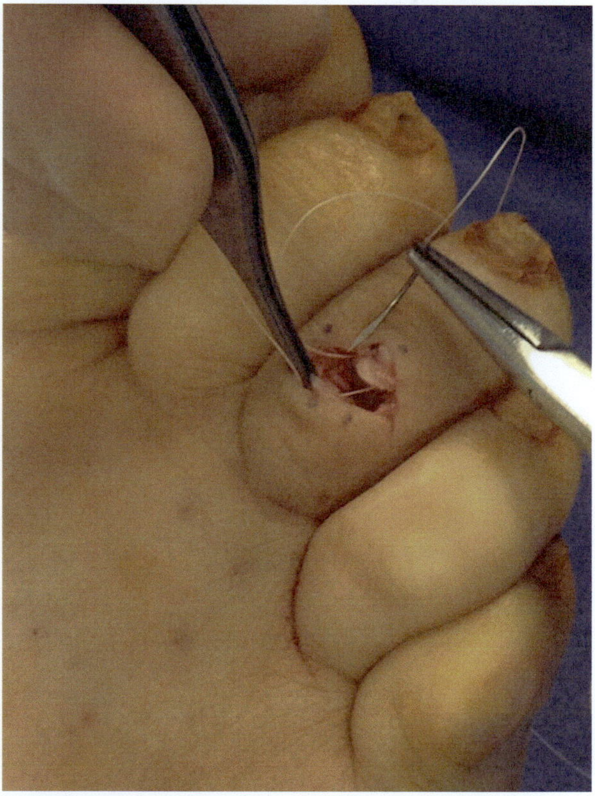

- Dorsiflex the toe to the corrected position as you complete the mattress suture.

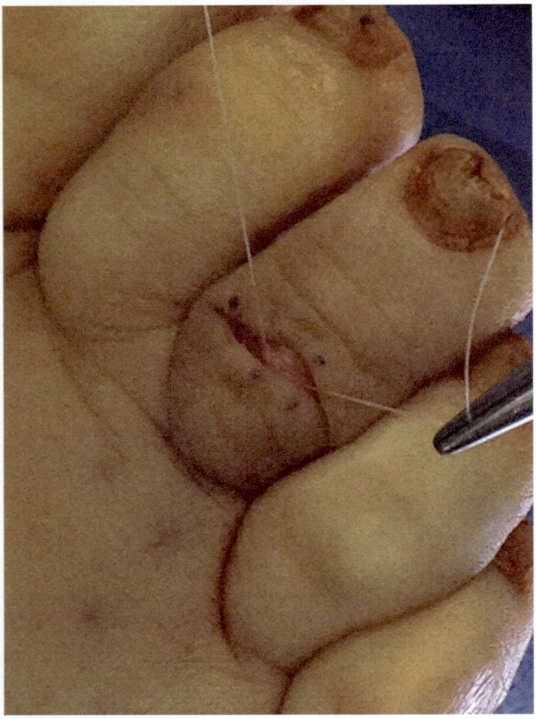

- Close the skin incision with a simple interrupted stitch.
- Bandage the toe in a splinted corrected position.

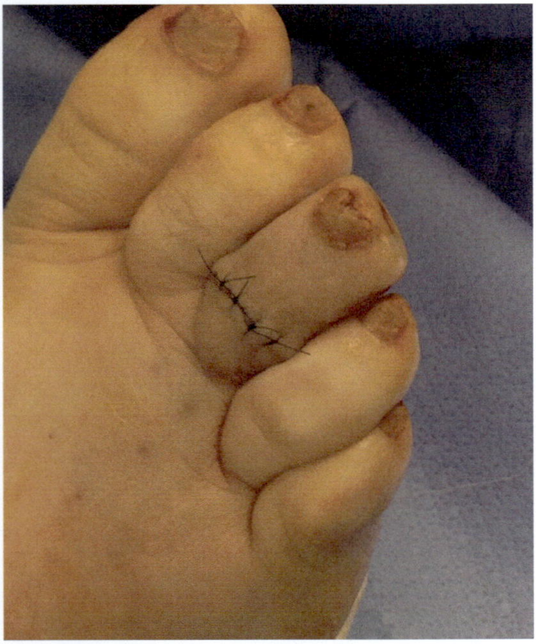

- Surgically corrected toe in the operating room

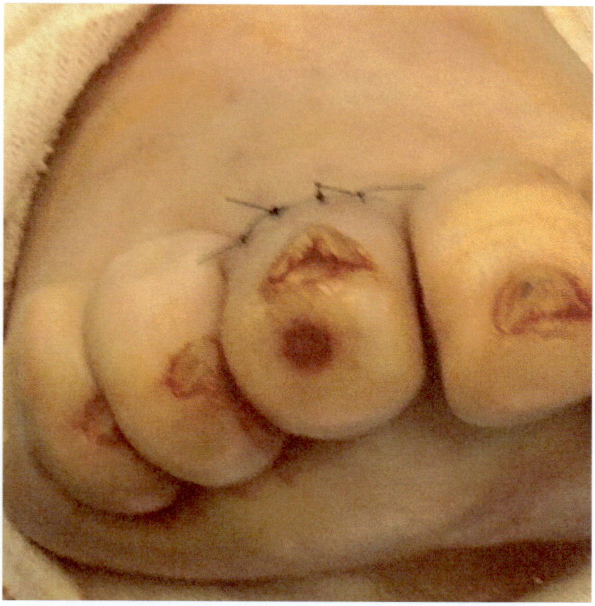

- Post-op day 3
- Lesion beginning to close over and fill in

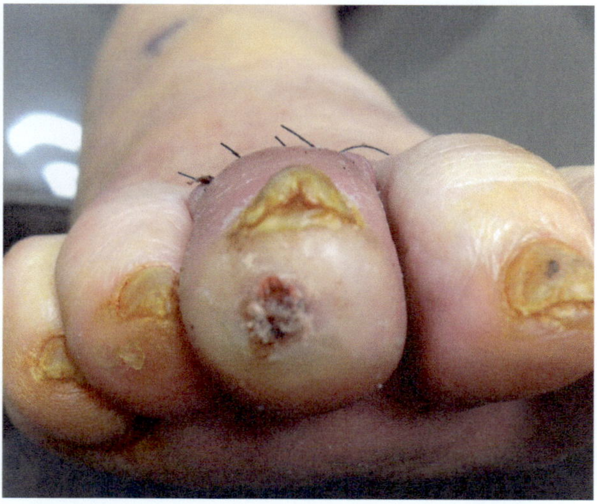

- Two weeks post-op
- Hyperkeratotic skin removed
- Pink tissue with shallow lesion
- No pressure on distal third toe

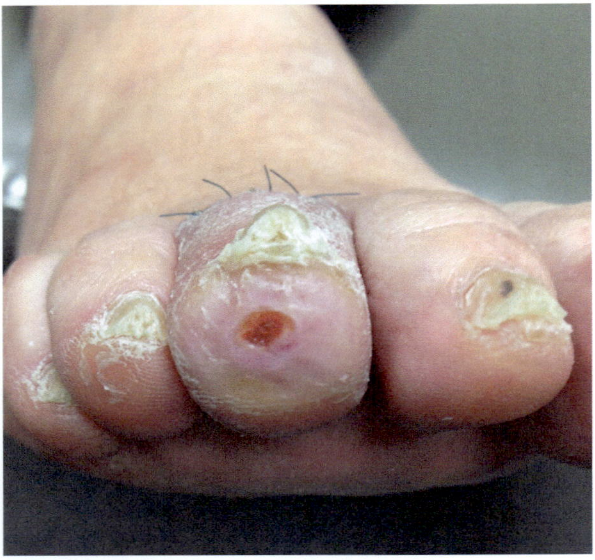

Pitfalls

- There is potential for a floppy digit (that can be minimized with Coban or other splinting).
- Potential for a new distal pressure lesion on an adjacent toe (can be managed by ongoing at-risk care).

Pearls

- Consider a flexor tendon release if needed.
- Use good postoperative bandaging and splinting to assist with alignment.

Chapter 5
PIPJ Interpositional Arthroplasty

Adam Landsman

Presentation/History

Hammertoe deformity can be classified in numerous ways, depending on the etiology, flexibility, and direction of deformity. Hammertoes may be flexible, semirigid, or rigid depending on whether it is reducible or not. The position may be adducted or abducted, varus or valgus, over- or underlapped with adjacent toes, and flexed to various degrees [1–4]. Although rare, hammertoes can be congenital [5]. More commonly, hammertoes are acquired as a result of imbalances from intrinsic and/or extrinsic muscles influencing the metatarsal phalangeal and interphalangeal joints.

Once developed, hammertoes can be quite painful. Joint contractures result in pressure points at the interphalangeal joints and tip of the toes and can lead to retrograde buckling and subsequent metatarsalgia [6]. Flexed joints frequently result in callous formation and may lead to painful porokeratosis, ulcerations, and bursitis. Degenerative changes can cause malpositioning and lead to joint spurs and arthritis.

Diagnosis/Assessment

Diagnosis and assessment begin with a physical examination to determine the location of any skin lesions, erythema, open wounds, callous, edema, pain, and interdigital maceration. Flexibility of the interphalangeal joints can be described by the ability to reduce a deformity. Flexible hammertoes are easily reduced, while rigid

A. Landsman (✉)
Division of Podiatric Surgery, Cambridge Health Alliance, Cambridge, MA, USA

Harvard University, School of Medicine, Cambridge, MA, USA
e-mail: alandsman@cha.harvard.edu

E. A. Cook, J. J. Cook (eds.), *Hammertoes*,
https://doi.org/10.1007/978-3-319-16552-3_5

hammertoes may be permanently flexed and even arthrosed in position. Radiographic images may demonstrate subluxation, dislocation, malpositioning, and arthritic changes.

Biomechanics is critical to the assessment of hammertoe deformity, and a proper evaluation should include static and dynamic examinations, as well as weight-bearing and non-weight-bearing measurements. Some common causes of hammertoe deformity include flexor substitution, flexor stabilization, and extensor substitution.

Treatment/Surgical Technique

The interpositional arthroplasty is an excellent treatment for contracted hammertoes when a simple soft tissue release is insufficient, and an arthrodesis of the proximal interphalangeal joint (PIPJ) is unnecessary. With this procedure, the proximal phalanx is transected at the level of the surgical neck (diaphyseal/metaphyseal junction), and the head is delivered from the operative field. However, instead of leaving the raw bone at the cut surface of the proximal phalanx exposed, the extensor tendon is flapped down into the interspace and sutured in place. With this procedure, the interposed tendon helps to separate the proximal and middle phalanx, retaining some flexibility in the joint (Figs. 5.1, 5.2, 5.3, 5.4, 5.5, 5.6, 5.7, 5.8, and 5.9).

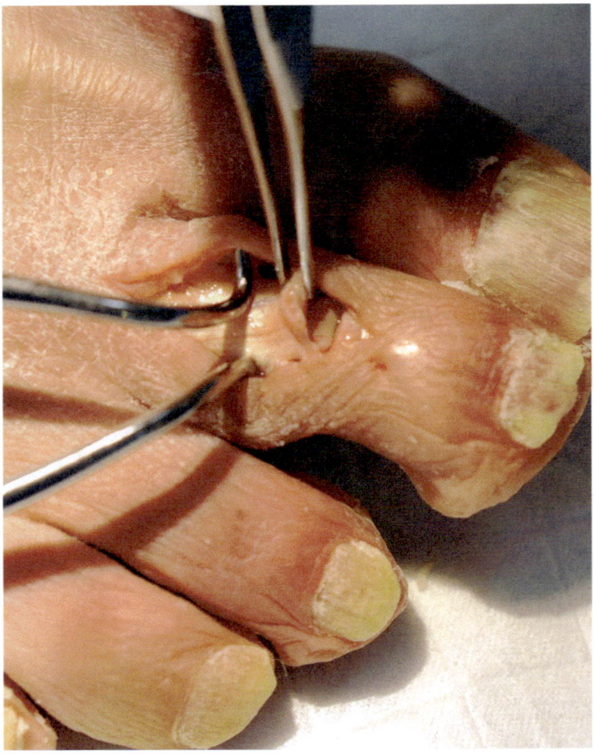

Fig. 5.1 After performing a longitudinal incision, dissection is deepened to the level of the extensor tendon. The tendon is transected distal to the proximal interphalangeal joint (PIPJ). The wing and sling are released on the medial and lateral sides of the joint, and the tendon is reflected proximally to the level of the surgical neck of the proximal phalanx

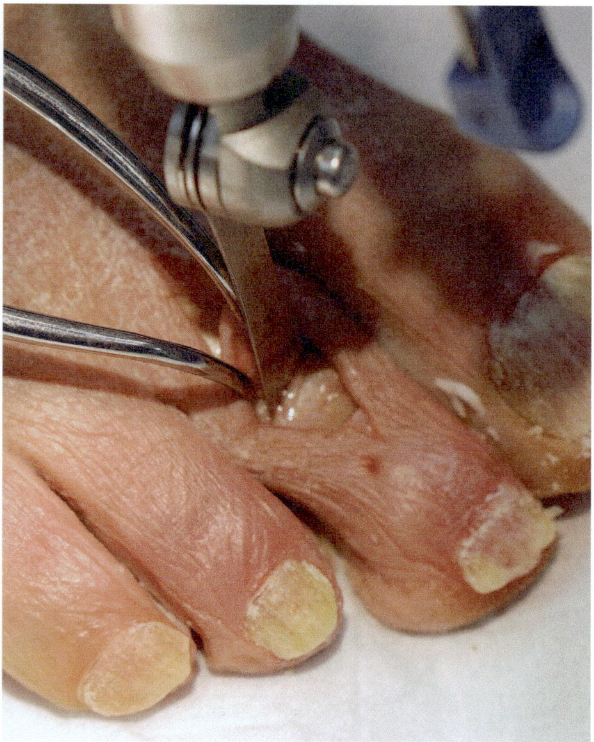

Fig. 5.2 The phalanx is transected at the level of the surgical neck

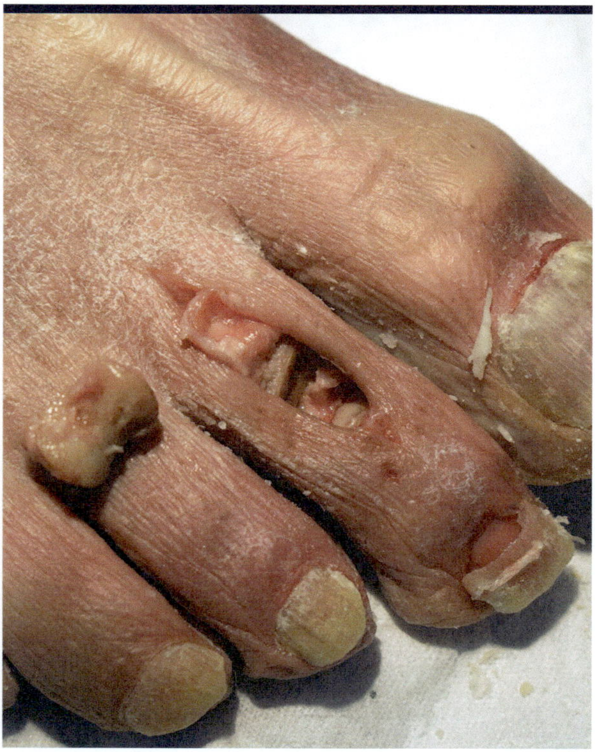

Fig. 5.3 The head of the proximal phalanx is delivered from the surgical field

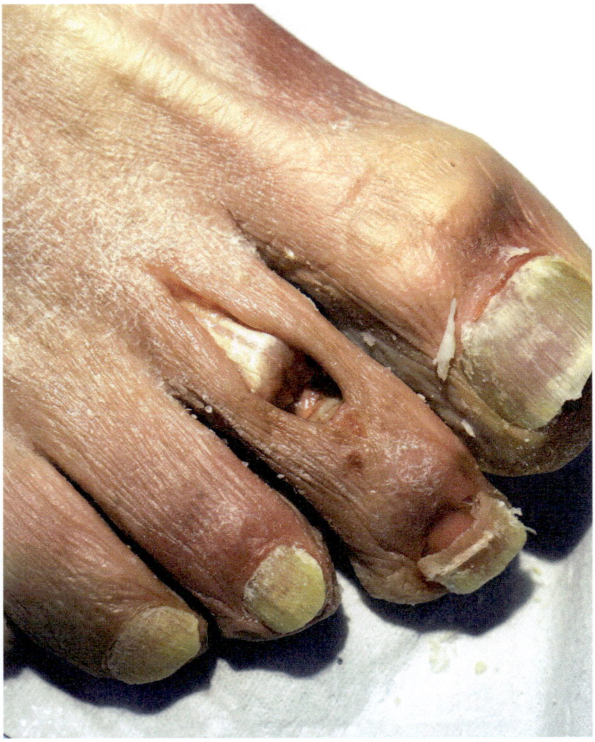

Fig. 5.4 The extensor tendon is extended distally and flapped over the cut end of the proximal phalanx

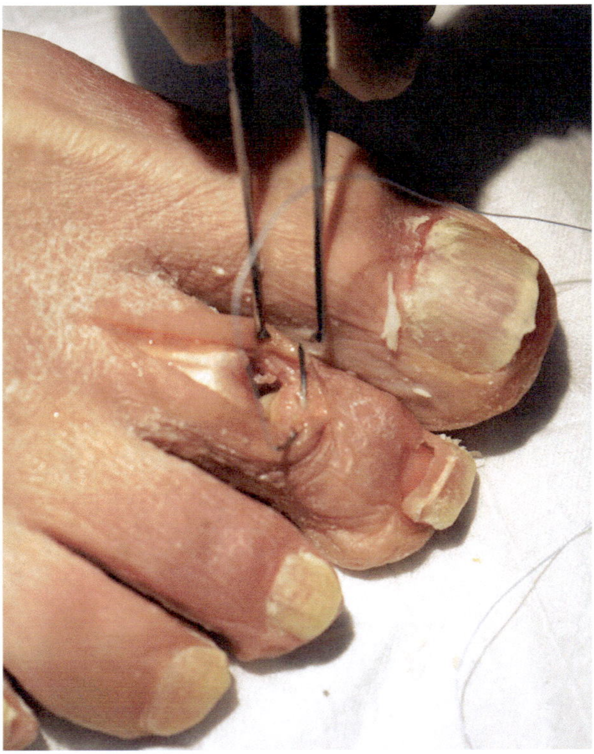

Fig. 5.5 The extensor tendon is re-approximated with a box stitch. First the suture is passed from lateral to medial through the portion of the tendon overlying the base of the middle phalanx

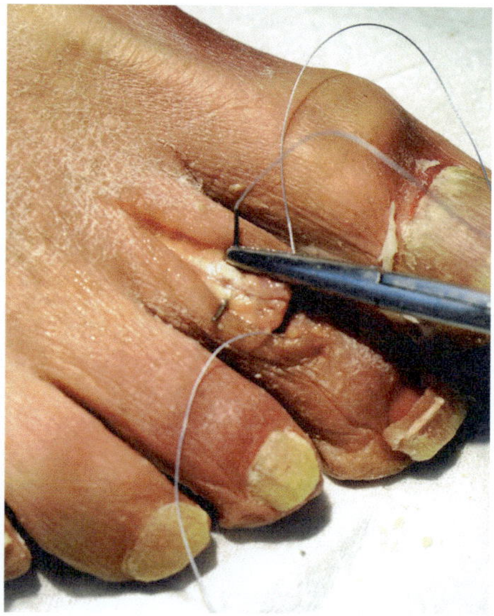

Fig. 5.6 Next, the proximal portion of the extensor tendon is draped over the distal end of the proximal phalanx, and the suture is passed from medial to lateral, just above the distal end of the proximal phalanx

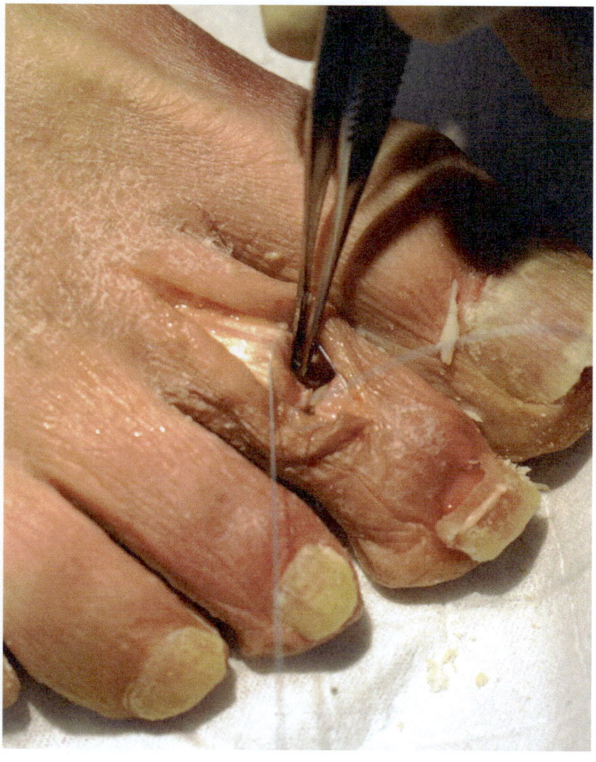

Fig. 5.7 The tip of the extensor tendon is held down with a forceps, between the phalanges

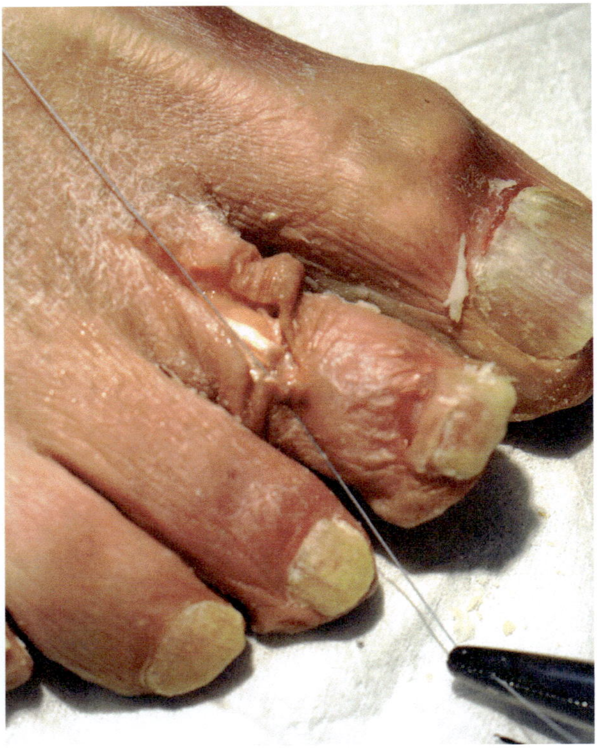

Fig. 5.8 While the tendon is held in place, the box stitch is tied snuggly, trapping the tip of the extensor tendon in the joint space

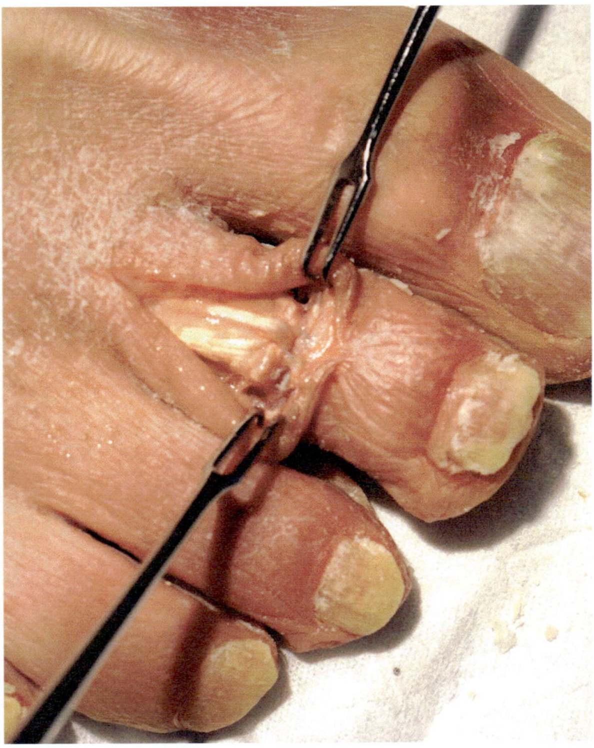

Fig. 5.9 Final result is seen. The extensor tendon is re-approximated with the tip of the extensor tendon secured in the space of the proximal interphalangeal joint

Outcomes/Case Resolution

This procedure results in a soft tissue buffer between the raw end of the proximal phalanx and the base of the middle phalanx. As a result, the patients report less pain and less stiffness with range of motion. Swelling is no different from the standard approach, and the use of the tip of the tendon as a spacer helps to retain length in the toe. Typically, I have these patients bearing full weight on the surgical foot on the day of surgery, provided that they wear a surgical shoe. After 1 week, I transition them to an athletic shoe, and they can return to full athletic activity 3 to 6 weeks after surgery. It is not uncommon to see some edema in the toe that can last up to 3 months, regardless of the procedure used to correct the deformity.

Clinical Pearls/Pitfalls

- With this procedure, there is a tendency to overtighten the extensor tendon, resulting in dorsiflexion at the PIPJ. It is recommended that the toe be held in a rectus or slightly plantarflexed position at the PIPJ while the suture is being secured to prevent this.
- In cases where there is an angular deformity to the toe, either a medial or lateral stitch can be added after securing the extensor tendon. This will have the effect of moving the toe medially or laterally. It also adds strength to the entire construct and so is recommended to help reinforce the repair.
- Finally, reinforced steri-strips can be placed longitudinally on the toe to help further stabilize the surgical repair. These can be used instead of percutaneous pins to help maintain alignment of the toe.

References

1. Jimenez AL, McGlamry ED, Green DR. Lesser ray deformities. In: McGlamry ED, editor. Comprehensive textbook of foot surgery. 1st ed. Baltimore: Williams & Wilkins; 1987. p. 71–3.
2. Turain I. Deformities of the smaller toes and surgical treatment. J Foot Surg. 1990;29(2):176–8.
3. Sorto LA. Surgical correction of hammer toes. J Am Podiatr Assoc. 1974;64(12):930–40.
4. Root ML, Orien WP, Weed JH. Normal and abnormal function of the foot. In: Clinical biomechanics. 2nd ed. Los Angeles: Clinical Biomechanics Corp; 1977. p. 442–60.
5. Yale I. Congenital and acquired deformities of the foot. In: Podiatric medicine. 2nd ed. Baltimore: Williams & Wilkins; 1980. p. 278–300.
6. Malay DS, Hillstrom H, Stanifer EG, Lefkowitz LR. The influence of digital stabilization on metatarsalgia. In: The Podiatry Institute, update 1990. Decatur: Podiatry Institute Publishing; 1990. p. 50–1.

Chapter 6
PIPJ Arthrodesis via Peg and Hole Technique

Amber M. Shane, Christopher L. Reeves, and Francesca Zappasodi

Presentation/History

The function of the lesser digits of the foot is based on a delicate balance of anatomic structures and their corresponding functions. Both intrinsic and extrinsic muscles alike contribute to the stability of the lesser digits. When this muscular balance is disrupted, it can result in various deformities such as hammertoes, claw toes, and mallet toes. These deformities are related to a person's inherited foot type as well as the specific biomechanics of a patient's foot. In general, these deformities are attributed to three different causes: flexor substitution, extensor substitution, and flexor stabilization [3]. In all of these instances, the balance between the functions of the flexors and extensors has been disrupted and leads to the development of the aforementioned digital deformities.

Patients typically present with complaints of contracted digits that cause discomfort from rubbing in closed shoe gear. Patients also can present with a heloma dura on the dorsal aspect of the PIPJ or at the distal tip of the digit, as a result of increased pressures to these areas in shoe gear. However, patients with hammered digits may not always initially complain about appearance or pain from the hammertoe itself. It is common that patients have metatarsalgia beneath the metatarsal heads of the corresponding hammered digits, since the toes are no longer fully contacting the ground and assuming the weight-bearing load. In addition, these

A. M. Shane (✉)
Orlando Foot and Ankle Clinic, Orlando, FL, USA

C. L. Reeves
Florida Hospital, Winter Park, FL, USA

F. Zappasodi
Foot and Ankle Associates, Mooresville, NC, USA

E. A. Cook, J. J. Cook (eds.), *Hammertoes*,
https://doi.org/10.1007/978-3-319-16552-3_6

patients tend to develop painful hyperkeratotic lesions under the affected metatarsal heads. This pain and increased plantar pressure to the area are a result of the retrograde subluxation that the hammered digits impose on their corresponding metatarsals.

Diagnosis/Assessment

Clinical assessment of digital deformities should begin with an overall assessment of the foot type. A pes cavus type foot structure lends itself to hammertoes with an etiology of extensor substitution. The increased declination of the lesser metatarsals results in passive pulling of the extensor tendons, resulting in metatarsophalangeal joint dorsiflexion. Prior to surgical intervention in these patients, hereditary motor-sensory neuropathies and other conditions commonly seen in patients with a cavus foot type should be ruled out. A pes planus foot type is more commonly associated with hammertoes caused by flexor stabilization, where the flexor digitorum longus or brevis muscles have gained mechanical advantage over the interossei [3]. Understanding the basic biomechanics associated with these foot types and the development of deformities can allow for a better understanding and the ability to treat the patient most effectively.

Radiographically, hammertoes can be evaluated on a lateral view where there is sagittal plane dorsal contracture at the proximal interphalangeal joint, when there is a fixed deformity (Fig. 6.1). On an AP (anterior-posterior) view, severe fixed digital contractures display a "gun barrel" sign at the interphalangeal joint. This radiographic sign is a result of the dorsiflexed proximal phalanx and plantarflexed middle phalanx overlapping, creating a hole analogous to the barrel of a gun. A peg and hole arthrodesis will particularly benefit hammertoes with a long second ray and an elongated middle or proximal phalanx (Fig. 6.2).

Treatment/Surgical Technique

There are multiple surgical procedures described in the literature that can be used to fix hammertoe deformities. The overall goals of these procedures are to create a rectus digit that has normal biomechanical function and to prevent recurrence of deformity. The repaired toe should participate in normal toe off during the gait cycle [3]. The peg and hole arthrodesis is particularly beneficial in reducing excessive digital length and providing a stable arthrodesis construct at the level of the PIPJ.

The peg and hole arthrodesis has been described in the literature for over 50 years. The advantages of this procedure include greater bone-to-bone contact, high union rate, and shortening of an excessively long digit. In addition, the peg and hole pro-

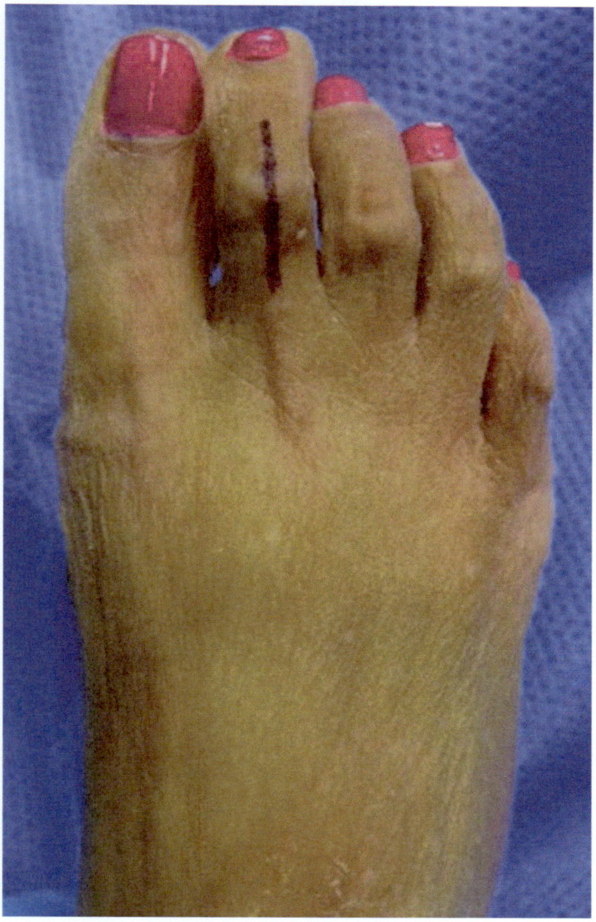

Fig. 6.1 Linear incisional approach for peg and hole arthrodesis

cedure doesn't necessitate fixation and offers superior strength with sagittal plane loading compared to end-to-end procedures [1, 2].

The incision for this procedure can be linear, transverse, or transverse semi-elliptical (Fig. 6.3). After the skin incision is made, blunt dissection is carried down until the long extensor tendon is visualized. The tendon is then transected transversely at the level of the PIPJ and the collateral ligaments released, allowing exposure of the interphalangeal joint. The extensor tendon is carefully reflected proximally allowing for exposure of the head and distal shaft of the proximal phalanx. Next, the medial, lateral, and plantar condyle resections are carefully drawn out on the head of the proximal phalanx (Fig. 6.4). These condyles are then resected from the head of proximal phalanx with a micro-oscillating saw to create the peg while preserving the dorsal cortex (Fig. 6.5). The cartilage on the distal tip of the

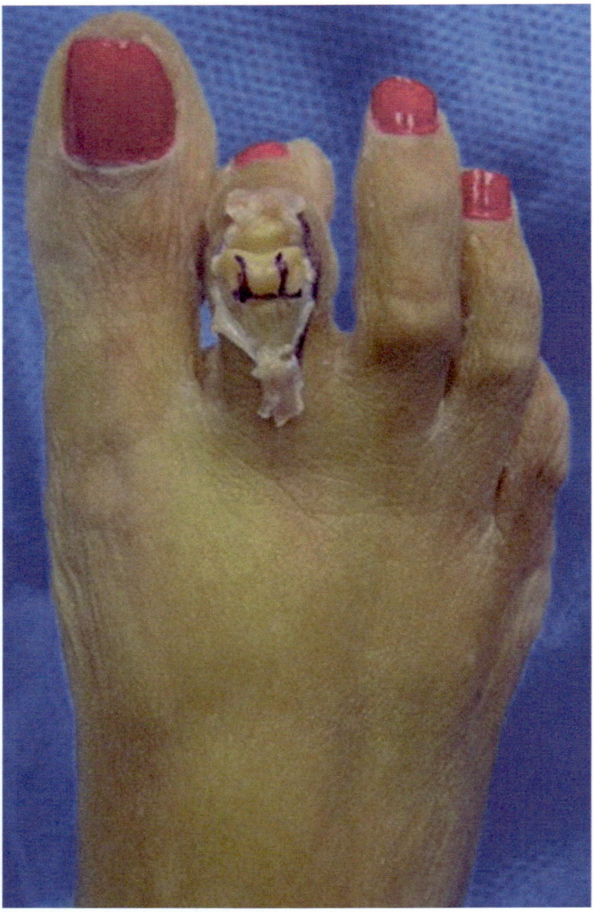

Fig. 6.2 Marking of the medial and lateral condyles on the proximal phalanx

remaining proximal phalanx is then resected (Fig. 6.6). A rotary bur can be used to further shape the peg to the desired size and shape. Next, a drill bit is used to create a hole in the base of the middle phalanx (Fig. 6.7). The hole is then subsequently reamed with a bur, to allow for seating of the peg (Fig. 6.8). Once the peg of the proximal phalanx fits into the prepared hole in the middle phalanx, an optional K-wire can then be placed in an anterograde fashion across the middle and distal phalanx, exiting the toe (Fig. 6.9). The K-wire is then advanced in a retrograde fashion across the PIPJ or MTPJ (metatarsophalangeal joint), while the joint is held in the reduced position (Fig. 6.10). Next, the K-wire is bent at a 90-degree angle to the toe; the tip of the wire is cut and appropriately capped. Redundant extensor tendon is excised and remaining tendon repaired with absorbable suture and the skin incision closed. The K-wire is left in place for 4–6 weeks duration postoperatively [3].

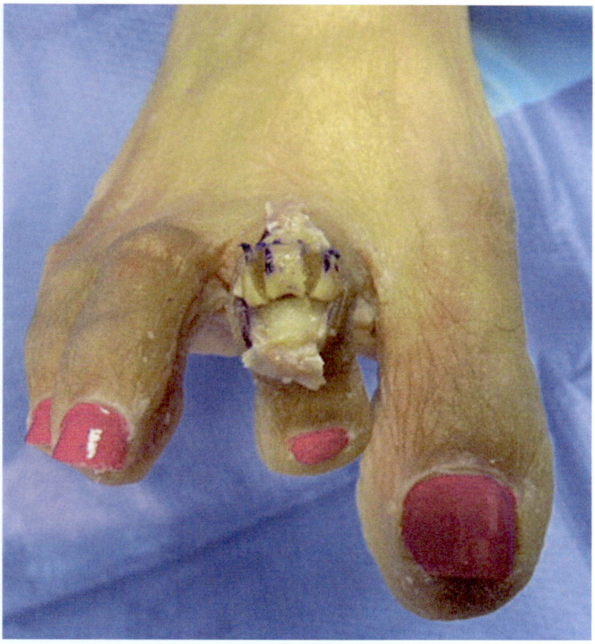

Fig. 6.3 Resection of the medial and lateral condyles with preservation of dorsal cortex

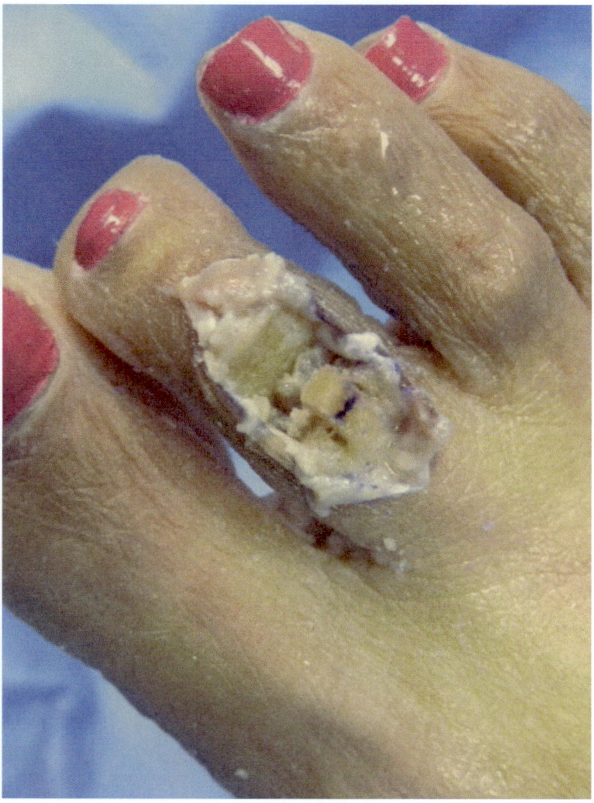

Fig. 6.4 Cartilage resected from the distal tip of proximal phalanx

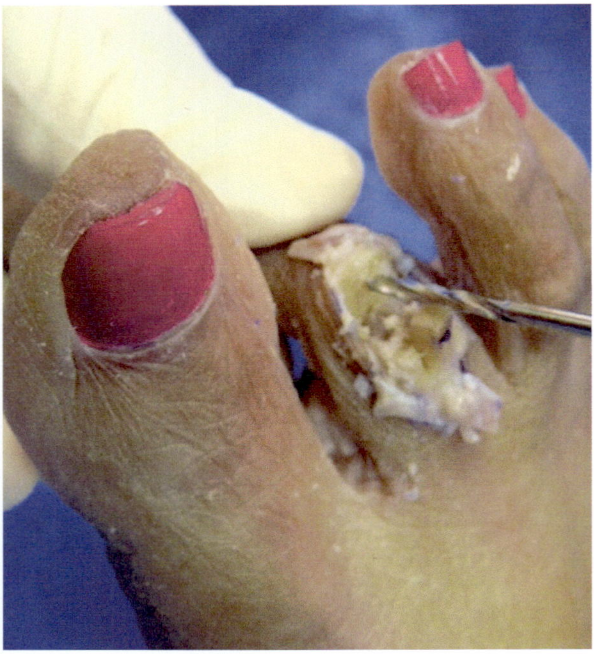

Fig. 6.5 Drilling of the middle phalanx to create hole to receive peg

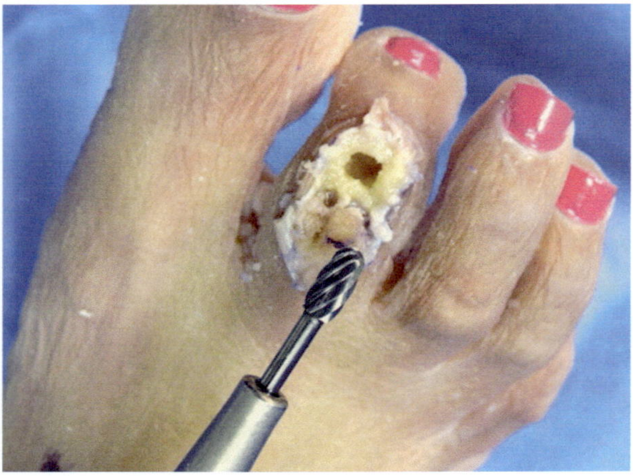

Fig. 6.6 A burr is used to expand the hole in the middle phalanx

Outcomes/Case Resolution

We present the case of a 52-year-old female who presented with complaints of a contracted right second toe. The patient reported that over the preceding two years, she had observed worsening contracture. She related that she was starting to have trouble wearing certain closed-toed shoes because they would rub and irritate the top of the toe. She had tried using over-the-counter padding and taping in her shoes to protect the toe and hold it down; however, she had no success or improvement in symptoms.

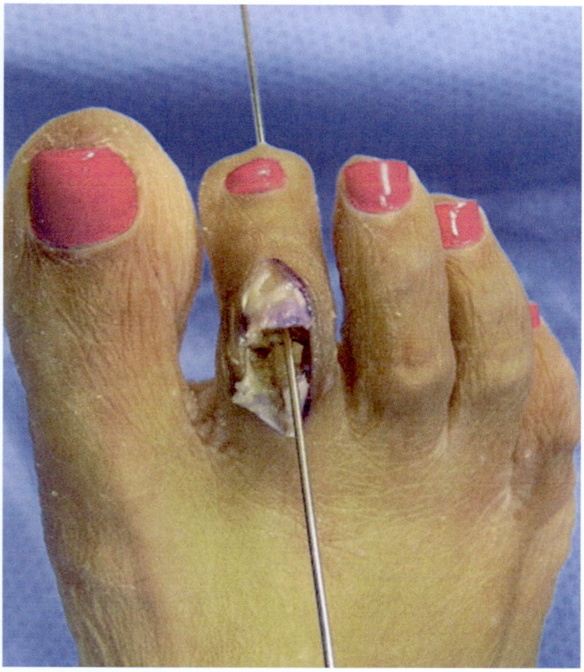

Fig. 6.7 A K-wire is inserted in an anterograde fashion across the middle and distal phalanx

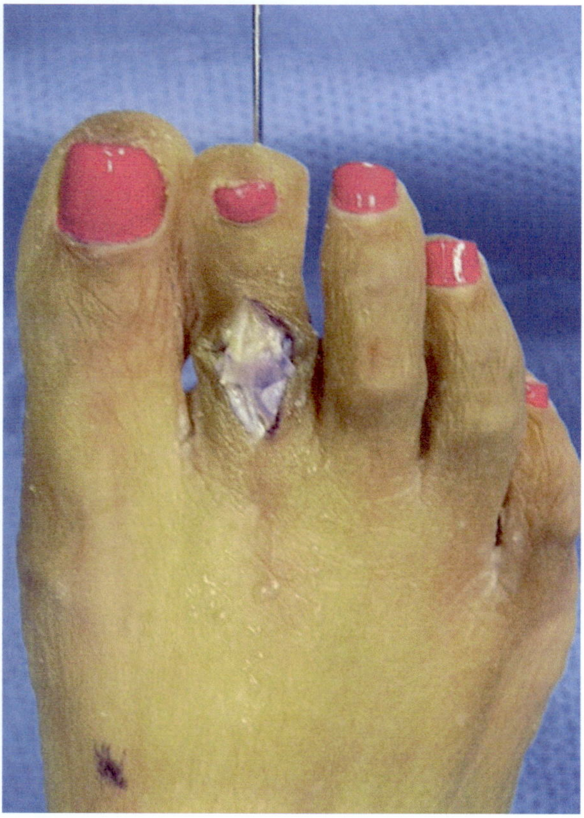

Fig. 6.8 The K-wire is advanced in a retrograde fashion across the peg and hole arthrodesis site

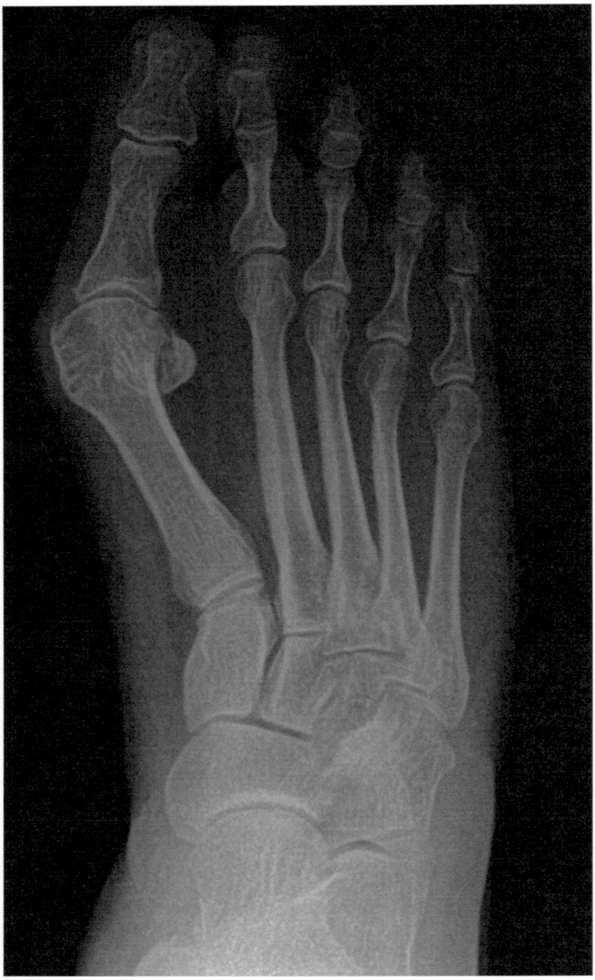

Fig. 6.9 An AP view demonstrating an elongated middle and proximal phalanx of the second toe

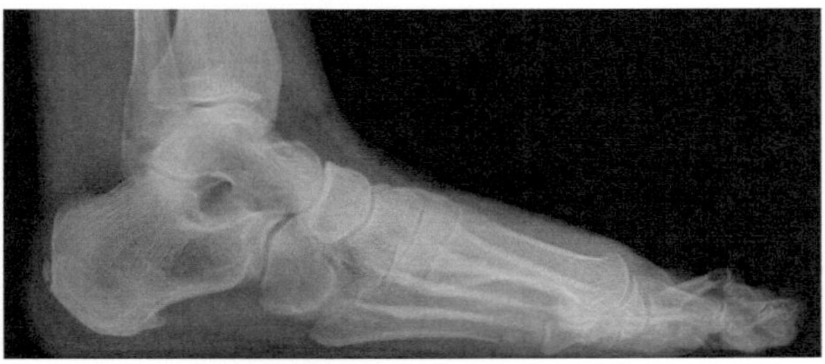

Fig. 6.10 A lateral view demonstrating the sagittal plane contracture of the second toe at the proximal interphalangeal joint

Physical exam revealed a rigid hammertoe contracture of the PIPJ of the right second toe that was painful to palpation. The AP radiograph demonstrated an elongated proximal and middle phalanx of the second toe (Fig. 6.9). The lateral radiograph showed a severely contracted second digit at the PIPJ with the middle phalanx plantar flexed on the proximal phalanx (Fig. 6.10).

Since the patient had failed initial conservative therapies, surgical intervention was discussed to address the hammertoe deformity. The patient was deemed a great candidate for the peg and hole arthrodesis due to her excessively long proximal and middle phalanx of the affected toe. The patient was counseled on surgical plans as well as the risks including nonunion, malunion, continued digital edema, and infection.

We proceeded forward with the planned peg and hole arthrodesis as described previously in our surgical technique. Postoperatively, the K-wire was left in place for 6 weeks and then removed in the office. She maintained rectus digital alignment throughout her entire postoperative course. She has been able to wear closed-toed shoes without difficulty or pain. She does relate some continued edema in the toe, worse at the end of the day. The patient was overall very satisfied with the procedure.

Clinical Pearls/Pitfalls

- When performing any surgical procedure, it is always important to address patients' primary concerns and expectations. With this procedure, patients should be educated on the long-term digital swelling they will experience and should be adequately prepared for the appearance of their toe with protruding K-wire fixation. While no K-wire fixation is technically needed with this procedure due to its stability, it is our recommendation to use K-wire fixation [3]. This procedure should be reserved for patients with PIPJ hammertoes that have a long middle and/or proximal phalanx where significant digital shortening is desired. Shortening of the toe is a clinical pitfall of the procedure. Performing a peg and hole procedure prevents gapping at the arthrodesis site when aggressive resection is needed and also prevents an internal hammertoe implant or K-wire fixation from pistoning at the arthrodesis site. This procedure should be avoided in elderly patients with poor bone stock, as the osseous integrity of the peg may not be preserved. Care must be taken when burring the hole in the base of the middle phalanx, as overaggressive burring may result in fracture. The procedure is more technically difficult than an end-to-end arthrodesis, and there is a risk of fracture of the dorsal cortex of the proximal phalanx [2]. However, the benefits of increased osseous union rates and greater stability at the arthrodesis sites make the peg and hole arthrodesis a viable option to be considered when surgically addressing an elongated hammertoe.

References

1. Lamm BM, Ribeiro CE, Vlahovic TC, Bauer GR, Hillstrom HJ. Peg-in-hole, end-to-end, and V arthrodesis, a comparison of digital stabilization in fresh cadaveric specimens. J Am Podiatr Med Assoc. 2001;91(2):63–7.
2. Lamm BM, Ribeiro CE, Vlahovic TC, Fiorilli A, Bauer GR, Hillstrom HJ. Lesser proximal interphalangeal joint arthrodesis, a retrospective analysis of the peg-in-hole and end-to-end procedures. J Am Podiatr Med Assoc. 2001;91(7):331–6.
3. McGlamry ED, Jimenez AL, Green DR. Lesser ray deformities. Part I: deformities of the intermediate digits and the metatarsophalangeal joint. In: Banks AS, Downey MS, Martin DE, Miller SJ. McGlamry's comprehensive textbook of foot and ankle surgery. Philadelphia: Lippincott Williams & Wilkins; 2001. 1. 3rd p. 253–304.

Suggested Reading

Jones PC, Robinette J, Hahn P. A new technique for cylindrical peg-in-hole arthrodesis of the interphalangeal joint. J Foot Ankle Surg. 2002;41(6):414–6.

Chapter 7
Proximal Interphalangeal Joint Arthrodesis via Kirschner Wire Fixation

Michelle Butterworth

Digital deformities are one of the most common entities we face as foot and ankle surgeons [1]. A hammertoe is a complex deformity, and throughout the years, various surgical procedures have been advocated for its correction. The proximal interphalangeal joint arthrodesis has stood the test of time and has been shown, when performed properly, that it produces a stable construct and affords for good long-term correction, high success rates, and a happy, satisfied patient [2]. Today, the most common digital arthrodesis technique is the end-to-end arthrodesis [3]. This technique has become the digital arthrodesis technique of choice mainly because it is easy to perform. Also, compared to the other digital arthrodesis procedures including the peg-in-hole and the V arthrodesis, the end-to-end procedure produces less digital shortening. One of the disadvantages of the end-to-end arthrodesis procedure, however, is that it renders the digit inherently unstable. One of the keys to success of this procedure then is obtaining stable fixation so that osseous union can be achieved.

Traditionally, the preferred form of fixation of lesser digital arthrodesis was with a percutaneous Kirschner wire (k-wire) [3–5]. In recent years, however, the number of fixation options for the correction of digital deformities has greatly expanded, mainly with internal implants. Advocates of these internal fixation devices state that they are more tolerable for the patient and easier to manage postoperatively and there is less risk for infection since there are no exposed wires [6]. The main disadvantage to these internal fixation devices is cost. Many of them are over a thousand dollars compared to a k-wire that costs just a few dollars. Also, although these internal fixation devices may have a higher patient acceptance rate, they really have not been shown to have a higher fusion rate or a higher patient satisfaction rate [7, 8]. So, the k-wire remains a cost-effective form of fixation for the proximal interphalangeal joint arthrodesis procedure, and its fusion rates and patient satisfaction rates remain comparable to other internal fixation devices [8].

M. Butterworth (✉)
Williamsburg Foot Center, Williamsburg Regional Hospital, Kingstree, SC, USA

E. A. Cook, J. J. Cook (eds.), *Hammertoes*,
https://doi.org/10.1007/978-3-319-16552-3_7

The k-wire is also versatile. The main disadvantage with k-wire fixation in the past has been exposed wires. This problem can easily be resolved by burying the k-wire. The k-wire can be buried and easily transformed into an internal fixation device, so that there are increased patient acceptance and decreased risk of infection, and it is cost-effective. The author will show the surgical technique of an end-to-end proximal interphalangeal joint arthrodesis with both percutaneous and buried k-wire fixation.

Surgical Technique

A standard dorsal linear incision is made on the digit. If a skin lesion is present, it is excised in an elliptical fashion. Either a transverse tenotomy or a Z-plasty lengthening is performed on the extensor tendon as warranted. Next, the medial and lateral collateral ligaments of the proximal interphalangeal joint are transected. Release of the extensor hood apparatus and capsulotomy of the metatarsophalangeal joint is then performed if deemed necessary to gain adequate correction of the deformity. Next, the cartilage on the head of the proximal phalanx is resected. The author prefers to use a bone-cutting forceps, but a power saw can be utilized as well (Fig. 7.1). Removal of the cartilage on the base of the middle phalanx is then performed with a rongeur (Fig. 7.2). This is easily done by grasping each corner of the phalanx with one jaw of the rongeur and then sliding the other jaw of the rongeur across the joint removing the cartilage. Again, the surgeon may utilize a power saw if desired. Care should be taken to maintain the extensor tendon that is attached at the dorsal aspect of the middle phalanx regardless of the device utilized for cartilage removal.

One of the keys to a successful fusion is to ensure complete removal of all cartilage with minimal osseous resection of the head of the proximal phalanx and base of the middle phalanx (Figs. 7.3 and 7.4). Fixation is then obtained with either a 0.045″ or a 0.062″ k-wire. The k-wire can be placed either percutaneously, or it can be buried. After fixation placement is achieved, appropriate tendon repair and wound closure then follow.

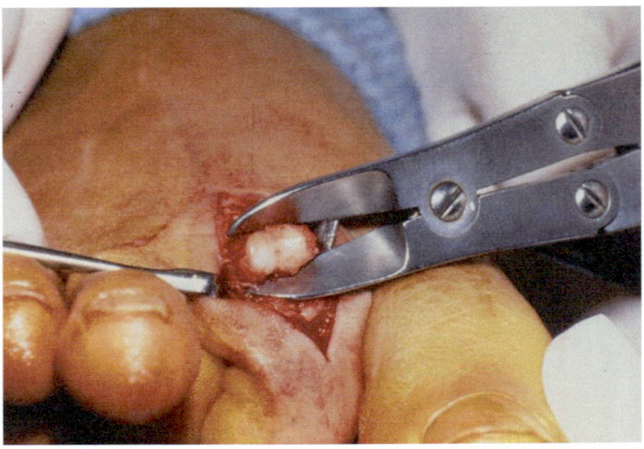

Fig. 7.1 A bone-cutting forceps is utilized to remove the cartilage on the head of the proximal phalanx. The surgeon should ensure appropriate alignment of the instrument, so a flat even surface is produced for good alignment of the fusion site

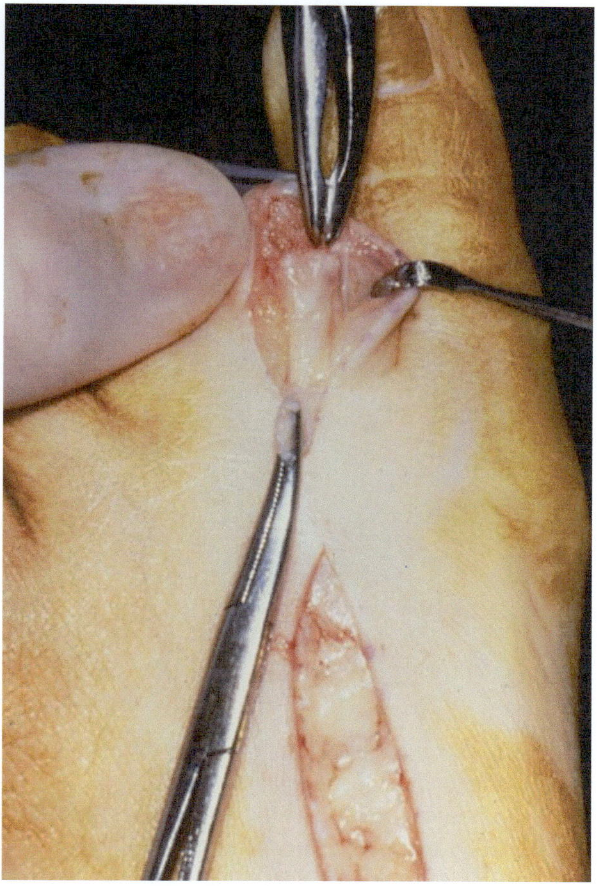

Fig. 7.2 A rongeur can be easily utilized to remove the cartilage on the base of the middle phalanx. One end of the rongeur is placed on one of the four corners of the bone, and then the other end is scraped along the content of the bone removing the cartilage. Depending on the size of the toe, this typically takes two to four swipes for complete cartilage resection

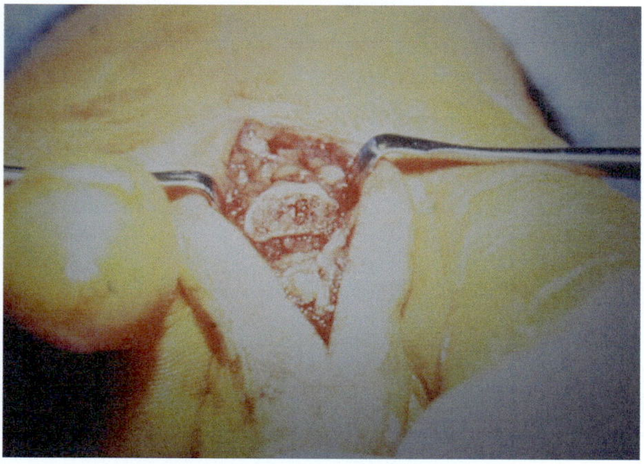

Fig. 7.3 Cartilage removal with minimal osseous resection has been performed on the proximal phalanx producing a good bleeding, flat surface

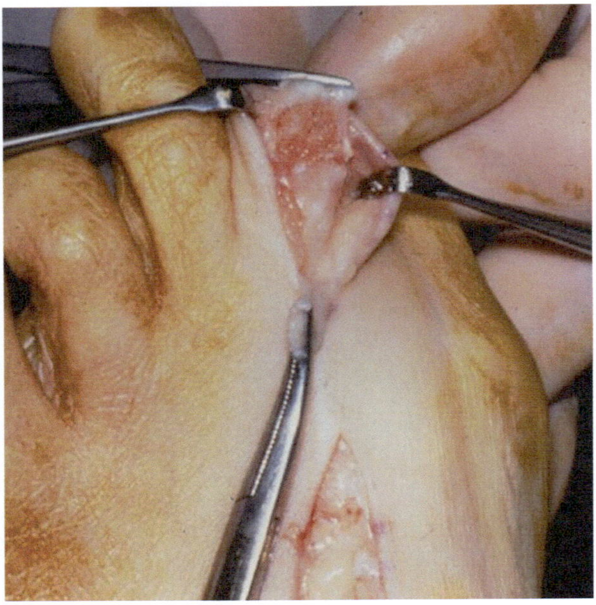

Fig. 7.4 All cartilage from the base of the middle phalanx has been removed producing a flat, bleeding surface to oppose the proximal phalanx for arthrodesis

Percutaneous K-Wire Placement

Prior to any fixation placement, the surgeon should ensure that all cartilage has been excised and that the opposing osseous surfaces are flat with good osseous apposition and appropriate alignment of the fusion site. The size of the k-wire utilized for fixation for this technique is surgeon preference. The 0.062″ k-wire is obviously larger; therefore, it is stronger and less likely to break. For smaller toes, however, or toes where there is a potential for a compromise in vascularity, the surgeon may choose the smaller 0.045″ k-wire.

To help ease the placement of the percutaneous k-wire fixation, the proximal phalanx is centrally reamed by hand, in a conical fashion, with a 0.045″ k-wire (Fig. 7.5). This creates a pilot hole and ensures adequate placement and alignment of the k-wire utilized for the final fixation. The k-wire is then placed into the center of the base of the middle phalanx and then run distally out the end of the toe with power instrumentation. The k-wire should exit in the center of the pulp of the toe inferior to the nail (Fig. 7.6). The best way to accomplish this is by holding the dorsal and plantar aspects of the toe with your thumb and forefinger and then aiming exactly between the two. The surgeon should also hold the distal interphalangeal joint in a slightly dorsiflexed position to ensure that the k-wire does not go through the nail or nail bed (Fig. 7.7). The k-wire is then run distally out the tip of the toe leaving a small portion still is exposed coming out of the base of the middle phalanx (Fig. 7.8). The tip of the k-wire is then placed into the pilot hole created previously in the proximal phalanx (Fig. 7.9). Next, the middle phalanx is compressed against the proximal phalanx, and the proximal interphalangeal joint is held in appropriate

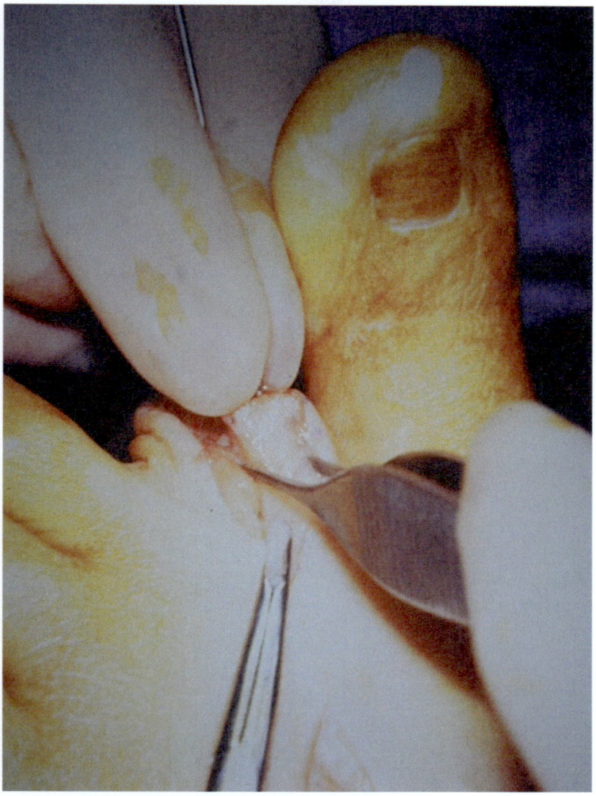

Fig. 7.5 A 0.045″ k-wire is utilized to create a pilot hole in the proximal phalanx. This is done by hand, moving it in a conical fashion. This helps to ensure adequate alignment of the k-wire utilized for final fixation

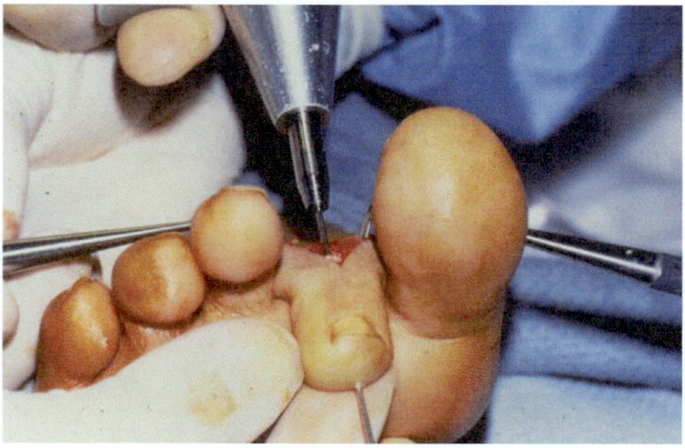

Fig. 7.6 The desired position for exit of the k-wire is in the center of the pulp of the toe

position, and the k-wire is retrograded back into the proximal phalanx. The k-wire will easily follow the path that has already been made by the pilot hole. Resistance will be met when the k-wire reaches the base of the proximal phalanx which is the desired end point. The surgeon can check the length of the implanted k-wire with an unloaded k-wire to ensure that it has not entered the metatarsophalangeal joint

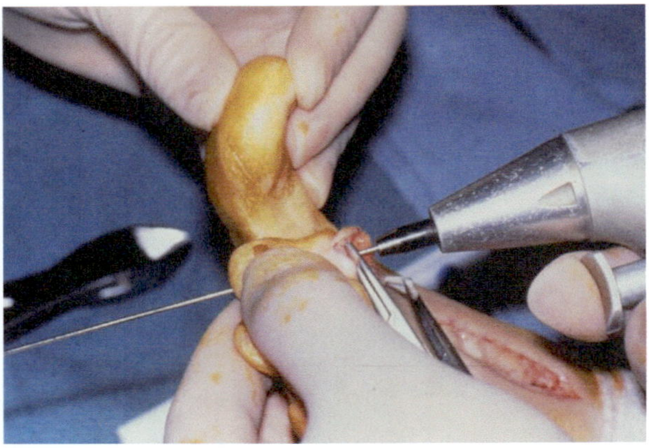

Fig. 7.7 The toe is stabilized by hand, and the distal interphalangeal joint is slightly dorsiflexed, while the k-wire is run distally out the end of the toe. This helps to ensure that k-wire does not exit through the nail or nail bed

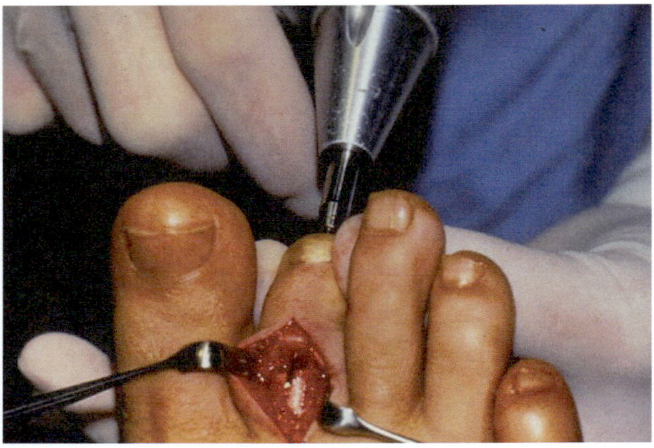

Fig. 7.8 The k-wire is retrograded distally out the end of the toe until only a small amount of wire is left exposed in the proximal interphalangeal joint

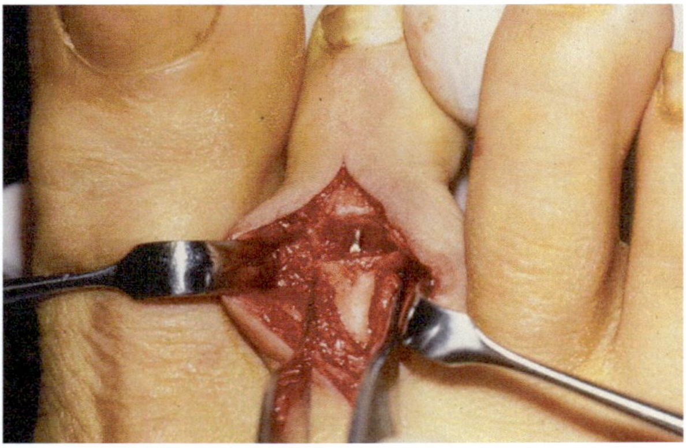

Fig. 7.9 The end of the k-wire is placed into the pilot hole in the proximal phalanx and run proximally until resistance is met upon reaching the base

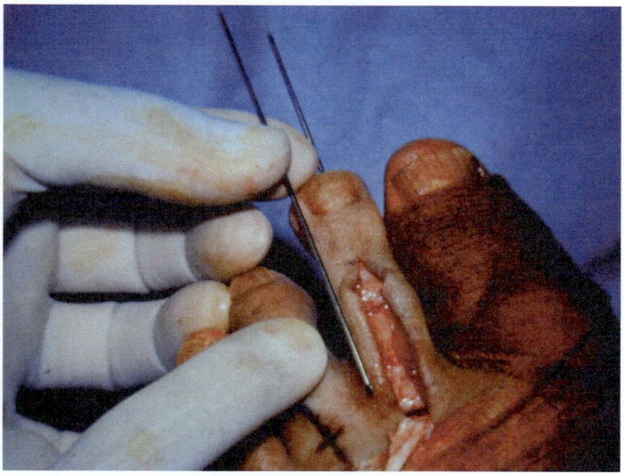

Fig. 7.10 Alignment and length of the k-wire are checked with an unloaded k-wire to ensure adequate placement

(Fig. 7.10). The toe can also be put through a range of motion to ensure that there is no resistance at the level of the metatarsophalangeal joint.

One of the disadvantages of the internal fixation devices is the inability to cross the metatarsophalangeal joint if needed. There are devices in which the k-wire may go through the implant to cross the metatarsophalangeal joint, but still an external k-wire must be used. So, if the surgery warrants crossing the metatarsophalangeal joint, an external k-wire is the best option. After the k-wire has reached the base of the proximal phalanx, the surgeon may penetrate the cartilage to visualize the k-wire in the metatarsophalangeal joint. The surgeon then manually holds the toe in the desired position at the metatarsophalangeal joint, and the k-wire is then run into the metatarsal head and shaft at the desired length.

Finally, the surgeon should check the fusion site intraoperatively at the proximal interphalangeal joint to ensure good alignment and osseous apposition. Gapping at the fusion site could result in nonunion or malunion. Once adequate position of the fixation and fusion site is achieved, the k-wire is bent and cut. A small amount of space between the tip of the toe and the bend in the wire should be maintained, so the wire is not directly up against the toe causing irritation. This is usually the width of the jaws of the wire bender. The bend in the wire also helps prevent the wire from retrograding below the skin. The pin is then cut level with the tip of the toe. This allows for placement of a pin cap. The pin cap keeps the end of the pin from getting caught on things and inadvertently pulled out, and it also protects puncture or scratching with the end of the exposed wire (Figs. 7.11 and 7.12).

One significant advantage of the percutaneous k-wire is that it can be easily removed after healing and the patient has no retained metal or hardware left in their body from the surgical procedure. K-wires are easily removed in the office once osseous union has been achieved. There is no need for anesthesia, and there is typically very little discomfort with removal (Figs. 7.13 and 7.14).

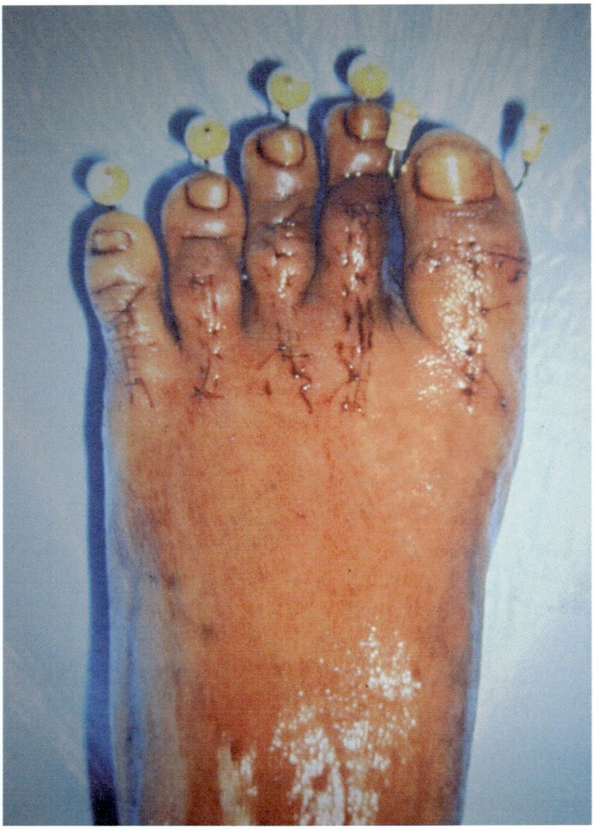

Fig. 7.11 Clinical image displaying proper placement and bending of the percutaneous pins. Adequate space is maintained between the bend of the pin and the end of the toe to avoid skin irritation. The bend in the pin is necessary to avoid the pin from retrograding underneath the skin

Buried K-Wire Placement

As with the percutaneous k-wire placement, first the surgeon must ensure that all cartilage has been successfully removed and the joint surfaces are flat and allow for appropriate alignment. The author recommends a 0.062″ k-wire for most of the toes utilizing the buried k-wire technique since it affords for more stability than the 0.045″ k-wire. For smaller toes, however, a smaller wire may be utilized. First, a pilot hole is created by hand with a 0.045″ k-wire as previously described for the percutaneous pin placement. Next, utilizing power instrumentation, the k-wire being placed for the permanent fixation is run down the pilot hole until resistance is met at the base of the proximal phalanx (Fig. 7.15). The surgeon must ensure that the k-wire does not go through the base of the proximal phalanx and enter the metatarsophalangeal joint.

The toe is then held in a rectus position at the proximal interphalangeal joint with the wire lying next to the middle phalanx. The length of the k-wire needed in the middle phalanx is then determined by direct visualization. There needs to be enough

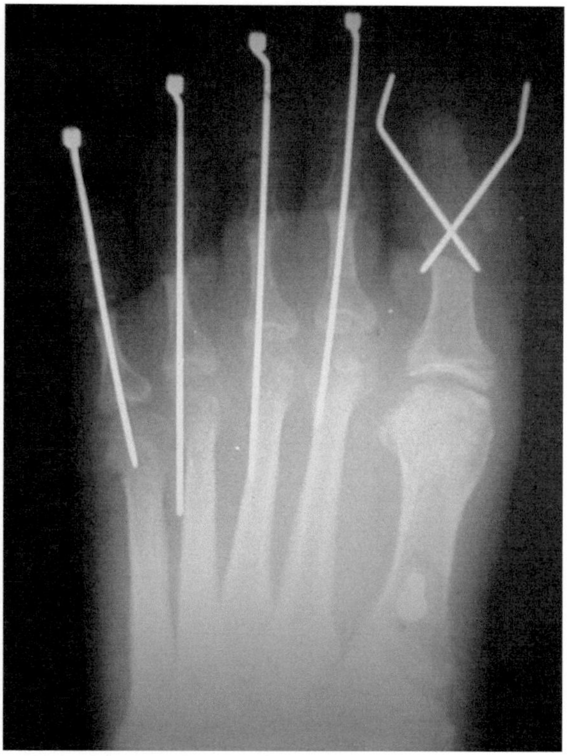

Fig. 7.12 Radiograph of percutaneous k-wires crossing the metatarsophalangeal joints. Proximal interphalangeal joint arthrodesis has been performed on toes 2, 3, and 4, and all appear in good alignment with good approximation of the joint surfaces

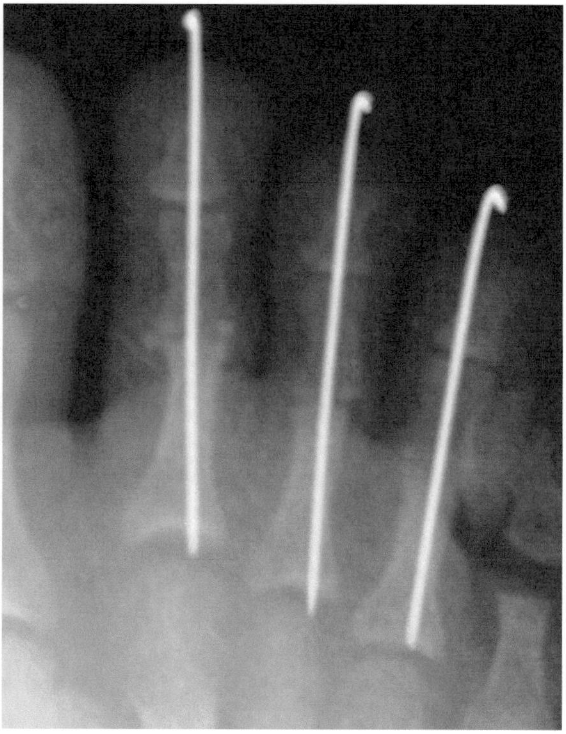

Fig. 7.13 Percutaneous k-wires utilized as fixation for the end-to-end proximal interphalangeal joint arthrodesis of toes 2, 3, and 4

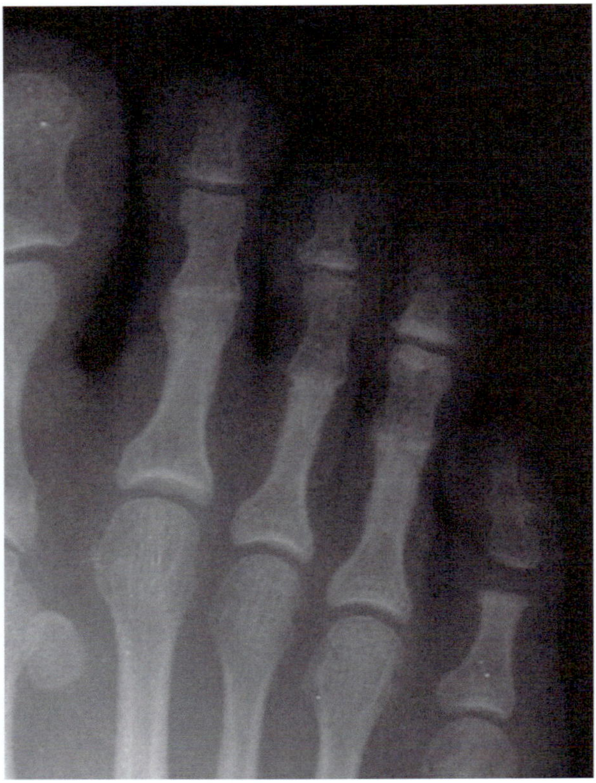

Fig. 7.14 The percutaneous k-wires were removed once osseous fusion was seen radiographically at the arthrodesis sites

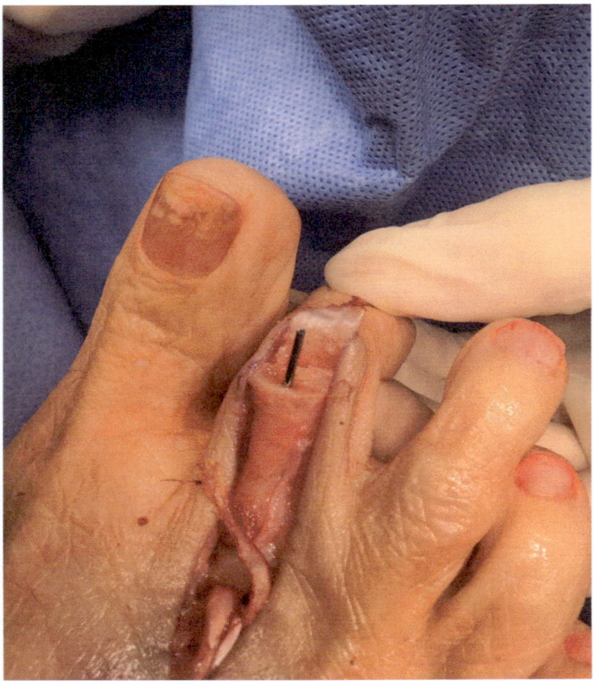

Fig. 7.15 The k-wire is run into the pilot hole in the proximal phalanx. The wire is then cut at appropriate length for placement into the middle phalanx

k-wire in the middle phalanx to afford for stability and to keep the joint from separating and gapping, but the wire cannot be so long that it exceeds the length of the middle phalanx or it prevents the middle phalanx from being reduced and placed over the end of the pin. Once the appropriate length is determined, the k-wire is cut (Fig. 7.16). The middle phalanx is then manipulated over the end of the k-wire. The wire should be placed in the central aspect of the base of the middle phalanx. The end of the toe is then compressed down on the wire, reducing the proximal interphalangeal joint (Fig. 7.17). The joint is checked after final pin placement to ensure good apposition and alignment of the joint surfaces.

If the toe cannot be manipulated over the end of the k-wire, the wire may need to be cut shorter. Prior to doing this, however, the surgeon should check the dissection to ensure that the nonreduction is not from inadequate soft tissue reflection. If the toe is unstable after placement of the buried k-wire, it is most likely because the

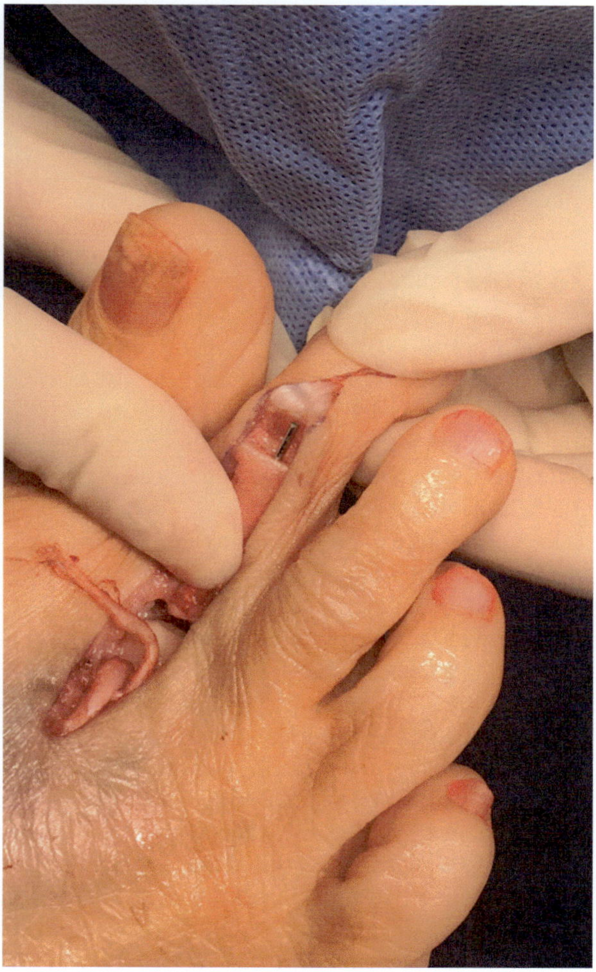

Fig. 7.16 The middle phalanx is manipulated over the end of the k-wire. The k-wire is placed in the center of the base of the middle phalanx to ensure good alignment

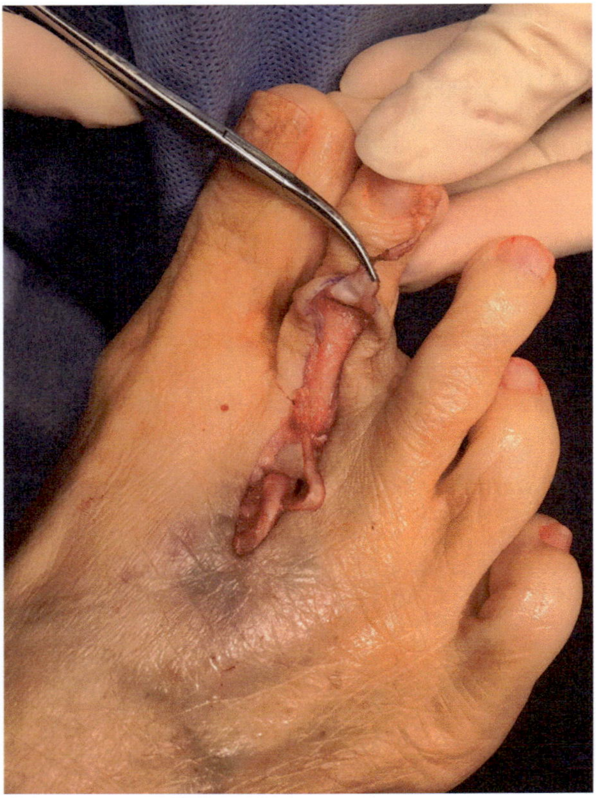

Fig. 7.17 The middle phalanx is then compressed onto the proximal phalanx producing good bone-to-bone contact at the arthrodesis site

distal end of the wire is not long enough. The lever arm of the wire in the middle phalanx needs to be long enough, so the toe cannot easily pop off of the wire. There is a slight learning curve in determining the appropriate length of the buried k-wire. Fortunately, however, the k-wire can be easily replaced intraoperatively if the fixation fails the first time.

In rare instances, the bone stock in the middle phalanx is poor and unable to stabilize the buried k-wire, or the middle phalanx is very small rendering the buried k-wire inadequate even at its maximum length. If successful fixation cannot be achieved with a buried k-wire for whatever reason, this procedure can easily be converted to a percutaneous k-wire placement.

One of the advantages of the internal implants is that most of the devices come with the option of a 10-degree angle to afford for some plantarflexion and bend to the toe if desired by the surgeon. This angle can be achieved with the buried k-wire also. After the k-wire is measured and cut to adequate length, it can simply be bent at the desired angle with a wire bender, prior to placing the middle phalanx over the end of it. This slight plantarflexed angle to the toe produces a more natural curl to the toe and allows the tip of the toe to purchase the ground more easily. It also keeps the toe from looking too straight, especially when compared to other toes not undergoing surgical reconstruction (Figs. 7.18, 7.19, and 7.20).

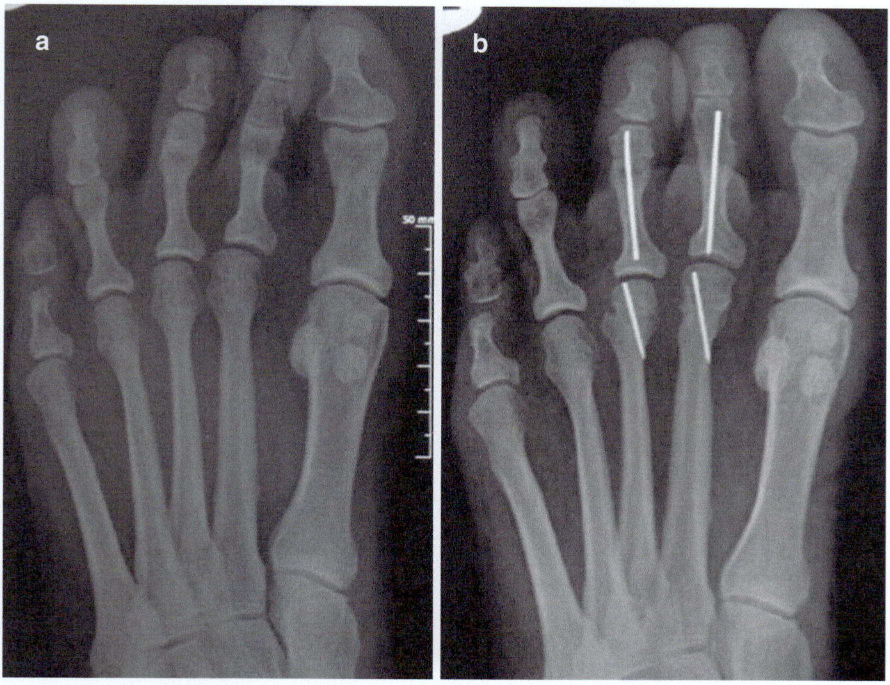

Fig. 7.18 (**a**) Preoperative radiographs and (**b**) postoperative radiographs showing buried k-wires for fixation of the proximal interphalangeal joint arthrodesis

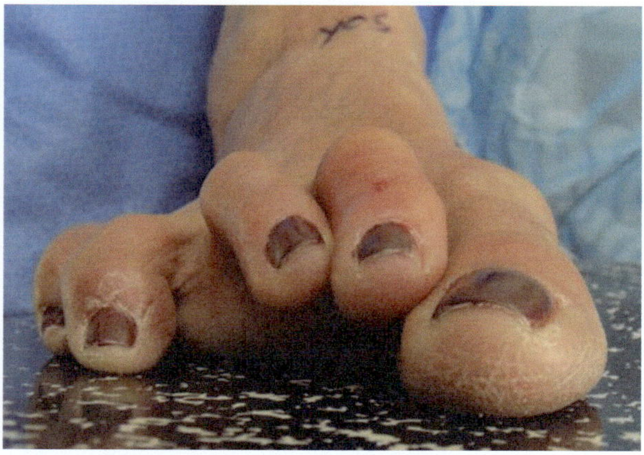

Fig. 7.19 Clinical presentation preoperatively of the hammertoe deformities seen radiographically in Fig. 7.18

Postoperative Course

Regardless of whether the fixation utilized for the proximal interphalangeal joint arthrodesis is with a percutaneous or buried k-wire, the postoperative course is similar. Patients are usually kept partial weight-bearing on their heel in a surgical shoe

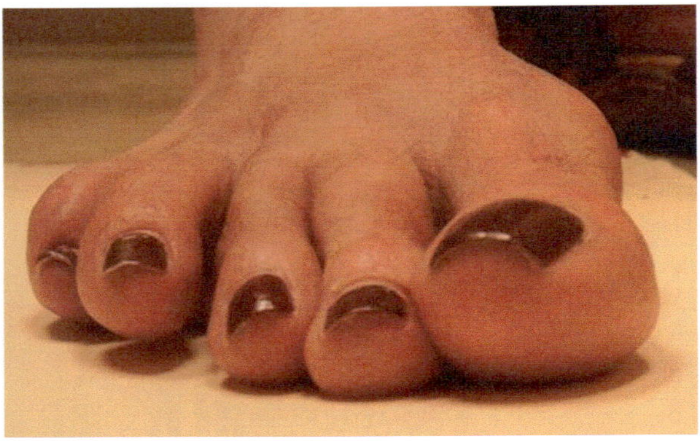

Fig. 7.20 Clinical presentation postoperatively of the hammertoes corrected with the proximal interphalangeal joint arthrodesis with buried k-wires

until adequate fusion of the joint is achieved. This is determined by radiographic osseous union. If k-wires cross the metatarsophalangeal joints, felt padding is placed in the surgical shoe to the level of the digital sulcus to decrease any chances of pin breakage. The percutaneous pins will need to be removed prior to returning to regular shoe gear. Patients with buried k-wires may be able to return to regular shoe gear sooner depending on their swelling and discomfort level. Patients with percutaneous k-wires cannot submerge their foot in water until after the pins have been removed and the pin holes have sealed over. Once the incisions are healed, however, they may clean their foot without introducing water along the pin sites. Antibiotic ointment is placed along the pin sites during their postoperative visits; however, the patient does not have to perform any other pin care on their own. For patients with the buried k-wires, they may begin bathing once their incisions are healed. Once patients have returned to normal shoe gear, they can return to normal activities as their pain and swelling permit. Of course, this protocol is followed for this specific surgical procedure. Often, other procedures are performed along with hammertoe correction which may warrant a different postoperative course and weight-bearing status.

Complications

Complications that may result from the proximal interphalangeal joint arthrodesis are not inherent to just k-wire fixation but really apply to digital arthrodesis in general, regardless of the type of fixation utilized. Possible complications for this procedure include malunion, nonunion, shortened toe, floppy toe, stiff toe, mallet toe, recurrent lesions, recurrent deformity, and vascular compromise which could lead to loss of the toe. Fixation problems could result as well including failure and breakage. Fortunately, when a k-wire fails, typically there is still enough bone and other fixation options for revisional surgery if needed. When some of the internal implants fail or break, however, there is often significant damage to the bone and limited revisional options. Of course, infection, scarring, numbness, and prolonged swelling may also occur as with any foot surgery.

Discussion

Despite the commonality of the end-to-end digital arthrodesis with k-wire fixation for correction of hammertoe deformity, there are few reported success rates. Coughlin et al. conducted a study with 118 toes on 63 patients with an average follow-up of 61 months. The deformity involved the second toe in 35%, the third toe in 21%, the fourth toe in 24%, and the fifth toe in 20%. They reported a fusion rate of the proximal interphalangeal joint in 81% of toes. A fibrous union resulted in the remaining 19% of cases. Subjective satisfaction was noted by 84% of patients. Minor complications occurred in 5%. Malalignment and numbness were the major factors associated with an unsuccessful result. They concluded that resection arthroplasty of the proximal interphalangeal joint with intramedullary k-wire fixation as a technique for correction of a fixed hammertoe deformity is a reliable technique that consistently gives a high level of satisfactory results [2].

Baig and Geary reviewed proximal interphalangeal joint arthrodesis with k-wire fixation in 19 patients and 42 toes. They assessed the results at 6 weeks and then again at 6 months and reported a fusion rate of 83% and infection rate of 7%. Postoperative mallet toe formation was a common finding in their study, and this was the biggest reason for patient dissatisfaction [5].

Recently, increased emphasis has been placed on developing internal fixation devices for the correction of digital deformities. Advocates of these internal implants profess that they are more tolerable for the patient since there are no exposed wires. They also claim to have fewer complications when utilizing these devices compared with k-wire fixation. In comparative studies, however, there has not been any significant difference between internal implants versus k-wires when evaluating fusion rates and patient satisfaction [7].

Ellington et al. performed a retrospective review on 38 toes in 27 patients treated with an intramedullary fusion device. The indications for surgery were primary deformity in 12 toes and recurrent deformities in 26 toes. The mean follow-up was 31 months. Union occurred in 23 of 38 toes (60.5%). The union rate was 9 of 12 for primary procedures and 14 of 26 toes for revisions. Including nonunion, the overall complication rate was 55.3%, 21 of 38 toes. There were 15 nonunions, 3 hardware failures, 1 intraoperative fracture, 1 requiring surgery, and 1 requiring a larger implant. Even though they report a high nonunion and complication rate, they state the intramedullary fusion device was efficacious in maintaining proximal interphalangeal joint alignment in the treatment of lesser toe deformities [8].

Scholl et al. did a comparative study on the Smart Toe implant versus buried k-wire fixation for proximal interphalangeal joint arthrodesis. Fifty-eight toes with the Smart Toe implant and 28 toes with buried k-wires were included in the study. Of the 86 total implants, 87.9% of the Smart Toe implants and 85.7% of the buried k-wire implants were in good position. Osseous union was achieved in 68.9% of the Smart Toe implants and 82.1% of the buried k-wires. Fracture of the fixation occurred in 12 of the Smart Toe implants (20.7%) and 2 of the buried k-wires (7.1%). Most of the fractures and malunions were asymptomatic, and the revisional surgery rate was 8.6% for the Smart Toe implants and 10.7% for the buried k-wires.

They concluded that there was no statistically significant difference between the Smart Toe implant and the buried k-wire in the rate of malunion, nonunion, fracture of internal fixation, and need for revisional surgery. They stated that both forms of fixation were a viable choice for digital arthrodesis when compared to other studies using other techniques [7].

Conclusion

Although digital surgery is very common for most foot and ankle surgeons, hammertoe deformities are complex and can be challenging. The end-to-end proximal interphalangeal joint arthrodesis with k-wire fixation affords for good long-term correction, high success rates, and happy, satisfied patients. The k-wire can be placed percutaneously leaving exposed wires out the tip of the toes. Although some will say this is very difficult for a patient to accept, there are no studies showing any significant difference between fusion rates and patient satisfaction with this technique compared to internal implants. However, if one prefers an internal implant, the k-wire is versatile and can simply be buried. This technique eliminates issues with patient acceptance, and it leaves nothing exposed, therefore minimizing the risk of infection. Internal implant devices can be very expensive. In our cost-conscious healthcare environment today, the buried k-wire is a cost-effective alternative for internal implantation. K-wires have been shown to be easy to use; they are cost-effective and produce similar results as other, more expensive internal implants. Regardless of the form of fixation utilized, the surgeon must appreciate all components involved with the digital deformity to achieve complete surgical success. The proximal interphalangeal joint arthrodesis has been proven to produce a stable toe; however, supplemental procedures may be warranted to gain full correction of the deformity.

Clinical Pearls

There are a few pearls for performing a successful proximal interphalangeal joint arthrodesis with k-wire fixation

- As with any arthrodesis procedure, ensuring that all cartilage has been removed from both sides of the joint is essential. Good bleeding osseous surfaces is crucial to achieve fusion.
- The proximal interphalangeal joint surfaces must be flat and well aligned after cartilage resection. The joint surfaces should afford for good bone-to-bone contact and place the toe in a corrected position. If not, malunion or nonunion can result.
- A pilot hole should be created in the proximal phalanx to allow for easy positioning of the final k-wire fixation. This is done by hand in a conical fashion.

- The k-wire should meet resistance at the base of the proximal phalanx. It should be stopped here before it goes through into the metatarsophalangeal joint.
- When performing the buried k-wire technique, if the middle phalanx cannot be manipulated over the end of the k-wire, cut it a little shorter, but not too short.
- If the middle phalanx is unstable, once placed over the end of the buried k-wire, try a longer wire. If it is still unstable, it can be easily converted to a percutaneous wire.
- The buried k-wire can be bent to afford for a slightly plantarflexed angle as some of the other internal implants offer. If this is desired, it is done after the k-wire is placed into the proximal phalanx and prior to the middle phalanx being placed over the wire.
- There is very little surface area of available bone within the proximal phalanx and middle phalanx of toes; therefore, there is little room for error with our surgical techniques. If the k-wire fails to provide adequate stability, it can be easily removed. There is typically minimal damage to the bone after utilizing a k-wire; therefore, the procedure can be easily converted to utilize other forms of fixation. This conversion is not so easy with the internal implants however. The learning curve for some of the internal implant devices is quite high. Poor surgical technique and poor placement of these internal implants can produce significant bone damage resulting in limited options for revisional surgery or fixation. Also, if the internal implants need to be removed, this often results in significant bone loss making revisional surgery quite challenging.

References

1. Good J, Fiala K. Digital surgery: current trends and techniques. Clin Podiatr Med Surg. 2010;27(4):625–8.
2. Coughlin MJ, Dorris J, Polk E. Operative repair of the fixed hammertoe deformity. Foot Ankle Int. 2000;21(2):94–104.
3. Hofbauer MH, Shane AM. Lesser digital surgery: arthroplasty, arthrodesis, and flexor tendon transfer. In: Chang TJ, editor. Master techniques in podiatric surgery: the foot and ankle. Philadelphia: Lippincott Williams and Wilkins; 2005. p. 35–47.
4. Lamm BM, Ribeiro CE, et al. Peg-in-hole, end-to-end, and V arthrodesis a comparison of digital stabilization in fresh cadaveric specimens. J Am Podiatr Med Assoc. 2001;91(2):63–7.
5. Baig AU, Geary NPJ. Fusion rate and patient satisfaction in proximal interphalangeal joint fusion of the minor toes using Kirschner wire fixation. Foot. 1996;6(3):120–1.
6. Angirasa AK, Augoyard M, Coughlin MJ, Fridman R, Ruch J, Weil L Jr, Section Editor. Hammer toe, mallet toe, and claw toe (roundtable discussion). Foot Ankle Spec. 2011;4(3):182–7.
7. Scholl A, McCarty J, Scholl D, Mar A. Smart toe implant versus buried Kirschner wire for proximal interphalangeal joint arthrodesis: a comparative study. J Foot Ankle Surg. 2013;52(5):580–3.
8. Ellington K, Anderson RB, Davis WH, Cohen BE, Jones CP. Radiographic analysis of proximal interphalangeal joint arthrodesis with an intramedullary fusion device for lesser toe deformities. Foot Ankle Int. 2010;31(5):372–6.

Chapter 8
PIPJ Arthrodesis with a One-Component Metallic Implant

Ryan T. Scott, Christopher F. Hyer, and Gregory C. Berlet

Presentation/History

Hammertoes are ubiquitous in the shoed population of modern society and a common malady of the foot. Hammertoe digital deformity is characterized by an extension deformity at the metatarsophalangeal joint (MTPJ) and flexion deformity at the proximal interphalangeal joint (PIPJ) [1, 2]. Digital deformity typically is associated with pain in the forefoot, difficultly fitting shoes, and unacceptable cosmetic appearance for the affected patients [2, 3]. Forefoot pain is typically accompanied by hyperkeratotic skin lesions, callosities, or ulcerations about the metatarsal-phalangeal joint, the PIP joint, and the distal interphalangeal joints and nail deformities secondary to the curling of the digits [4]. Loss of purchase of the digit overloads the MTP joint as well as the surrounding digits ultimately changing the gait pattern. This altered gait may aggravate other biomechanical ailments of the lower extremity.

Treatment options are guided by the patient's discomfort as well as the reducibility of the affected digit. A digit where it is possible to actively correct the deformity is considered flexible, whereas a hammertoe that maintains its pathologic posture despite a reduction attempt is considered fixed. Conservative management of a fixed hammertoe includes shoe gear modification with a high and wide toe box, toe sleeves, foam cushioning devices, orthotics, or offloading pads such as a metatarsal bar. If these nonoperative management strategies fail to alleviate symptoms, then discussion of surgical correction is warranted.

Kirschner wires (K-wires) have long been the gold standard for hammertoe digital repair. K-wires were initially introduced to orthopedics in 1909 by Martin

R. T. Scott (✉)
The CORE Institute, Phoenix, AZ, USA

C. F. Hyer · G. C. Berlet
Orthopedic Foot and Ankle Center, Westerville, OH, USA

E. A. Cook, J. J. Cook (eds.), *Hammertoes*,
https://doi.org/10.1007/978-3-319-16552-3_8

Kirschner utilizing surgical-grade stainless steel for fixation of fractures. Taylor was the first surgeon to introduce K-wires for fixation of hammertoe repairs in 1940 [5]. Today the most commonly used sizes for K-wire fixation in the foot and ankle are 0.9 mm (0.035 inch) to 1.6 mm (0.062 inch). Introduction of K-wire fixation for hammertoe correction was initially popularized to help prevent flail toe, which is the most common complication secondary to excessive bone resection [1].

Although K-wires are simplistic to use as fixation, they carry inherit risks such as pin tract infections, migration, and breakage [3]. Zingas et al. noted a 2.5% failure rate when the 1.1 mm (0.045 inch) K-wire was used for fixation of the lesser digit hammertoe deformity [6]. Reece et al. reported as much as 18% pin tract infections in digital arthrodesis fixed by K-wires [7]. The average incidence of non-union following PIP joint arthrodesis fixed by intramedullary K-wire was about 20% [8].

In the authors' experience, the biggest concern our patients have about externally protruding K-wires is the anxiety with the removal of the K-wire in the office, as well as accidental "trauma" within their home. Another concern in the use of K-wires was the potential damage that may occur to the articular cartilage, in the case that the K-wire crosses the MTP joint. Galli et al. evaluated the disruption of the cartilage as the K-wire was passed into the metatarsal in a cadaveric model [9]. It was noted that 1.8% of the surface area of the articular cartilage was damaged during this procedure.

In recent years, there has been a move away from the percutaneous K-wire to other forms of fixation for digital correction in foot surgery. This has been spearheaded by the desire of surgeon and patient alike to avoid the risks and pain of percutaneous fixation and offer long-term internal stabilization of the corrected deformity. As technology has advanced, there have been a multitude of options in the management of this deformity, both surgical technique and implant technology. These include resection arthroplasty, tendon transfers, and arthrodesis with pins, wires, screws, bone dowels, bioabsorbable pins, and metallic intramedullary implants [2, 10–16].

Material development of memory metal, optimization of thread caliber and pitch, and internal compression strategies have moved the material science of hammertoe correction ahead significantly and have been corroborated by the literature. Utilization of an internal implant for hammertoe correction was found safe and provided acceptable alignment, pain reduction, and improved function at the final follow-up in two recent studies [17, 18].

Today there are at least five different one-component implants commonly utilized by the foot and ankle surgeon. The implants that will be discussed include PROTOE (Wright Medical Technologies – Arlington, TN), PhaLinx (OrthoPro/Wright Medical Technologies – Arlington, TN), Smart Toe (Stryker – Mahwah, NJ), HammerLock (BME – San Antonio, TX), and cannulated screws.

This chapter will discuss the clinical application, surgical technique, and pearls/pitfalls of the one-component metallic implant.

Treatment/Surgical Technique

PROTOE™ (Wright Medical Technologies – Arlington, TN)

The PROTOE™ device is one of the latest implants released to the market for the management of hammertoes. As an intramedullary implant, the risk of digital infection is low. The PROTOE™ is a stainless steel single-piece hammertoe implant. The implant design utilizes a proximal threaded section that is screwed into place within the medullary canal of the proximal phalanx (Fig. 8.1). The distal serrated flanges are then impacted into the base of the middle phalanx (Fig. 8.2). There are currently ten unique implants available. Five variable-sized implants (2.0, 2.4, 2.8, 3.2, 4.0 mm) come with a 0-degree or 10-degree angulation. The angulation gives the surgeon the ability to position the digit in both mechanically and cosmetically appropriate positions during the procedure. The 2.8 mm implant has been designed with a shortened proximal segment (9 mm) for use in the fifth toe. The 2.0 mm implant carries a 13 mm proximal thread, whereas the larger implants have a 16 mm thread. The angulation gives the surgeon the ability to position the digit in both mechanically and cosmetically appropriate positions during the procedure.

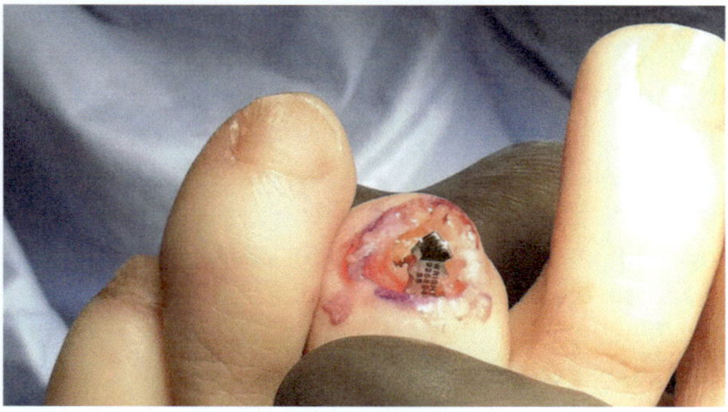

Fig. 8.1 Insertion of the PROTOE into the proximal phalanx

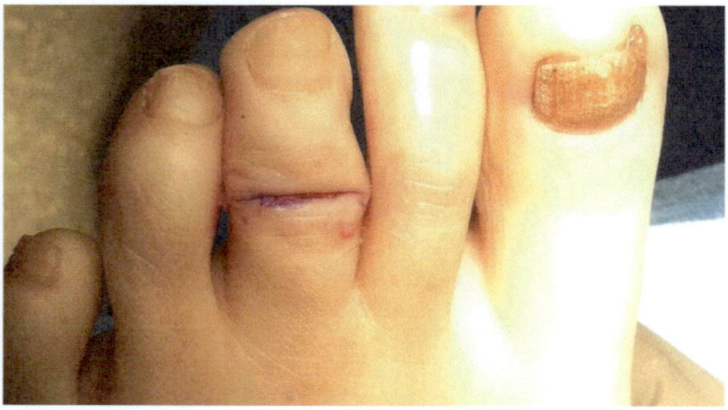

Fig. 8.2 Overall posture of the toe following impaction of the implant into the middle phalanx

In our practice, another noted advantage of these internal devices is the absence of exposed hardware, leading to decreased anxiety. We have also noted very little chronic swelling of the surgical digit [19, 20]. This has also been noted with the other similar intramedullary devices listed.

The PROTOE C2™ and PROTOE VO™ cannulated implants are second-generation devices that are cannulated for the management of digital contractures. These devices are similar to the first generation in the fact that it is an intramedullary implant. However, the major advantage of the PROTOE C2™ and PROTOE VO™ cannulated implants is the ability to cannulate a 0.045/0.062″ wire through the implant and across both the distal interphalangeal (DIP) joint and the metatarsophalangeal (MTP) joint. In doing so, this allows stability and splintage of the DIP and MTP as the surgically corrected toe heals. The versatility of being able to stabilize the MTP joint helps to reduce the risk of a "floating toe" and/or recurrence of the extensor contracture. The PROTOE C2™ is a bipolar threaded implant, which allows for compression across the IP joint as the distal threads of the implant engage the middle phalanx.

PhaLinx (OrthoPro/Wright Medical Technologies – Arlington, TN)

PhaLinx is a one-piece titanium implant that is screwed into the middle phalanx (Fig. 8.3). It is then impacted into the proximal phalanx. This implant was designed as one of the first cannulated hammertoe implants on the market. Insertion of the implant can be completely performed with cannulated instrumentation. The cannulated implant allows for a K-wire to be used for stabilization of the DIP joint and across the MTP joint if the surgeon desires. The implant comes in extra small, small, medium, and large sizes. Straight-cannulated and 10-degree angulated options are available. 0.9 mm, 1.1 mm, and 1.4 mm K-wires are, respectively, used for the extra small/small, medium, and large straight implants. One of the greatest advantages of PhaLinx is the cannulated option for stability.

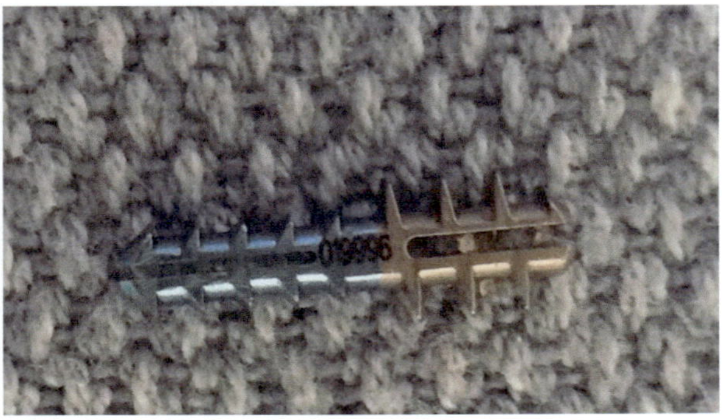

Fig. 8.3 PhaLinx implant

Smart Toe (Stryker – Mahwah, NJ)

The Smart Toe implant is a memory-based nitinol implant that compresses across the PIP joint as it warms to body level (Fig. 8.4). As a one-piece implant, there are no interconnecting parts, which allows for easy insertion [21]. The newest generation comes in both neutral and 10-degree plantarflexed implants allowing for further correction of the digital deformity. The new implant also comes with a "grenade pin" which is placed into the central aspect of the implant prohibiting migration of the implant too proximal during implantation. The Smart Toe has a large variety of sizes among all the implants on the market: 15 mm, 16 mm, 19 mm, 20 mm, 21 mm, and 22 mm. A DIP joint implant is also available. A drawback to this implant is the fact that it is a thermally reactive implant. Once the implant begins to warm, compression is noted. Therefore, there is limited working time and "playability" to change the position of the implant/digit if the surgeon doesn't approve of the initial correction.

Fig. 8.4 Smart Toe

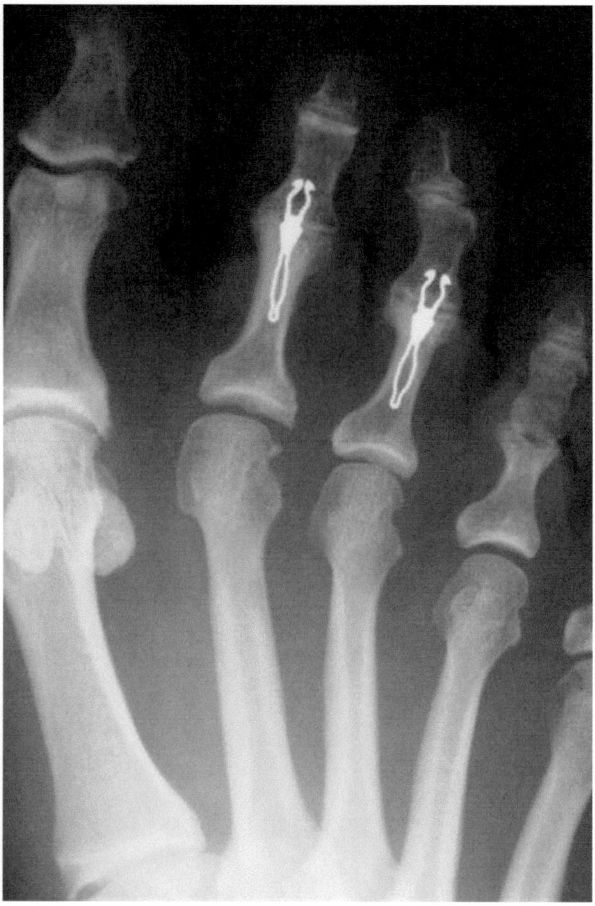

Scholl et al. compared hammertoe correction with the Smart Toe versus a buried K-wire and noted complete osseous union in 68.9% within the Smart Toe subset [22]. They also noted an 8.1% surgical revision rate in cases where there was symptomatic malunion/union. Angirasa noted similar findings with the effectiveness of the implant and concluded that the Smart Toe has comparable outcomes to surgically corrected toes with K-wire fixation [23].

HammerLock (BME – San Antonio, TX)

The HammerLock implant is similar to the Smart Toe implant in the fact that it too is a nitinol-based implant. The "X"-shaped design allows for purchase in both the proximal and middle phalanges giving compression across the IP joint (Fig. 8.5). This implant must be stored in a freezer as it uses body temperature to create the compression. The implant comes in a petite (14 mm length), small (16 mm), medium (19 mm), and large (22 mm) with neutral and 10-degree angulation. The angled implant is only available in the small-, medium-, and large-sized IP joint implant. Hallux and DIP joint implants are also available.

Cannulated Screws

Recently, small-cannulated screws have also been used for fixation (Fig. 8.6). Although this surgical procedure sacrifices the DIP joint to treat the PIP joint, it significantly reduces the risk of residual toe angulation, the risk of mallet toe deformity, and the risk of nonunion of the PIP joint and, finally, reduces postoperative shoe restrictions. Disadvantages of this technique are the risks of a second operation related to persistent pain at the tip of the toe, caused by the head of the screw, and the breakage of the screw [8]. Another disadvantage is the lack of bone purchase in

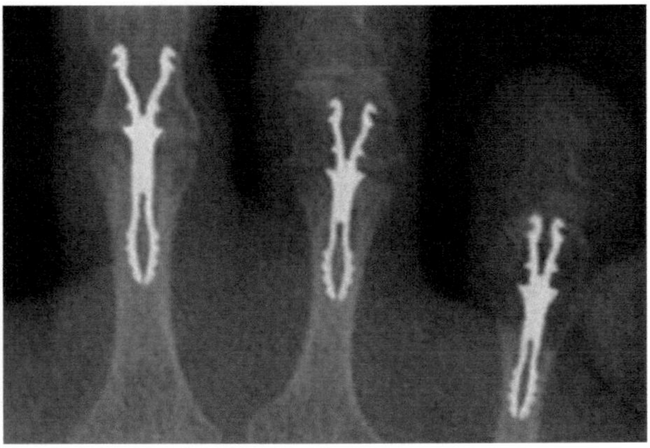

Fig. 8.5 HammerLock

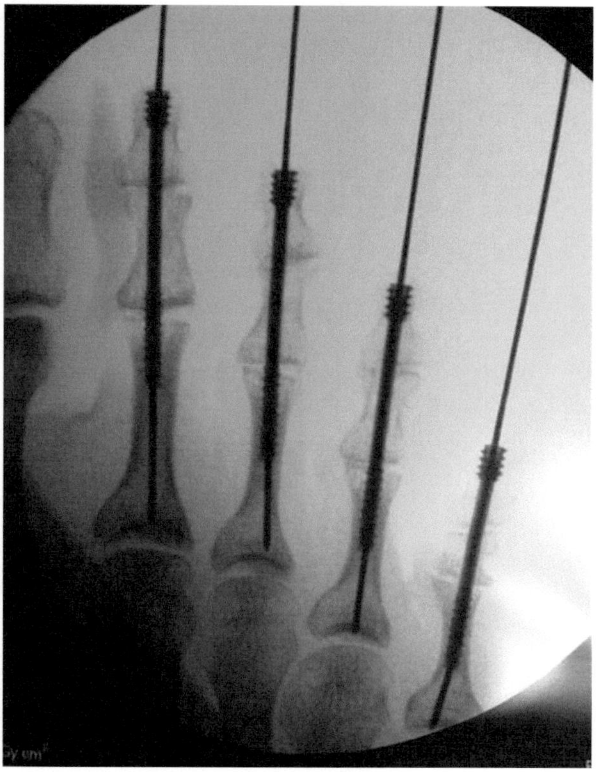

Fig. 8.6 Cannulated screws with optional K-wire fixation

larger proximal phalanges. This may cause pistoning of the screw and/or backing out of the implant, which increases the amount of swelling present in the digit, as well as increasing the risk of infection. We have also found that screw length can pose a significant problem. In a few cases, we have noted screw threads in either the DIPJ or PIPJ distracting the joint. When this occurs, we leave the guide wire in place and driven into the proximal aspect of the phalanx. It should be noted that these wires should not be driven across the MTPJ as there is a high risk of breakage due to the small diameter of the wire.

Surgical Technique

The surgical approach for hammertoe correction is based on the surgeon's preferred approach. We prefer the transverse elliptical incision over the proximal interphalangeal (PIP) joint. This allows a skin plasty to be performed of redundant tissue at the PIP joint and also hides the surgical scar within the tension lines above the joint. Another advantage is that the extensor mechanism can be tightened and imbricated as another reinforcement against recurrent deformity. A DuVries condylectomy, usually at the metaphyseal/diaphyseal junction, is performed on the head of the proximal phalanx with a sagittal saw. Removal of the cartilage of the base of the middle phalanx is then performed with a rongeur. The proximal phalanx is K-wire pre-drilled with the included wire. K-wire pre-drilling several small holes in the base of the middle phalanx centrally will allow the broach to be inserted in a much easier centered fashion. The base of the middle phalanx is then broached. Implantation of the hardware is then performed under standard protocol. The proximal aspect of the implant is screwed into the proximal phalanx. Once the implant is full seated, confirm that the implant is rotated in the proper orientation if using an angled implant. Gentle longitudinal traction is then placed on the digit, and the digit is impacted onto the serrated fins. Manual axial compression firmly seats the device into the medullary canal of the middle phalanx. Fluoroscopic exam is utilized to ensure adequate seating of the implant.

The surgical approach for the PROTOE C2™ and PROTOE VO™ cannulated implants is similar in fashion to that of the first-generation PROTOE™ with the addition of a cannulated system. A 1.1/1.6 mm wire is then passed through the middle phalanx and out the distal aspect of the toe based on the respective implant selected. Following the condylectomy and preparation of the cartilaginous surfaces, the middle phalanx is countersunk. The implant is first screwed into the proximal phalanx. The K-wire is then docked in the PROTOE VO™ cannulated implant, and compression of the toe from distal to proximal seats the device into the middle phalanx.

Similarly, with the PROTOE C2™, a hexalobe/trocar wire is passed from proximal to distal through the middle phalanx. The hexalobe is then docked into the distal end of the implant. The toe is relocated, allowing the distal end of the implant to seat into the middle phalanx. Several reverse turns (counterclockwise) will engage the middle phalanx, and compression at the IP joint will be noted. The K-wire can then be advanced across the MTP joint with the toe held in the desired position.

Several advantages have been realized using a retained intramedullary device versus K-wire fixation. First, the absence of exposed hardware has led to significantly decreased anxiety and improved patient satisfaction with the procedure. Second, we have also noted less chronic swelling of the surgical digit. Lastly, since the implant is retained and not removed, we have seen far less recurrence of the hammertoe deformity or other malalignments.

Case Presentation

1. A 62-year-old female underwent a bunionectomy with hammertoe repair (first-generation PROTOE™ 10-degree angled implant) in 2012 (Fig. 8.7). Although pleased with her bunion, she was disappointed with her second toe posture. The second toe implant began to cut out the medial aspect of the toe causing a lateral drift at the IP joint leading to discomfort. Surgical revision was discussed with her using the PROTOE C2™ cannulated implant.

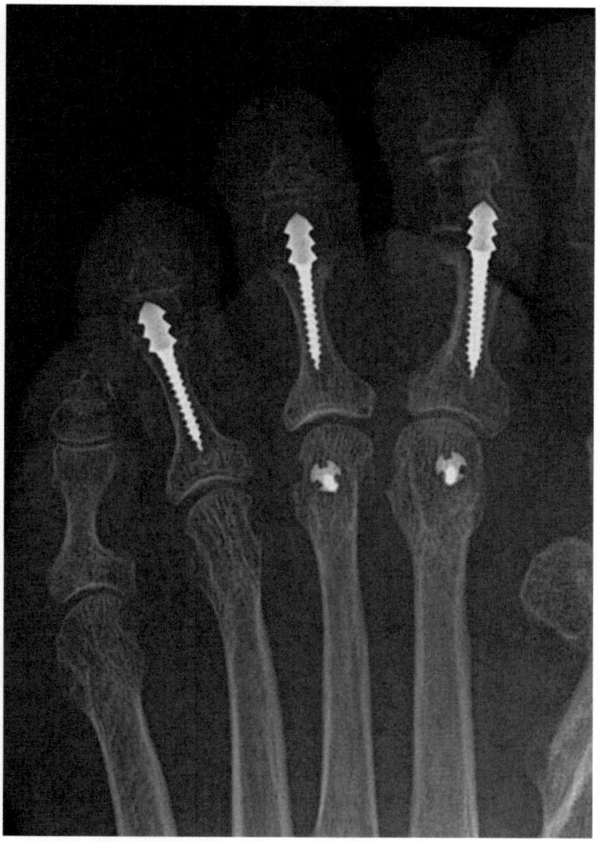

Fig. 8.7 Original implant with medial drift

The original implant was removed by distracting the toe, releasing the distal aspect of the device. The device was then removed. The PROTOE C2™ implant was then inserted following the standard protocol. The 1.6 mm K-wire was then passed across the metatarsophalangeal joint for stability (Figs. 8.8 and 8.9).

Clinical Pearls

- Ensure you have straight bone cuts to eliminate abduction/deformity of the toe.
- Preoperatively consider the amount of desired shortening of the toe to guide your intra-op bone resection from the proximal phalanx.
- Adequate bone prep of the proximal and middle phalanx to increase fusion rate.
- Re-approximation of the extensor tendon over the surgical site.
- Consider a transverse incision versus the standard longitudinal incision.
- Repair of the extensor mechanism, including imbrication, for soft tissue stability.
- Consider a plantar plate repair or ligament rebalancing for a subluxed/dislocated toe.

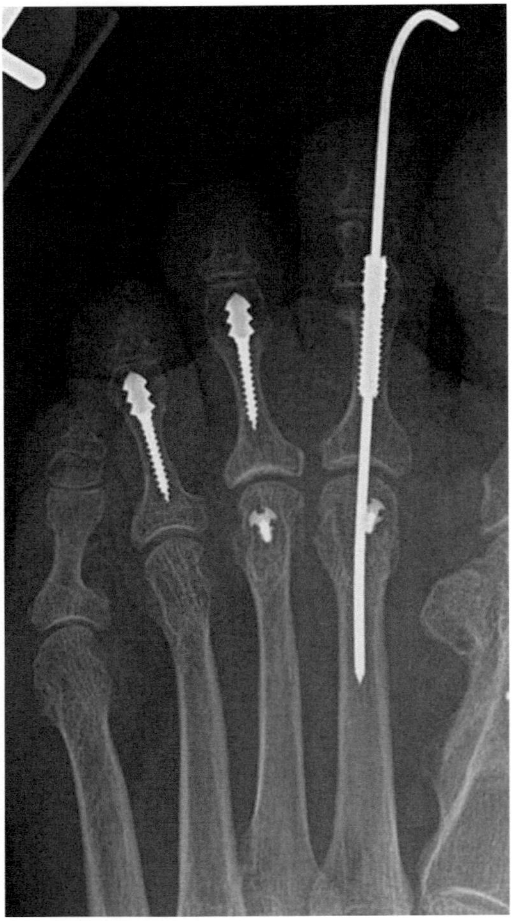

Fig. 8.8 Revision to a cannulated implant with K-wire fixation across the MTP joint

Conclusion

Hammertoe deformity is one of the most common surgical procedures performed in the United States annually. Successful hammertoe surgery is defined as a stable, straight toe that allows for comfortable shoe wear.

The maintenance of correction with hammertoe surgery has only recently entered the modern era of implant technology. One-piece implants, for maintenance of surgical correction of hammertoes, offer the advantages of multiple choices of implant design and metallurgy and an intuitive and reproducible technique.

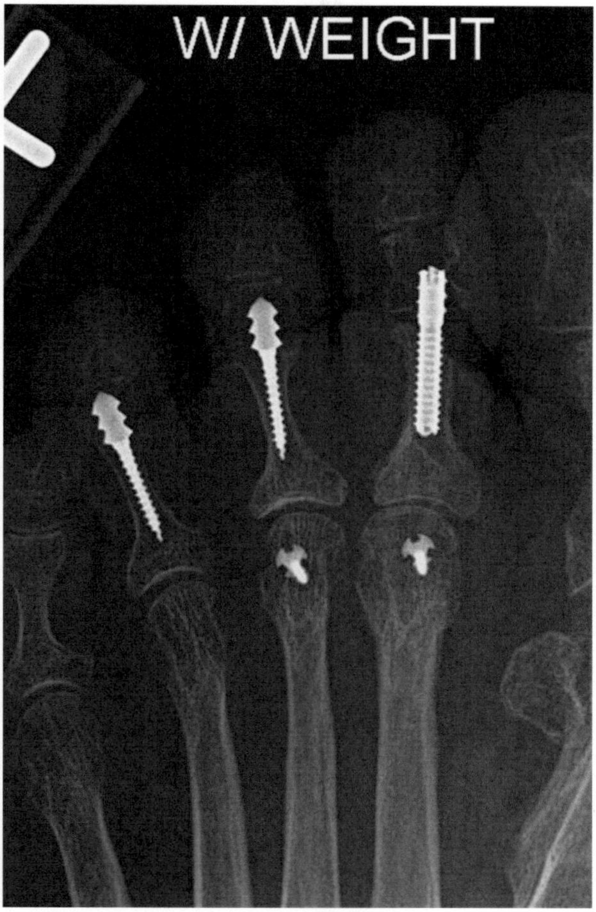

Fig. 8.9 Final implant with more stable fixation in the middle phalanx reducing medial drift

References

1. Coughlin MJ. Operative repair of the mallet toe deformity. Foot Ankle Int. 1995;16(3):109–16.
2. Harmonson JK, Harkless LB. Operative procedures for the correction of hammertoe, claw toe, and mallet toe: a literature review. Clin Podiatr Med Surg. 1996;13(2):211–20.
3. Coughlin M. Lesser toe deformities. In: Coughlin MJMR, Saltzmann CL, editors. Surgery of the foot and ankle. 8th ed. Philadelphia: Mosby; 2007. p. 389–90.
4. Alvine FG, Garvin KL. Peg and dowel fusion of the proximal interphalangeal joint. Foot Ankle. 1980;1(2):90–4.
5. Taylor RG. An operative procedure for the treatment of hammer-toe and claw-toe. J Bone Joint Surg Am. 1940;22(3):608–9.
6. Zingas C, Katcherian DA, Wu KK. Kirschner wire breakage after surgery of the lesser toes. Foot Ankle Int. 1995;16(8):504–9.
7. Reece AT, Stone MH, Young AB. Toe fusion using Kirschner wire. A study of the postoperative infection rate and related problems. J R Coll Surg Edinb. 1987;32(3):158–9.

8. Caterini R, Farsetti P, Tarantino U, Potenza V, Ippolito E. Arthrodesis of the toe joints with an intramedullary cannulated screw for correction of hammertoe deformity. Foot Ankle Int. 2004;25(4):256–61.
9. Galli MM, Brigido SA, Protzman NM. Pinning across the metatarsophalangeal joint for hammertoe correction: where are we aiming and what is the damage to the metatarsal articular surface? J Foot Ankle Surg. 2014;53(4):405–10.
10. Coughlin MJ. Lesser toe deformities. Orthopedics. 1987;10(1):63–75.
11. Ellington JK, Anderson RB, Davis WH, Cohen BE, Jones CP. Radiographic analysis of proximal interphalangeal joint arthrodesis with an intramedullary fusion device for lesser toe deformities. Foot Ankle Int. 2010;31(5):372–6.
12. Konkel KF, Menger AG, Retzlaff SA. Hammer toe correction using an absorbable intramedullary pin. Foot Ankle Int. 2007;28(8):916–20.
13. Lehman DE, Smith RW. Treatment of symptomatic hammertoe with a proximal interphalangeal joint arthrodesis. Foot Ankle Int. 1995;16(9):535–41.
14. Pietrzak WS, Lessek TP, Perns SV. A bioabsorbable fixation implant for use in proximal interphalangeal joint (hammer toe) arthrodesis: biomechanical testing in a synthetic bone substrate. J Foot Ankle Surg. 2006;45(5):288–94.
15. Shaw AH, Alvarez G. The use of digital implants for the correction of hammer toe deformity and their potential complications and management. J Foot Surg. 1992;31(1):63–74.
16. Taylor RG. The treatment of claw toes by multiple transfers of flexor into extensor tendons. J Bone Joint Surg Br. 1951;33-B(4):539–42.
17. Catena F, Doty JF, Jastifer J, Coughlin MJ, Stevens F. Prospective study of hammertoe correction with an intramedullary implant. Foot Ankle Int. 2014;35(4):319–25.
18. Coillard JY, Petri GJ, van Damme G, Deprez P, Laffenetre O. Stabilization of proximal interphalangeal joint in lesser toe deformities with an angulated intramedullary implant. Foot Ankle Int. 2014;35(4):401–7.
19. Scott RT, Hyer CF, Berlet GC. The PROTOE intramedullary hammertoe device: an alternative to Kirschner wires. Foot Ankle Spec. 2013;6(3):214–6.
20. Witt BL, Hyer CF. Treatment of hammertoe deformity using a one-piece intramedullary device: a case series. J Foot Ankle Surg. 2012;51(4):450–6.
21. Roukis TS. A 1-piece shape-metal nitinol intramedullary internal fixation device for arthrodesis of the proximal interphalangeal joint in neuropathic patients with diabetes. Foot Ankle Spec. 2009;2(3):130–4.
22. Scholl A, McCarty J, Scholl D, Mar A. Smart toe(R) implant versus buried Kirschner wire for proximal interphalangeal joint arthrodesis: a comparative study. J Foot Ankle Surg. 2013;52(5):580–3.
23. Angirasa AK, Barrett MJ, Silvester D. SmartToe(R) implant compared with Kirschner wire fixation for hammer digit corrective surgery: a review of 28 patients. J Foot Ankle Surg. 2012;51(6):711–3.

Chapter 9
PIPJ Arthrodesis with a Thermal-Activated Metallic Implant

Michael A. Rivera and Thomas J. Chang

Hammertoe deformity is a common pathology seen by today's foot and ankle surgeons. The deformity of the lesser digits is a frequently encountered pathology in foot and ankle clinics. Arthrodesis is accepted as the gold standard for hammertoe correction. Surgeons performed this by removing the adjacent articular surface of the proximal interphalangeal joint to allow osseous fusion. Soule first described the procedure in 1910, and Jones later modified it to utilize a more straightforward dorsal approach [1]. In 1940, Taylor added the use of a Kirschner wire fixation for stabilization [2]. This is a simple and effective method of arthrodesis which remains a steadfast most common technique and practice despite its anterior weaknesses [3–6]. With modern intramedullary fixation systems, the goal is to address or remove the concerns surgeons encounter with K-wire fixation. Specifically, in a study involving 149 toes and 99 patients, Richman and colleagues noted positive results for intramedullary devices over K-wires for hammertoe fixation [5]. In discussing proximal interphalangeal joint arthrodesis for hammertoe correction, Ellington indicated a preference for intramedullary devices in order to avoid complications with K-wires [7].

Innovative Hammertoe Memory Devices

Nickel titanium, also known as nitinol (part of shape-memory alloy), is a metal alloy of nickel and titanium. Nitinol alloys exhibit two closely related and unique properties: shape-memory effect (SME) and superelasticity (SE, also called pseudoelasticity

M. A. Rivera
Memorial Hospital West, Pembroke Pines, FL, USA

T. J. Chang (✉)
Redwood Orthopedic Surgery Associates, Santa Rosa, CA, USA
e-mail: ThomasChang14@comcast.net

E. A. Cook, J. J. Cook (eds.), *Hammertoes*,
https://doi.org/10.1007/978-3-319-16552-3_9

(PE)). Shape memory is the ability of nitinol to undergo deformation at one temperature and then recover its original, undeformed shape upon heating above its "transformation temperature." Superelasticity occurs at a narrow temperature range just above its transformation temperature; in this case, no heating is necessary to cause the undeformed shape to recover, and the material exhibits enormous elasticity, some 10–30 times that of ordinary metal. The word nitinol is derived from its composition and its place of discovery: Nickel-Titanium-Naval Ordnance Laboratory. William J. Buehler [8] along with Frederick Wang [9] discovered its properties during research at the Naval Ordnance Laboratory in 1959 [10, 11]. Buehler was attempting to make a better missile nose cone, which could resist fatigue, heat, and the force of impact.

Several varieties of a nitinol metal implants have been utilized as an intramedullary fixation device. These implants require specialized instrumentation for insertion, and certainly a learning curve exists before a surgeon is able to insert the device in a uniform and predictable manner and also in an efficient amount of time. These implants do allow the surgeon to select a device that will stabilize the arthrodesis perfectly straight or one that allows for a small degree of flexion, thus allowing for a more anatomic configuration to the toe.

Variations of the above discussed implants have also been presented. One- and two-piece designs are marketed that incorporate threaded or barbed ends. One design incorporates a threaded screw-like portion that is initially inserted within the proximal phalanx. Distally, this implant possesses a barbed spade-like configuration that pierces and maintains position within the middle phalanx. Certainly, the question comes up of whether compression is necessary for successful hammertoe repair.

Screws are devices which provide more predictable purchase and compression. However, the majority of single-piece constructs required an additional incision to the distal tuft for insertion. Two-piece screw-in devices avoided the additional incision but added to complexity, not to mention an increased fear of tissue handling such as small implant components. In addition, there may be possible disengagement of the two-piece implant with the complication and failure of union at the PIPJ.

Prior studies have identified nearly more than 70 different products available over the past few years with notable progressive improvement in material quality, design, and ease of use for the hammertoe implants [12]. Early generation products were simple, often composed of static metallic of or absorbable composites that acted as positional fixation. The disadvantages were the lack of pullout strength providing no compression and inability to conform to the naturally variable anatomy of the osseous proximal phalanxes prompting increased design improvement. Later, new generation devices incorporated threads or winged arms to provide additional stability and compression across the fusion site. The devices commonly required storage in a frozen state prior to direct application and implantation. This limitation posed inherent difficulties as it added an urgency for insertion once the device was exposed to room temperature and began early expansion, in addition to occasionally providing a freeze-dried state that required warmth activation (Fig. 9.1a,b).

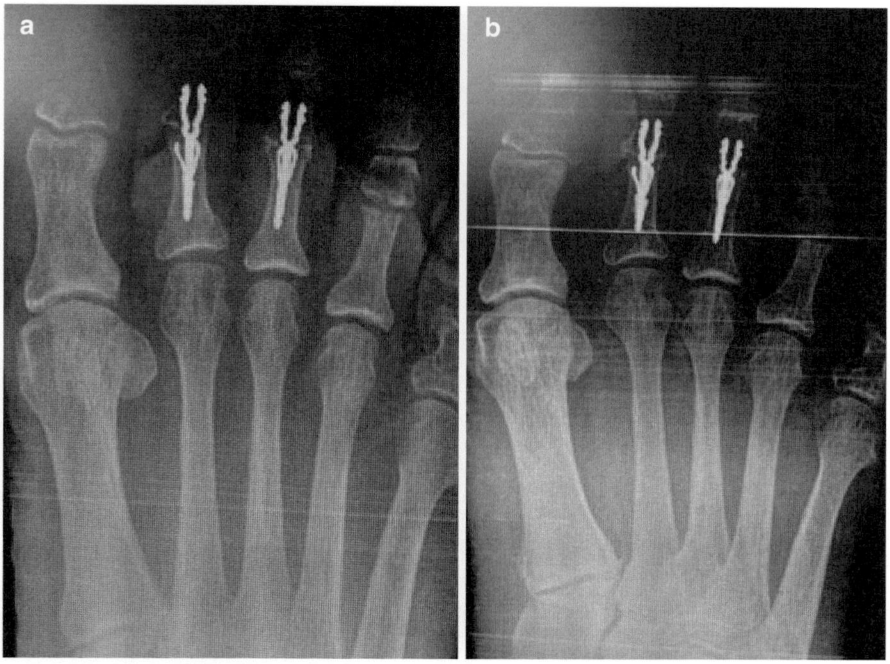

Fig. 9.1 (**a**) The HammerLock II implant and 2 weeks with good alignment. (**b**) The Hammerlock implant with arthrodesis at 6 weeks with full return to shoes and activity

Amiot, R.A. and Nowak, J. in a retrospective review looked at the use of HammerLock internal implant for fixation of PIPJ arthrodesis in the correction of fixed hammertoe deformities of the lesser digits. The osseous union in 20 out of 21 toes was 95% with an overall ACFAS-modified forefoot score improvement. Successful arthrodesis was achieved with a stable, asymptomatic pseudoarthrosis in one patient overall and one toe. The conclusion was that overall, there was extremely high fusion rates and a statistically significant improvement in pain and function scores postoperatively with very low complication rates (Fig. 9.2a, b, c).

Sandu, J.S.; DeCarbo, T. W.; and Hofbauer, H.M., in a retrospective study showed overall 93.8% fixation rate was noted in 35 patients who underwent surgical correction with the use of 65 implants for correction of hammertoes. The arthrodesis of the PIPJ utilized a one-piece memory nitinol intramedullary fixation device in which 27 presented in the follow-up study. Complications were identified in four patients for a 6.1% finding, including one asymptomatic non-union (1.5%), two hardware failures (3%), and one implant displacement (1.5%). None of the patients required revisional surgery.

Colliard, Jean-Yves; Gianfranco, John Petri; Van Damme, Geert; Deprez, Patrick; and Laffenetre, Olivier in a prospective multicenter study used an angulated intramedullary fixation for PIPJ fusion with the use of the IPP-ON implant. This study by Integra included 117 patients where 156 had hammertoe digital corrections

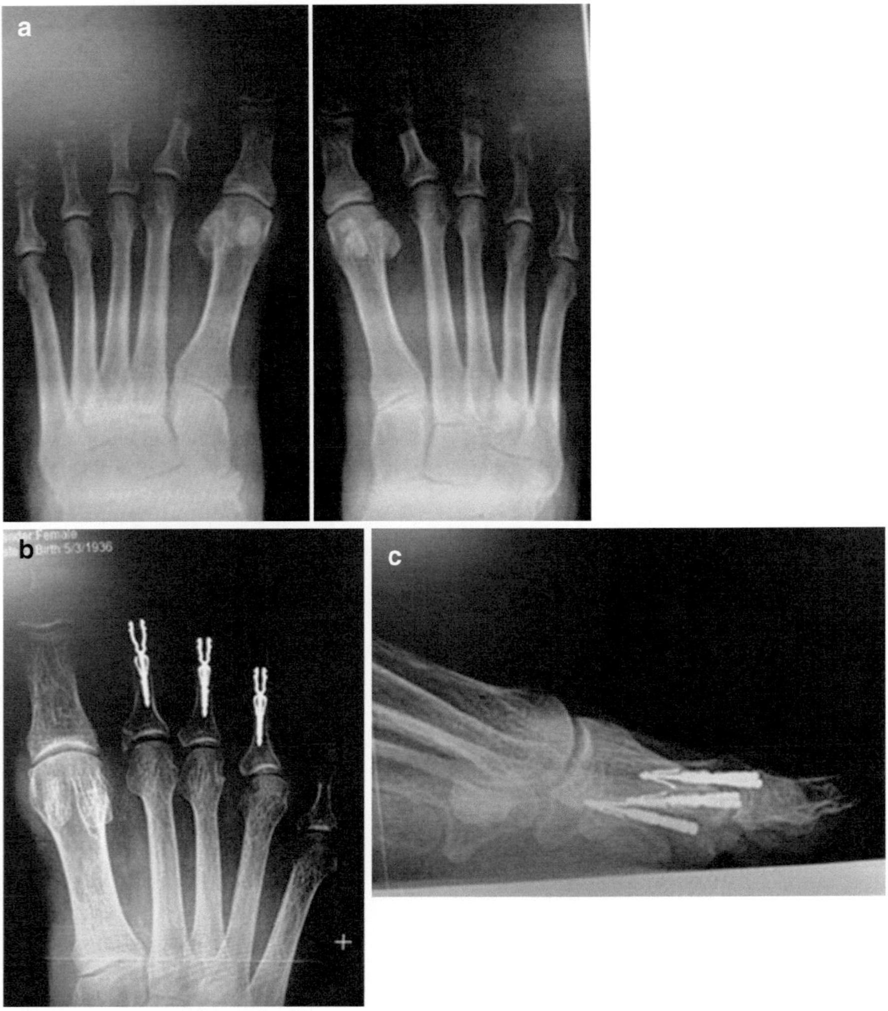

Fig. 9.2 (**a**) Preoperative anteroposterior projections of second, third and fourth hammertoe contractures. (**b**) Anteroposterior projection showing good alignment of memory nitinol intramedullary hammertoe correction involving toes 2, 3, 4. (**c**) Lateral projection demonstrating good sagittal plane alignment of memory nitinol intramedullary hammertoe correction involving toes 2, 3, 4

and concluded an 83.8% arthrodesis rate after 12 months. There were five post-op complications (3.2%), two cases were treated intraoperatively, and one case required revision.

What Advantages Do Intramedullary Hammertoe Devices Offer

Intramedullary devices have various benefits over the standard percutaneous Kirschner wire fixation [12].

Typically, the distal interphalangeal joint is not violated with the placement of most intramedullary systems in comparison with K-wires. Beyond sparing uninvolved joints, intramedullary devices provided multi-planar resistance to rotational forces with the majority of intramedullary implants providing a source of compression across the fusion site. This compression is lacking with the standard percutaneous Kirschner wire fixation.

A recent retrospect review of 136 s PIP joints in 114 patients found improved postoperative radiograph alignment with the use of intramedullary implants in comparison to traditional K-wire [12]. Addiotionally, the placement of internal fixation in the intramedullary canal neglects the risks of pin-tract infection associated with percutaneous exiting of the Kirschner wire fixation. Elimination of percutaneous fixation alleviates anxiety and complications associated with pin site care and the appearance of percutaneous pins including cosmesis. The placement of internal fixation also lessens the concern for traumatic disruption of exposed fixation. The use of modern memory nitinol implants often simplifies the postoperative course as opposed to Kirschner wire fixation. K-wire patients are likely to have pins extruding from their toes as opposed to recommended intramedullary fixation devices which pose less pain, increased osseous fixation, and improved clinical appearance. Ultimately, patient's satisfaction is more important regardless of radiographic or clinical appearance, and high satisfaction rates have occurred with intramedullary fixation devices [4, 13].

In a retrospective study of 30 PIPJ fusions using nitinol in 10 patients with diabetic neuropathy, Roukis cited a 93% success fusion rate with the remaining patients having a stable non-union [4].

Important Considerations in Surgical Planning

Surgical planning for hammertoes is far more complex than what we have learned over the years, especially as residents. Once examination and testing are complete, one has to consider not only the hammertoe correction but the stability and alignment of the MPJ in all planes as well. It is also imperative to evaluate the plantar plate, especially if there is a positive drawer sign (positive Lachman's maneuver). The clinical exam also calls for suspicion of interdigital neuromas between the second and third interspace. X-ray examination, as well as MRI or 3-D CTs, may be obtained to further assess the clinical planning and surgical correction of toes.

It is often necessary to explain the potential need for plantar plate repair, metatarsal osteotomy, hallux valgus correction, and different hammertoe correction options prior to surgery. If there are flexible hammertoes on adjacent digits, attention should be considered for surgical correction on these adjacent digits simultaneously, as arthrodesis for one digit may necessitate a substitution phenomenon of the other subsequent toes. It is also important to adjust the staging and categorizing of the flexibility of the toe. If one toe has more extensor substitution and flexor substitution exhibited, definitive arthrodesis should be performed. This allows for better positioning of the toes, less swelling, and the more long-term standardized outcome.

Equally important is a thorough evaluation of the plantar plate. If the plantar plate rupture or injury does exist, repair it accordingly. If the plantar plate is not repaired, a resulting crooked toe or loss of purchase is noted often with a shift medially or laterally. Surgeons may perform the plantar plate repair unilaterally or completely. Finally one may shift the metatarsal slightly medial or lateral during the procedure to allow for some correction of the toe position with an osteotomy.

Fixation Method and Surgical Technique

We recommend performing associated procedures for any forefoot surgery prior to addressing the hammertoe deformity. This includes a bunionectomy, tailor's bunionectomy, and possible neuroma excision. This also decrease the stress on the toe and possible MPJ correction during the other procedures. Furthermore, consider the MPJ positions and metatarsal parabola with regard to the position of corrected first and fifth metatarsals.

The memory implants usually come in a straight design as well as 10-degree angle. Both have been used with a good cosmetic and functional result. The angled design assumes a "flexed fusion" position which may be more cosmetically pleasing to some, rather than a toe which is too straight. The large and medium sizes are usually placed within the second digit and medium and small implants placed within the third and fourth toes. It is uncommon to fuse the fifth toe yet more commonly seen within the orthopedic community. This is often seen in neurologic conditions as well as revisions.

A standard dissection technique for the arthrodesis is identical to that of the arthroplasty with regard to joint exposure. Standard dissection is carried down to the extensor tendon. Next a transverse or Z-lengthening extensor tenotomy is performed, releasing the extensor wing and sling mechanism both medially and laterally and across the MPJ. The IPJ capsulotomy is performed slightly proximal to the dorsal apex of the joint. The soft tissues are freed from the head of the proximal phalanx and the base of the middle phalanx. The head of the proximal phalanx is then resected recommending distal to the surgical neck and proximal to the articular cartilage. The oscillating saw blade is then reversed, and resection of the base of the middle phalanx is performed. Care should be taken to remove any bony fragments or ledges in the depths of the proximal phalanx cortex or middle phalanx cortex with no prominence. The bone ends are then manually opposed to assess sagittal, frontal, and transverse plane correction with bony apposition. Any transverse or sagittal plane osseous deformities can be corrected with angled cuts using the oscillating saw and soft tissue balancing. Next assessment of soft tissue correction with Kelikian testing at the metatarsophalangeal joint should be performed to assess any contractures in a sagittal, transverse, or frontal plane position.

The metatarsal osteotomies should be performed in conjunction to the correction of the digit if there is abnormal metatarsal parabola with structural elongated second or third metatarsals (Fig. 9.3a-f). It is imperative to assess the integrity of the plantar plate clinically, prior to doing the surgical correction of the second digit. It may be

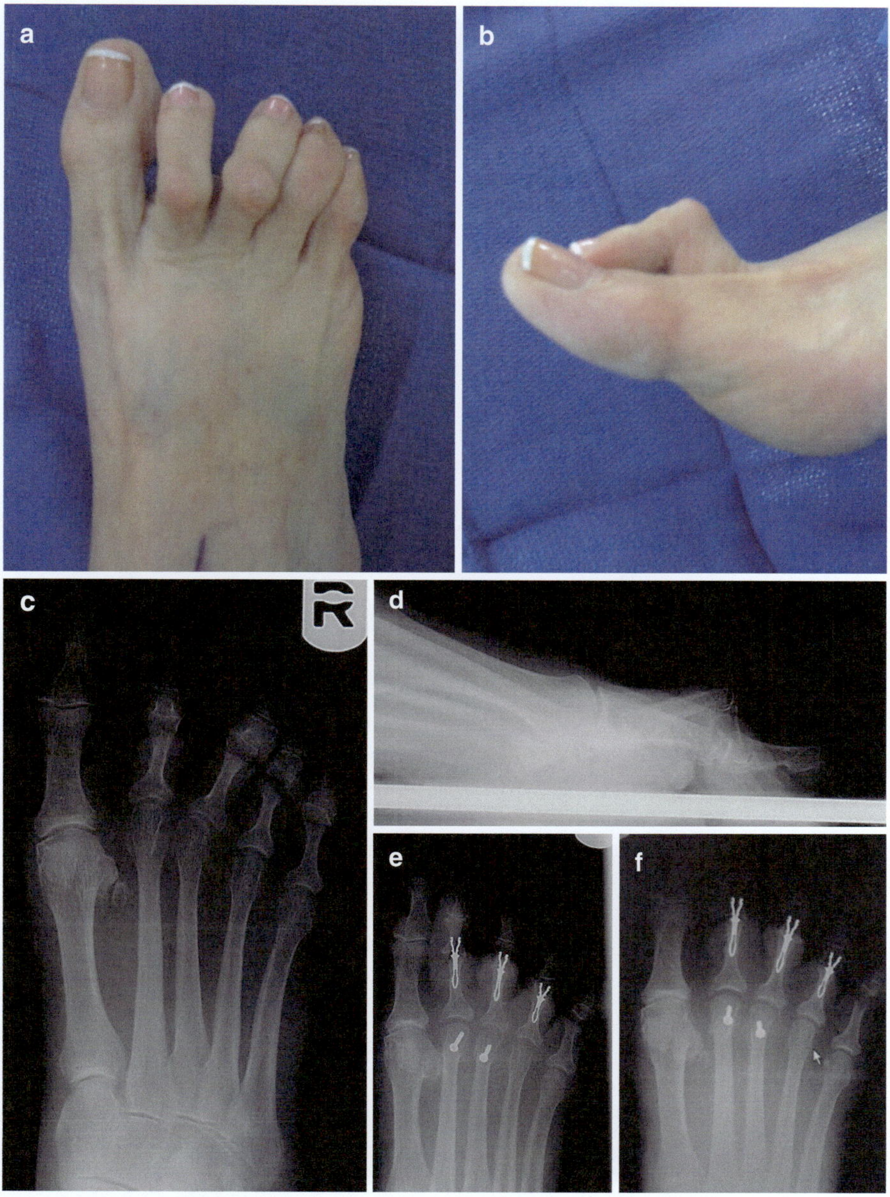

Fig. 9.3 (**a**) Presentation of classic hammer toes with structural elongated metatarsals 2,3 right foot. (**b**) Lateral projection of rigid contracture of toes. (**c**) Preoperative anteroposterior projection of hammertoes involving the second and third toes. (**d**) Preoperative lateral projection of second and third hammertoe contractures. (**e**) Postoperative X-rays at 4 weeks with good alignment HammerLock fixation and 2,3 met osteotomies. (**f**) Postoperative X-rays at 6 weeks with arthrodesis and with return to activities

helpful to utilize a MRI prior to addressing the correction of these toes, especially the second MPJ. Next the correct size implant is selected with the assistance of fluoroscopy, and the corresponding drill bit is used to create a pilot hole in the proximal and middle phalanges. The drill bit is advanced in a retrograde fashion from distal to proximal into the medullary canal of the proximal phalanx, allowing for 75% of the cutting flutes to pass into the canal. Secondly the same drill bit is then passed in an antegrade fashion from proximal to distal into the medullary canal of the middle phalanx, allowing for 25% of the cutting flutes to pass into the canal. The current HammerLock II kit also has automatic stops designed into the drill system, so proper depth is easily achieved for each side. While stabilizing each phalanx, the corresponding broach is then used to broach the proximal and middle phalanges. Care must be taken not to rotate the phalanx or misalign the broach during the process. Pay special attention to assessing the medial lateral translation of the middle phalanx on the proximal phalanx when broaching the middle phalanx. Ideally, the medial and lateral cortices of the adequate phalanges should align to avoid symptomatic bony prominences once the joint is fused with the internal implant. Be sure to leave the middle tab in place. The exposed proximal end of the implant is then inserted into the prepared medullary canal of the proximal phalanx and advanced proximally until the clamshell/tab assembly makes contact with the distal bony surface of the proximal phalanx. A mallet may be used to gently seat the implant fully into the proximal phalanx. The forceps were then removed, along with the clamshell, exposing the distal portion of the implant. Be sure to leave the middle plastic tab and placed during this portion of the procedure. The exposed distal portion of the implant was then inserted into the prepared medullary canal of the middle phalanx; advancing the implant onto contact is made with the plastic tab. The plastic tab was then removed, and the arthrodesis site is manually compressed axillary for approximately 1–2 min to allow body heat activation. Manual compression is removed, and the arthrodesis site was then assessed directly under fluoroscopy for both excellent bone anastomosis and implant position (Fig. 9.4a–f).

In the earlier designs, the surgeon was required to hold the two phalanges together after implantation for 1–2 min to allow for the implant to warm up and then expansion of the device to occur before there was enough stability to release the toe. In patients with osteoporotic bone, this often took longer for stability to occur. With the newer generation of implants, there is a significant difference in perceived stability almost immediately upon phalangeal impaction and placement. It is a noticeable difference which seems to equate to better overall outcomes.

A C-arm (fluoroscopy) can be used to confirm that the component is properly engaged and the toe is well aligned. If there is slight gapping of the implant at the proximal interphalangeal joint, compression of the middle phalanx onto the proximal phalanx should be performed to improve placement position, making sure the arms are distracting along the internal cortex. Extensor tendon closure is now performed with simple interrupted 3–0 absorbable suture, and the skin is then closed in a simple interrupted-type fashion.

The nitinol implants provide proportional sizing for better fit, with straight and angled versions and multiple sizes. The second-generation Hammerlock II design provides for higher strength with more aggressive barbs providing solid fixation and flexible legs to minimize stress on cortical walls. Most implants provide fast and easy insertion systems in the self-contained sterilized packs.

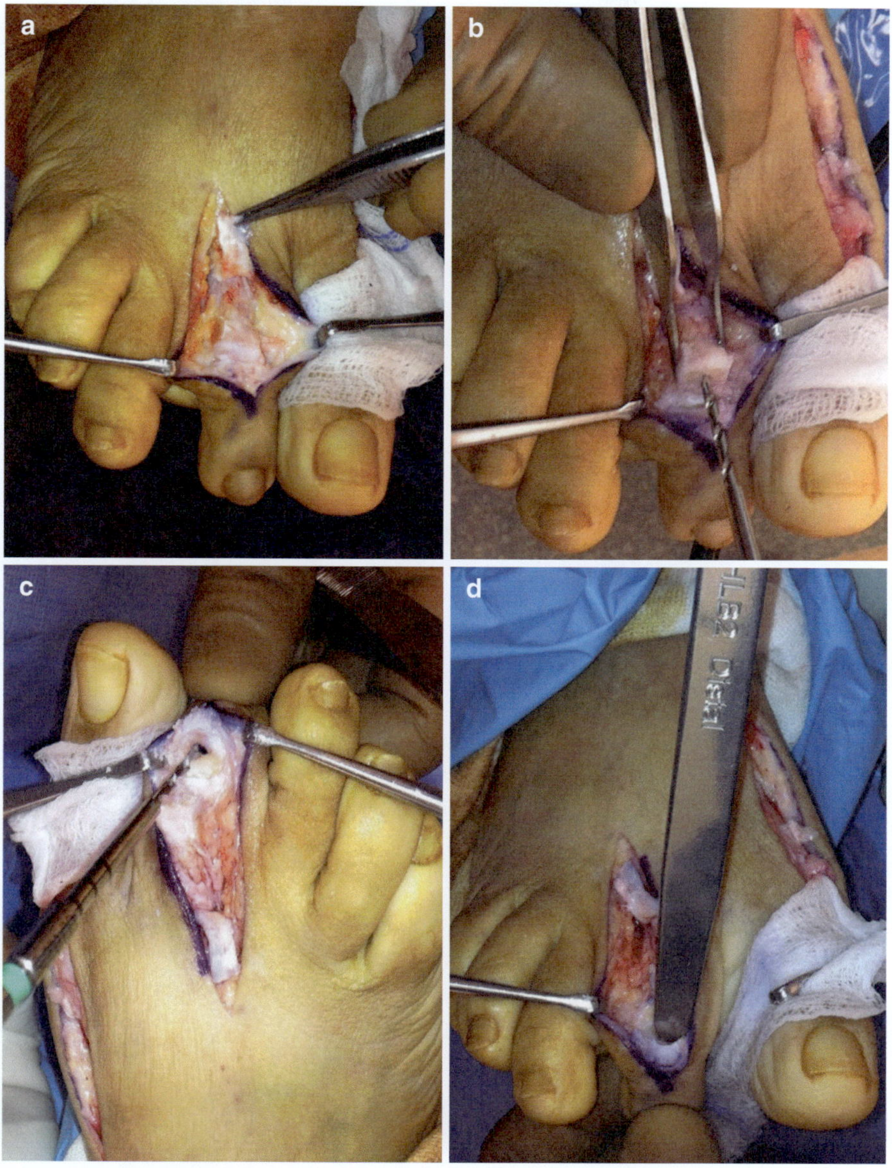

Fig. 9.4 (**a**) Preparation of the proximal phalanx with dissection of the extensor tendon. (**b**) Resection of the proximal phalanx head with dissection of the extensor tendon. Intramedullary drill with accurate alignment plane. (**c**) Middle phalanx is drilled and prepped, intramedullary canal is centered in good alignment and planes. (**d**) Middle phalanx is broached in accurate plane. (**e**) Insertion of the proximal phalanx implant with remaining exposed distal portion of the implant. This is then introduced into the medullary canal of the middle phalanx, advancing it forward and then removal of the central tab and manually compressing for 1–2 minutes. (**f**) Toe with implant properly seated. Proximal interphalangeal joint arthrodesis using the HammerLock implant

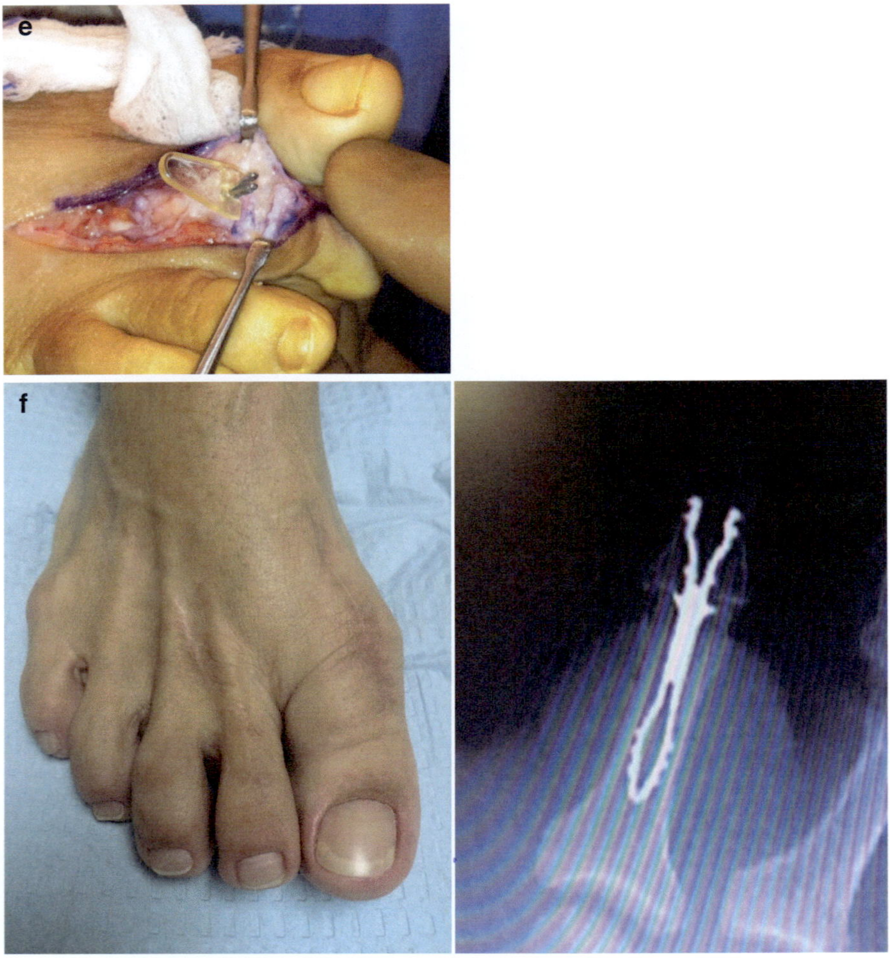

Fig. 9.4 (continued)

How to Avoid Complications

As with all implants, there are apparent weaknesses and potential complications. The superficial postoperative infections are among the most common postoperative complication as Roukis determined in a study of intramedullary fixation with a one-piece nitinol implant [4]. Due to the intramedullary nature of these implants, removal of the implant is often a concern for surgeons. I have not observed this to be a practical concern clinically. When the bone is well healed and solid, there is never a need to remove the implant deep within the bone. The material is nickel/titanium and is extremely biocompatible. The reasons to remove the implant usually stem from painful post-op problems, such as infection or non-union. When this is the case, there is relative ease in separating the two phalanges from each other and removing the implant manually. In several cases where the arms have broken thru the phalangeal wall, these patients have been asymptomatic, and implant removal was not required. The PIP joint space still was able to heal. Another case was stabilized with a K-wire from distal and placed across the MTPJ to provide stability for 6 weeks.

Prior experience with some of the first-generation memory hammertoe implants shows a fairly narrow waist. This is the area between the proximal and distal arms and acts as a point of directed stress with range of motion and excessive movement. Often the waist is located right in the joint space and is vulnerable to weight-bearing stresses when bone healing is delayed. When the waist fatigues and breaks, there is resultant instability often leading to a fibrous malunion. At times, bone healing did occur yet often with a slight deviation. This is not always symptomatic. The advent of the second-generation implants has provided much improved stability which does not appear to fatigue and fail like the earlier designs. Just a minor increase in the diameter of the arms provides tremendous increase in overall stability as well as adding more metal arms. The waist in the newer designs has been shifted slightly proximal, so now the weakest portion of the implant is resting within the proximal phalanx and is not prone to early movement and metal failure.

When implant loosening occurs, one must really analyze the cause. Perhaps the implant was not the proper size or too small, allowing unnecessary motion due to lack of osseous purchase. Cortical disruption may be seen once surgical drilling, broaching, and impaction of the implant. These are also potential pitfalls, increasing the risk of failure. Often manual impaction with splinting in the office setting may suffice. However, if there is failure to form a solid union or satisfactory fibrous union in shoes, then a revision may be required. The benefits from using an expanded implant which extends into the middle or proximal phalanx within the canals account for better compression and minimal loss of bone. Although we do not often think of intramedullary devices as an ideal fixation in the case of a failed index K-wire, a study by Ellington noted that fixation revision with intramedullary devices may be the best [7].

At times, technical difficulty with intramedullary implants is the other common concern. Given the lack of osseous volume and surface of the proximal and middle phalanges, this may require more initial precision with drill holes and preparation of the canals, especially when there is osteopenia, or poor bone quality. Excessive osseous distraction with multiple guide pins and drills will result in a loss of implant purchase and the potential need to resort to traditional K-wire fixation placement. Sung and co-workers noted superior alignment postoperatively in patients with implants and attributed the alignment to the increased need for precision and accuracy when using implants over the traditional wire fixation [12] (Fig. 9.5a, b).

There are some limitations of the implants available. The short or stubby intermediate phalanx does not always allow for complete settling of the distal prongs of the implants to lie within the phalanx. This may cause DIPJ injury or pain with

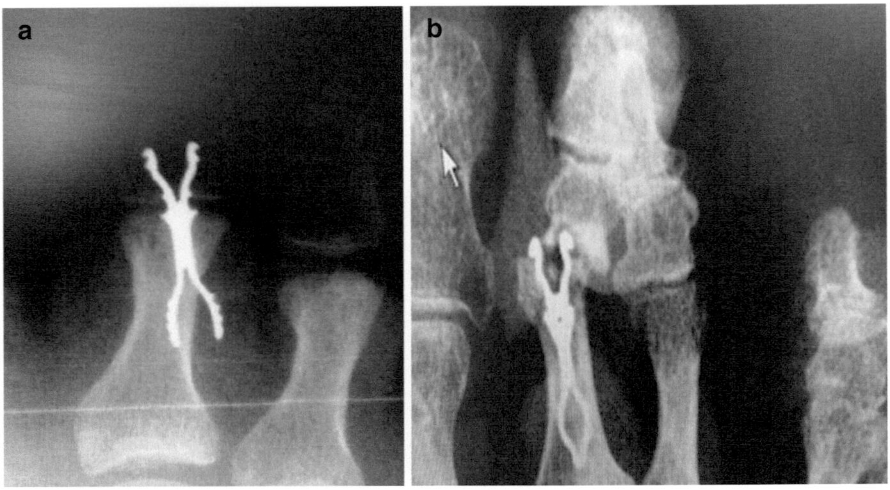

Fig. 9.5 (**a**) Extraosseous fixation of the proximal legs, due to inaccurate drilling and alignment with technique and an undersized implant. (**b**) Less than accurate alignment with the implant placed too proximal into the proximal phalanx and overdrilling

intra-articular placement. A narrow proximal phalanx is also a possible concern for placement and expansion. Soft bone may also be a concern as the expansive nature of the device upon placement and deployment may possibly break through the stiffness of the phalangeal wall.

Postoperative Care

Postoperatively, we have utilized memory nitinol intramedullary devices in over 500 procedures, and patients are weight-bearing as tolerated in a surgical shoe with a splint-type dressing along the surgical performed toes. We have found with increased stability, there is less pain using these implants which allows easier postoperative pain management recovery. The patient is evaluated at 1 week postoperatively for the first dressing change and again at 2–3 weeks to remove the sutures depending on their healing rate. The toes are then splinted with digital splinted devices or Coban taping techniques. These devices are usually worn for an additional 2–4 weeks. It is not uncommon to see arthrodesis at a faster rate with osseous fusion at 4–6 weeks which would allow a quicker recovery. If a metatarsal osteotomy or MPJ release is performed, patients are still in a surgical shoe for approximately 6 weeks followed by transition to an athletic shoe gear at 5–6 weeks postoperatively. Weight-bearing is performed as tolerated, and exercise is limited for approximately 6–8 weeks or when arthrodesis occurs clinically and radiographically (Fig. 9.6a-d).

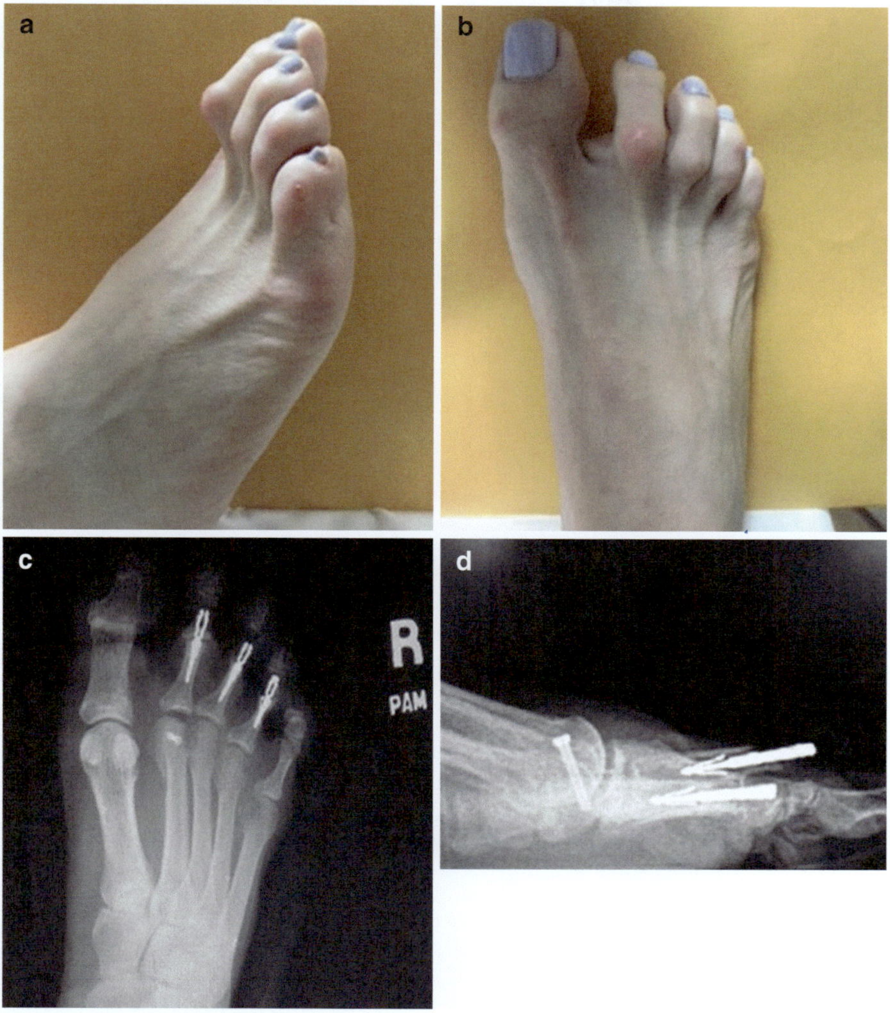

Fig. 9.6 (**a**) Lateral view of the foot showing painful hammertoes of toes 2, 3, 4. (**b**) Dorsal view of the foot with painful hammertoes of toes 2, 3, 4. (**c**) Anteroposterior view showing postoperative correction of hammertoes 2, 3, 4. (**d**) Lateral view with adequate sagittal plane correction of hammertoes 2, 3, 4

Conclusion

Innovations in foot and ankle surgery are advancing quickly with intramedullary hammertoe implants. Although current research evidence supports effectiveness and superiority in healing, the implant costs are highly variable, and ultimate cost-benefit studies are needed.

There are low complication fusion rates in comparison to the traditional wire fixation. It is our opinion these fusion rates and effectiveness of the nitinol implants provide the static continuous compression to allow effective arthrodesis and alignment in all planes. The inherited benefits of these nitinol devices clearly demonstrate their efficacy in place of hammertoe corrective surgery. Larger prospective studies and randomized control trials may offer future concrete answers and accepted gold standards of these implants. Nitinol implant fixation will likely become the new gold standard in years to come in arthrodesis of digital surgery. Lastly, with cost being a large concern, implant cost is highly variable, and ultimate cost-benefit studies are needed.

References

1. Soule R. Operation for the correction of hammer toe. New York Med. 1990;91:649–50.
2. Taylor R. An operation procedure for the treatment of hammertoe and claw-toe. J Bone Joint Surg. 1940;22:608–9.
3. Trethowan WH. The treatment of hammertoe, part 1- general considerations: conservative measures prophylaxis. Lancet. 1925;205(1):1257–8.
4. Roukis TS. A-1 piece shape-metal nitinol intramedullary internal fixation device for arthrodesis of PIPJ in neuropathic patients with diabetes. Foot Ankle Spec. 2009;2(3):129–34.
5. Richman S, Siqueira M, McCullough K, Berkowitz M. Correction of hammertoe deformity with novel intramedullary PIP fusion device versus K-wire fixation. Foot Ankle Int. 2017;38(2):174–80.
6. Ellington J. Hammertoes and clawtoes: proximal interphalangeal joint correction. Foot Ankle Clin. 2011;16(4):547–58.
7. Ellington JK, Anderson RB, Davies WH, Cohen BE, Jones CP. Radiographic analysis of proximal interphangeal joint arthrodesis with intramedullary fusion device for lesser toe deformities. Foot Ankle Int. 2010;31:372–6.
8. Buehler WJ, Gilfrich JW, Wiley RC. Effects of low-temperature phase changes on the mechanical properties of alloys near composition TiNi. J Appl Phys. 1963;34(5):1475–7.
9. Wang FE, Buehler WJ, Pickart SJ. Crystal structure and a unique martensitic transition of TiNi. J Appl Phys. 1965;36(10):3232–9.
10. "The Alloy That Remembers", Time, 1968-09-13.
11. Kauffman GB, Mayo I. The story of nitinol: the serendipitous discovery of the memory metal and its applications. Chem Educ. 1997;2(2):1–21.
12. Sung W, Weil L, Weil L. Retrospective comparative study of operative repair of hammertoe deformity. Foot Ankle Spec. 2014;7(3):185–92.
13. Moon JL, Kihm CA, Perez DA, Dowling LB, Adler DC. Digital arthrodesis: current fixation techniques. Clin Podiatr Med Surg. 2011;28:768–83.

Chapter 10
The Use of Allogenic Bone Implant in Proximal Interphalangeal Joint Arthrodesis

William T. DeCarbo and Joshua D. Thun

Introduction

The hammertoe deformity is one of the most common forefoot pathologic conditions encountered by foot and ankle surgeons. When nonoperative treatments such as strapping devices, splinting, modified orthotics, toe pads, anti-inflammatories, or specialized shoe gear have failed, surgical intervention may be indicated [1–6]. Surgical options include arthroplasty or arthrodesis of the proximal interphalangeal joint (PIPJ), PIPJ capsulotomy and tendon release, tendon transfers, phalangectomy, interpositional implant arthroplasty, or amputation [1, 7–21]. When PIPJ arthrodesis is performed, internal fixation with close contact between phalanges is required to achieve a stable union. Traditionally, fixation has been achieved utilizing Kirschner wire (K-wire) transfixation and remains an effective option [1, 9, 19]. Despite being a popular option due to ease of insertion and removal, complications such as pin-tract infection, toe migration, and patient dissatisfaction have been documented [1, 22].

A myriad of lesser digit PIPJ implants have been designed and introduced to offer a more optimal fixation construct. Most designs have shown to be effective with favorable results and can be broadly classified as absorbable and nonabsorbable. The focus of this chapter will be on the use of an allograft implant to achieve PIPJ arthrodesis in hammertoe correction. This implant's history, concept, and surgical technique will also be discussed in detail. Currently, the only allograft implant specifically designed for hammertoe correction is the TenFUSE™ PIP Allograft (Wright Medical Technology, Arlington, TN).

W. T. DeCarbo (✉)
St. Clair Orthopedic Associates, Pittsburgh, PA, USA

J. D. Thun
Western Orthopedics and Sports Medicine, Grand Junction, CO, USA

E. A. Cook, J. J. Cook (eds.), *Hammertoes*,
https://doi.org/10.1007/978-3-319-16552-3_10

Allograft Use in Hammertoe Correction

PIPJ arthrodesis by means of end-to-end fusion, peg-in-hole arthrodesis, or K-wire fixation has shown fusion rates ranging from 73% to 95% [23–30]. Published literature on the use of allograft for PIPJ arthrodesis is fairly limited. In 2002, Miller [31] reported achieving rigid internal fixation across the PIPJ using a 2.4-mm-diameter pin fashioned out of freeze-dried allogenic cortical bone in 26 toes. After an average of a 15-month follow-up, 25 of 26 toes went on to osseous union. Two of the implants fractured during the bone-healing process; however, only one required revision surgery, while the other continued on to fusion. He also noted that even in toes with a postoperative gap at the arthrodesis site of 1–4 mm, eventual fusion across the joint occurred. He accredits this to the cortical bone allograft pin across the fusion site.

Kominsky and colleagues [32] performed PIPJ arthrodesis on 63 toes in 32 patients by way of allograft implant with a 97% fusion rate and no complications. The average allograft resorption time was observed at 4 months with radiographic signs of fusion occurring at 14 weeks. They concluded that bone matrix allograft provided a suitable alternative fixation method for correction of hammertoe deformity.

Keller and Thun [33] performed a retrospective chart and radiograph review on 21 patients who underwent PIPJ fusion utilizing allogenic implants of the second through fourth digits. A total of 28 toes were included in the study with a mean follow-up of 13.7 months. They observed an 82.2% fusion rate with 5 asymptomatic non-unions identified, none of which required a revision surgery. They concluded that the use of allograft for PIPJ fusion was safe and effective with high patient satisfaction and was comparable to other forms of fixation.

Hofbauer and colleagues [34] performed a similar study on 12 patients including 19 toes using the allogenic implant on digits 2–5. They reported a fusion rate of 84.2% with three asymptomatic non-unions. No revision surgery was required for any of the 19 toes. They concluded that allograft intramedullary implant is comparable to other forms of fixation for hammertoe correction and negates the use of external K-wire fixation.

Overall, PIPJ arthrodesis by means of intramedullary allograft implant has shown fusion rates comparable to that of other forms of fixation.

Allograft Advantages

One significant advantage to utilizing an allograft implant for PIPJ arthrodesis is that it is completely internal and avoids any sort of external K-wire fixation through the postoperative course. A major complaint of patients who undergo hammertoe correction is that of unsightly external pin fixation. Not only does internal fixation increase patient satisfaction; it also avoids potential complications such as pin-tract infections and accidental or premature removal of a K-wire before fusion across the joint is achieved. Although many of the hammertoe implants are entirely internal, failure or painful implants often require removal through a subsequent surgical procedure. Required removal of metallic or other synthetic type implants can cause significant boney deficits and voids that are extremely difficult to revise and manage. The use of an allograft implant all but removes the need for implant removal for any reason. If the implant breaks or fails during the postoperative course, removal is not needed because the implant is an allograft. The few implants that we have seen fracture postoperatively have fully incorporated into the host bone. Although the authors have not encountered the need for revision surgery after using this allograft, a revision surgery would be relatively benign because removal of a previous implant is not necessary and graft incorporation will have likely occurred.

Implant Preparation and Design

When allograft is harvested from its cadaveric donor, it must undergo strict protocols of preparation and sterilization in order to be acceptable for implant into a recipient site. A sterility assurance level or SAL of 10^{-6} must be achieved before implantation. SAL is a term referring to the probability of a non-sterile implant occurring on a microscopic level and describes the microbial population that was destroyed during the sterilization process. For every log reduction (10^{-1}), a 90% reduction in the overall microbial population takes place. Therefore, a SAL of 10^{-6} theoretically provides a one in one million probability of having an unsterile implant. A 10^{-6} SAL is the orthopedic industry sterility standard for implants. SAL for this allograft is achieved by means of a validated gamma irradiation process. During the sterilization process, the bone is partially demineralized to maintain important inductive and conductive properties.

The allograft implant is manufactured using a computer numerically controlled machining technology which allows for dimensional reproducibility and conforming fit within the bone space. The graft is designed to be implanted into the intramedullary canal of both the proximal and medial phalanx of the toe and comes in four different sizes. Available diameters include both a 2.0 mm and a 2.7 mm option (Fig. 10.1). The 2.0-mm-diameter implant is 15 mm in length, while the 2.7-mm-diameter implant is 18 mm. Both size options are available in either a straight or angled construct. The angled allograft has 10 degrees of plantar flexion achieved at the PIPJ level. Proximally, the allograft is tapered to promote ease of insertion by the surgeon. The design includes an octagonal diameter with built-in ridges to resist frontal plane rotation and axial pistoning postoperatively. A built-in depth stop (Fig. 10.2) is located two-thirds of the distance distal on the graft and aids the surgeon in accurate intramedullary placement.

Intraoperative complications are also easily managed with this particular implant and will be discussed in detail later in this chapter.

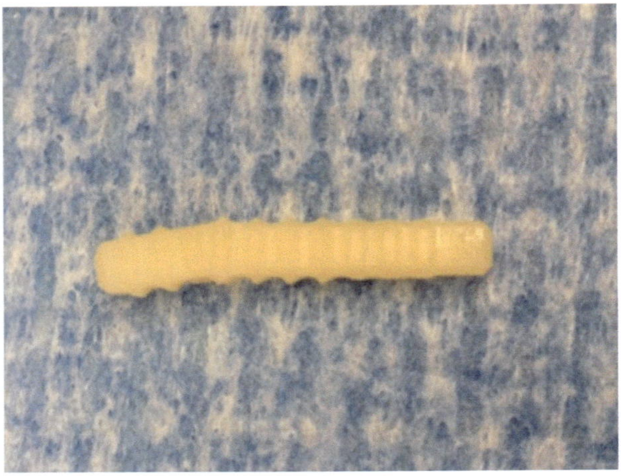

Fig. 10.1 Allograft implant

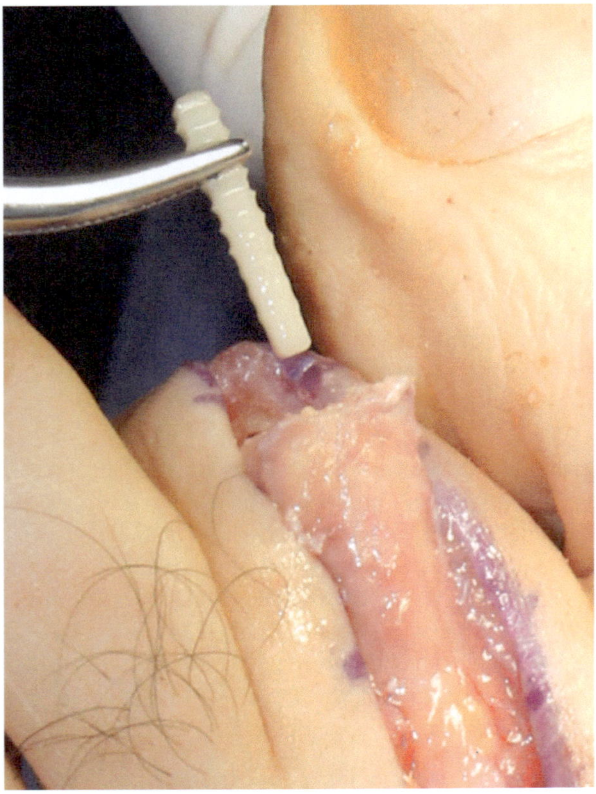

Fig. 10.2 Hemostat holding implant at depth stop for implantation

Surgical Technique and Considerations

Surgical dissection can either be performed through a standard dorsolinear or transverse incision at the level of the PIPJ. A transverse extensor digitorum longus tenotomy at the PIPJ is then achieved exposing the joint capsule. The joint capsule is then entered with a 15 mm blade with transection of the medial and lateral collateral ligaments allowing the head of the proximal phalanx to be delivered dorsally out the incision site. Head resection of the proximal phalanx is then performed either with an oscillating/sagittal saw or manually with a bone cutter or rongeur. Careful consideration must be given to the level at which the head is removed. As more of the phalangeal head is resected, the cortical shell becomes thinner while the medullary canal becomes wider. This can cause the arthrodesis site to be unstable or allow pistoning of the graft within the medullary canal (Fig. 10.3). Aggressive resection may also lead to unwanted shortening of the digit. Attention is then directed toward preparing the base of the middle phalanx. Minimal base resection should be achieved by either manual curettage or oscillating/sagittal saw. The authors recommend that the subchondral plate should be left intact. By doing so, the ribbed construct of the graft tends to achieve a more stable press fit into the medullary canal of the phalanx. Once the joint surfaces have been properly prepared, the next step is to prepare the phalanges for implant. If a 2.0-mm-diameter implant is used, the proximal and middle phalanx should be reamed with a 2.0-mm-wide reamer, while a 2.7 mm implant will first require a 2.0 mm reamer followed by a 2.7 mm reamer. The reamers have two distinct laser lines to aid the surgeon during the reaming process. The proximal phalanx should be reamed to the level of the second laser line, while the middle phalanx should only be reamed to the depth of the first laser line. During this process, the reamer should be 90 degrees to the prepared joint surface and centered down the medullary canal. Improper positioning can lead to a malpositioned toe

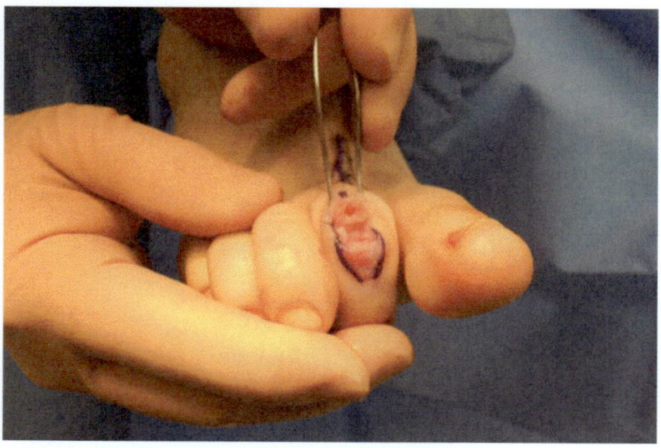

Fig. 10.3 Preparation of proximal medullary canal

after graft implantation. It is the author's experience that reaming with power instrumentation can lead to overaggressive widening of the intramedullary canal, causing unwanted pistoning of the phalanx on the implant both intraoperatively and postoperatively. To avoid this complication, the authors recommend the use of a hand reamer. While hand reaming, greater tactile and surgical control is achieved allowing the surgeon to sense a chatter of the reamer within the canal. Once the desired depth is achieved, immediately remove the reamer to avoid inadvertent over-widening of the intramedullary canal. At this point, the joint is fully prepared for allograft insertion. Using forceps or a hemostat, the graft is gripped just distal to the depth stop. Specialized forceps have been designed specifically for this implant which include a bowed nose tip to reduce weakening of the graft through aggressive squeezing and tightening of the forceps. Insertion of the graft into the proximal phalanx is then performed to the level of the depth stop. Care must be taken to avoid any frontal, transverse, or sagittal plane torque as it may lead to fracture of the phalanx or graft. With the tapered design and ridged construct of the graft, a press fit should be achieved. If the implant is not seeding properly to the level of the depth stop, do not force the implant. Carefully remove the implant, and use the designated hand reamer to slightly widen the hole followed by reinsertion of the graft. At this point, pistoning of the graft within the canal should not be observed. With the forceps remaining in place, the surgeon can then manually reduce the middle phalanx over the distal end of the implant (Fig. 10.4). Do not apply excessive force or torque

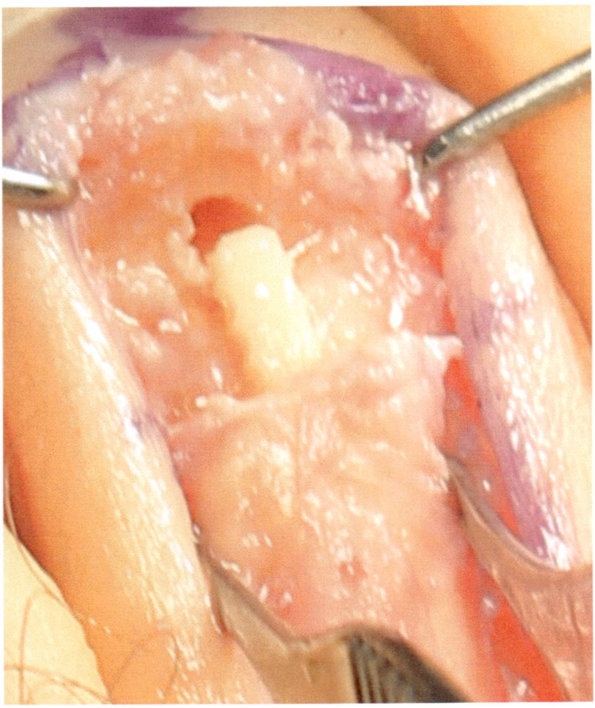

Fig. 10.4 Implant being inserted into middle phalanx

especially in the transverse or sagittal planes when reducing the middle phalanx over the graft as this subjects it to higher likelihood of fracture. Once the middle phalanx is reduced properly, axial compression is performed to achieve the desired press fit. Proper reduction is then observed with intraoperative image intensifier.

Surgical Pearls and Addressing Intraoperative Complications

The authors' allograft dimension choice is a 2.7 mm × 18 mm implant with a 10-degree angle. While the use of a straight versus an angled implant is usually made intraoperatively after observing the specific toe anatomy, we have found that patients are more satisfied postoperatively with a slight anatomical plantar flexion. With a straight implant, patients are more likely to complain that their toe is slightly elevated while weight-bearing and therefore utilize the 10-degree plantar flexed implant to allow toe purchase. The advantage of the 2.7 mm graft diameter is that it takes up more of the medullary canal allowing the ridged outer construct of the implant to grip the cortical edges of the phalanx. The 2.0-mm-diameter seems to be too narrow in larger toes, especially the second and third digits, and does not have required interaction with the cortical surface of the phalanx to achieve a stable construct. On very few occasions, we have noticed a highly porous intramedullary canal with little cancellous bone present. After insertion of a 2.7 mm implant, pistoning was still observed with the graft. In this rare occasion, we have either secured the joint with a K-wire (Fig. 10.5) or removed the graft, morsalized it into bone chips, and reinserted these chips back into the canal. A K-wire was then inserted across the arthrodesis site to stabilize the procedure.

The authors prefer to leave the subchondral plate of the middle phalanx intact when preparing the joint surfaces. By doing so, the ribbed construct of the allograft has better purchase of this hard subchondral bone once reduction has been performed. If the subchondral plate is fully removed, the medullary canal of the middle phalanx is often too wide, and postoperative pistoning occurs at the arthrodesis site. When considering the use of this implant, careful examination of preoperative radiographs should take place. Examine the middle phalanx carefully. Our general observation has shown two shapes of this bone: either short with a square block shape or a long tapered anatomy. The short block type of bone is more prone to complication both intraoperatively and postoperatively. Overaggressive joint resection and removal of the subchondral bone plate will reveal a large intramedullary canal and cause pistoning of the graft. Aggressive resection will also shorten this already small bone leaving little area to receive the graft implant.

Reduction of the middle phalanx over the graft is the most critical portion of the procedure, and the surgeon may encounter some obstacles in doing so. The authors have experienced both difficulties in getting the middle phalanx to reduce over the implant and graft fracture. If the surgeon is having difficulty in reducing the middle phalanx, a few steps can be taken to aid in the process. First, there may be a need for further soft tissue release around the phalanges. Second, the surgeon may resect

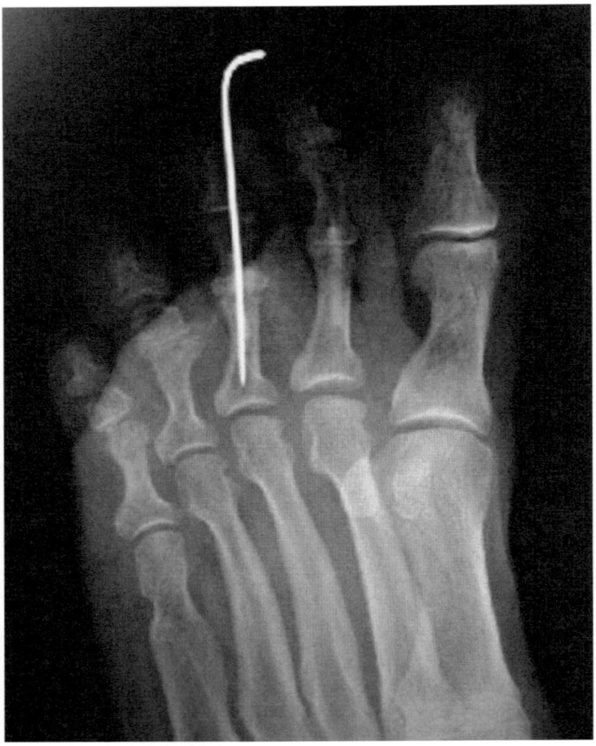

Fig. 10.5 K-wire inserted with implant for increased stability

more bone from the head of the proximal phalanx or base of the middle phalanx. Third, if a Weil osteotomy is to be performed, making this cut may decompress the joint enough to allow reduction. Fourth, we have found that a 10-degree angled implant allows for easier reduction of the middle phalanx over the graft. And finally, because the implant is allograft, a small portion of the distal allograft may be removed to allow the base of the middle phalanx to be reduced over the implant. If the allograft breaks during the process, removal of the implant can be performed with insertion of a new graft. If on occasion the graft cannot be removed from the canal due to the firm press fit, a percutaneous K-wire can be placed across the joint and removed at a later date. If this occurs, the K-wire can be placed through or alongside the graft to achieve digit stabilization. Re-drilling over the graft can also be performed but is technically difficult because the graft is usually denser than the surrounding bone and is therefore easy for the drill to slip and blow out the adjacent cortical shell of the phalanx. While these situations are extremely rare, it is important for the surgeon to be cognizant of its possibility and how to respond if they arise. The advantage of the implant being allograft is that removal is not required if complication arises.

Finally, we encourage the surgeon to take a final intraoperative radiograph once the tourniquet has been deflated. If gapping is observed, apply gentle axial compression at the site to reduce the graft. Extreme care must be taken at this point to not

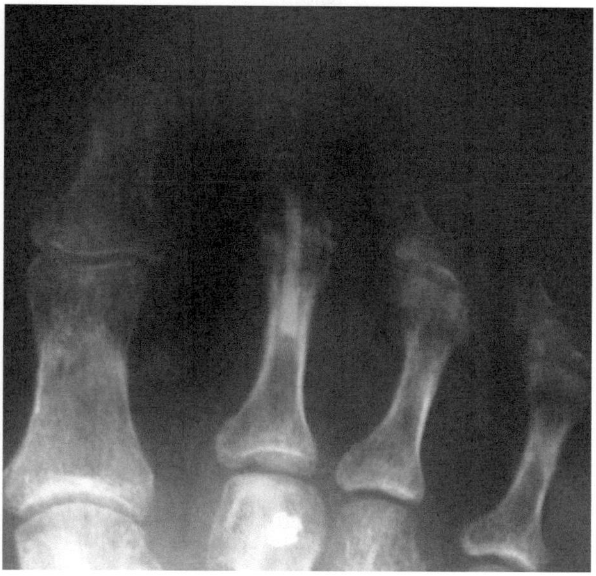

Fig. 10.6 Allograft implant with complete PIPJ fusion

apply transverse or sagittal pressure to the graft. It has been the author's experience that even when slight gapping has been noted in the immediate postoperative course, eventual trabeculation usually occurs across the fusion site as creeping substitution and incorporation of the allograft take place (Fig. 10.6).

Conclusion

Hammertoe correction by means of PIPJ arthrodesis has shown to be effective with fusion rates of 73–95%. The reported use of an intramedullary allograft implant to achieve PIPJ arthrodesis has had similar fusion rates ranging from 84.2% to 97%. The allograft's ease of use, decreased complication rate, and ability to manage potential intraoperative and postoperative complications make it an excellent option for surgical correction of hammertoe deformity.

References

1. Coughlin MJ, Dorris J, Polk E. Operative repair of the fixed hammertoe deformity. Foot Ankle Int. 2000;21:94–104.
2. Yu GV, Vincent AL, Khoury WE, Schinke TL. Techniques of digital arthrodesis: revisiting the old and discovering the new. Clin Podiatr Med Surg. 2004;21:17–50.
3. Coughlin MJ. Lesser toe deformities. Orthopedics. 1987;10:63–75.
4. Mann RA, Coughlin MJ. Lesser toe deformities. Instr Course Lect. 1987;36:137–59.

5. Unsdorfer GL, Unsdorfer KM. Proximal phalangeal osteotomy with proximal interphalangeal joint arthrodesis for multiplanar deformities of the second toe: historical perspectives and review of a case series. J Foot Ankle Surg. 2011;50:687–94.
6. Yu GV, Judge MS, Hudson JR, Seidelmann FE. Predislocation syndrome: progressive subluxation/dislocation of the lesser metatarsophalangeal joint. J Am Podiatr Med Assoc. 2002;92:182–99.
7. Lehman DE, Smith RW. Treatment of symptomatic hammertoe with a proximal interphalangeal joint arthrodesis. Foot Ankle Int. 1995;16:535–41.
8. Scheck M. Etiology of acquired hammertoe deformity. Clin Orthop Relat Res. 1977;(123):63–9.
9. Higgs SL. Hammer Toe. Postgrad Med J. 1931;6:130–2.
10. Lamm BM, Ribeiro CE, Vlahovic TC, Bauer GR, Hillstrom HJ. Peg-in-hole, end-to-end, and V arthrodesis: a comparison of digital stabilization in fresh cadaveric specimens. J Am Podiatr Med Assoc. 2001;91:63–7.
11. Baig A, Geary NPJ. Fusion rate and patient satisfaction in proximal interphalangeal joint fusion of the minor toes using Kirschner wire fixation. Foot. 1996;6:120–1.
12. Trethowan W. The treatment of hammer toe. Lancet. 1925;205:1312.
13. Post A. Hallux valgus with displacement of the smaller toes. Med Rec. 1882;22:120–1.
14. Newman RJ, Fitton JM. An evaluation of operative procedures in the treatment of hammer toe. Acta Orthop Scand. 1979;50(6, pt 1):709–12.
15. DuVries H. Deformities of the proximal phalanx. Chir Record. 1933;16:5–6.
16. McConnell BE. Hammertoe surgery: waist resection of the proximal phalanx, a more simplified procedure. South Med J. 1975;68:595–8.
17. Sgarlato TE. Implants for lesser toes. J Foot Surg. 1983;22:247–50.
18. Cracchiolo A III, Kitaoka HB, Leventen EO. Silicone implant arthroplasty for second metatarsophalangeal joint disorders with and without hallux valgus deformities. Foot Ankle. 1988;9:10–8.
19. Taylor RG. The treatment of claw toes by multiple transfers of flexor into extensor tendons. J Bone Joint Surg Br. 1951;33:539–42.
20. Cahill BR, Connor DE. A long-term follow-up on proximal phalangectomy for hammer toes. Clin Orthop Relat Res. 1972;86:191–2.
21. Sung W, Weil L Jr, Weil LS Sr. Retrospective comparative study of operative repair of hammertoe deformity. Foot Ankle Spec. 2014;7(3):185–92.
22. Reece AT, Stone MH, Young AB. Toe fusion using Kirschner wire: a study of the postoperative infection rate and related problems. J R Coll Surg Edinb. 1987;32:158–9.
23. Shaw AH, Alvarez G. The use of digital implants for the correction of hammertoe deformity and their potential complications and management. J Foot Surg. 1992;31(1):63–7.
24. Roukis T. A 1-piece shape-metal nitinol intramedullary internal fixation device for arthrodesis of the proximal interphalangeal joint in neuropathic patients with diabetes. Foot Ankle Spec. 2009;2(3):130–4.
25. Konkel KF. Hammer toe correction using an absorbable intramedullary pin. Foot Ankle Int. 2007;28(8):916–20.
26. Caterini R, Farsetti P, Tarantino U, Potenza V, Ippolito E. Arthrodesis of the toe joints with an intramedullary cannulated screw for correction of hammertoe deformity. Foot Ankle Int. 2004;25(4):256–61.
27. Pietrzak WS, Lessek TP, Perns SV. A bioabsorbable fixation implant for use in proximal interphalangeal joint (hammer toe) arthrodesis: biomechanical testing in a synthetic bone substrate. J Foot Ankle Surg. 2006;45(5):288–94.
28. Ellington JK, Anderson RB, Davis WH, Cohen BE, Jones CP. Radiographic analysis of proximal interphalangeal joint arthrodesis with an intramedullary fusion device for lesser toe deformities. Foot Ankle Int. 2010;31(5):372–6.
29. Harris W, Mote GA, Malay DS. Fixation of the proximal interphalangeal arthrodesis with the use of an intraosseous loop of stainless-steel wire suture. J Foot Ankle Surg. 2009;48(3):411–4.

30. Witt BL, Hyer CF. Treatment of hammertoe deformity using a one-piece intramedullary device: a case series. J Foot Ankle Surg. 2012;51:450–6.
31. Miller SJ. Hammer toe correction by arthrodesis of the proximal interphalangeal joint using a cortical bone allograft pin. J Am Podiatr Med Assoc. 2002;92:563–9.
32. Kominsky SJ, Bermudez R, Bannerjee A. Using a bone allograft to fixate proximal interphalangeal joint arthrodesis. Foot Ankle Spec. 2013;6(2):132–6.
33. Keller MC, Thun JD. Use of allogenic bone implant in proximal interphalangeal joint arthrodesis: a case series. ACFAS Annual Scientific Conference 2014, Orlando, FL.
34. Hofbauer M, Stasko P, Decarbo W. Digital arthrodesis with use of allograft implant: a retrospective review. ACFAS Annual Scientific Conference 2013, Las Vegas, NV.

Chapter 11
Proximal Interphalangeal Joint (PIPJ) Arthrodesis with a Poly-etheretherketone (PEEK) Implant

Jeremy J. Cook and Emily A. Cook

Material and Implant Overview

Poly-etheretherketone (PEEK) has several properties which make it ideal for an implantable material and particularly in the setting of digital arthrodesis [1–3]. As a physiologically inert material, it doesn't elicit an inflammatory response from the host that would increase the likelihood of nonunion. Since the implant material has a modulus of elasticity very similar to bone, there is minimal stress shielding at the arthrodesis site and again reduces risk factors that would disrupt normal bone healing [2, 3]. Yet another benefit to PEEK as an implantable material is its radiolucency which makes radiographic assessment easier during the postoperative phase. Finally, the fact that PEEK requires no special handling such as refrigeration or heat activation reduces the ancillary costs of this material [1–3].

From a design perspective, the implant discussed in the subsequent case has several unique qualities. The implant is buried and therefore doesn't suffer from the exposure issues that a traditional Kirschner wire suffers from. Moreover, since the implant specifically targets the PIPJ, there is no damage or overcorrection to the DIPJ that other implants suffer via implantation. The design is press fit that yields a very stable compression at the arthrodesis site. Two-part implants are helpful as they impart greater flexibility to size each piece to the individual segment of bone.

J. J. Cook (✉) · E. A. Cook
Harvard Medical School, Division of Podiatry,
Department of Surgery, Mount Auburn Hospital, Cambridge, MA, USA
e-mail: jeremycook@post.harvard.edu

E. A. Cook, J. J. Cook (eds.), *Hammertoes*,
https://doi.org/10.1007/978-3-319-16552-3_11

Presentation/History

Case 1: A 59-year-old female presents with metatarsalgia, hallux valgus, and painful hammertoe deformity. All issues have been present for several years, and she has been conservatively managed with treatments ranging from orthotics to injections. She reports that the hammertoe and metatarsalgia symptoms appeared first. Over time, the hallux valgus deformity becomes more prominent, and the second toe became more contracted and started to cross over the hallux.

Clinical and radiographic evaluations prompt surgical intervention in the form of Kalish bunionectomy, second metatarsal distal wedge osteotomy, plantar plate reconstruction, and hammertoe correction with a PIP fusion (Fig. 11.1).

Diagnosis/Assessment

Clinical and weight-bearing radiographic assessment should be correlated with symptoms. The decision to proceed with arthrodesis is largely based on reducibility of the deformity, the need for long-term stability, and possibly evidence of arthritic changes. The presence of neurologic dysfunction and connective tissue disorders are also important considerations but are beyond the scope of this chapter. Permanent implant arthrodesis should be avoided in the setting of infection.

Surgical Technique

Over the past decade, we have employed a variety of fixation methods for arthrodesis of a PIPJ. In all instances, we have relied on intramedullary fixation covering a spectrum of materials and designs. The focus here is the PIP fusion implant (Smith

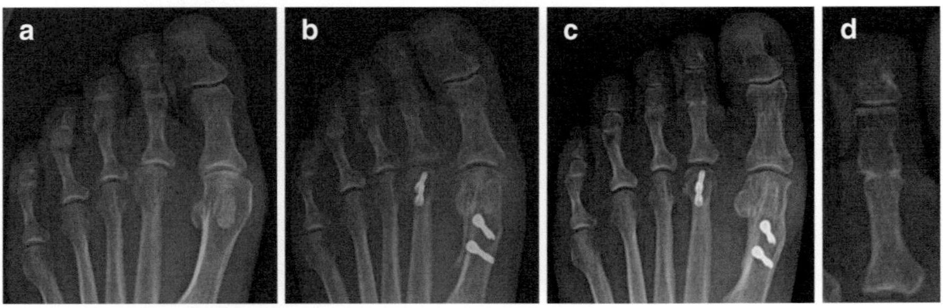

Fig. 11.1 Anterior-posterior weight-bearing radiographs of the patient. (**a**) Preoperatively with evidence of plantar plate compromise with hammertoe and hallux valgus deformity. (**b**) 8 weeks following Kalish osteotomy, second metatarsal distal wedge osteotomy, plantar plate reconstruction, and PIP fusion is doing well showing excellent healing of the hammertoe site. (**c**) 6 months postoperatively with complete healing and no indication of recurrence of the second ray deformity. (**d**) Magnifed view of fusion site 6 months postoperatively

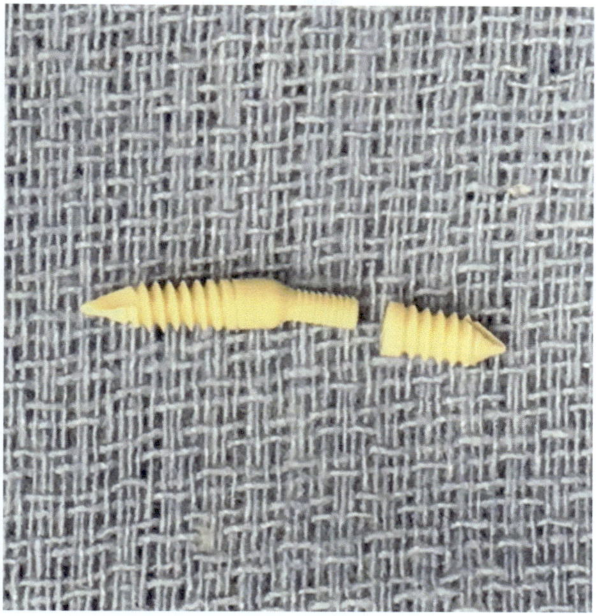

Fig. 11.2 PIP fusion implant (Smith and Nephew Orthopedics)

and Nephew Orthopedics) (Fig. 11.2). As discussed above, it is a two-component design made of poly-etheretherketone. The overall arthrodesis procedure is largely the same regardless of fixation preference. The greatest change relates to the implant insertion technique specifically. Depending on the concomitant procedures, we rely on either a linear or transverse converging semielliptical incision. Dissection passes through ligamentous and tendinous structures at the level of the proximal interphalangeal joint. The capsule is incised to access the joint, and then the collateral ligaments are reflected both medially and laterally along the head of the proximal phalanx. With the proximal phalanx head exposed, we may proceed with joint preparation. The orientation of the ostectomy of the proximal phalanx head is traditionally oriented neutral within all three cardinal planes. The PIP fusion implant comes in two sagittal plane options: 0° or 10° of plantar flexion. Selection of the most appropriate configuration is based on surgeon preference. In our experience, the 10° implant is used most frequently to ensure a more natural digital purchase. In this case, the ostectomy cut is made ~10° off the frontal plane which optimizes fixation and bone-to-bone contact specific to this implant design. Resection is performed traditionally at the metaphyseal-diaphyseal junction using a bone cutter or power instrumentation based on surgeon preference. Regardless of which type of intramedullary implant used, we always assess if this ostectomy location is ideal. In some cases, the flare of the proximal phalanx metaphyseal-diaphyseal junction is so wide that many intramedullary implants, which are designed to rely on cortical purchase, are instead forced to rely on cancellous bone which is less stable. The PIP fusion implant is less vulnerable to this issue because its threads engage the cancellous bone as well. A slightly more proximal cut will ensure that the implant engages with more of the internal cortical bone of the isthmus of the proximal phalanx. Next the cartilage of the base of the intermediate phalanx is removed; we prefer to contour the margins of the bone so that the final configuration is flat and contacts the proximal phalanx evenly. Irrigation is performed prior to implantation.

Implantation proceeds with first inserting the included 1.6 mm drill into the medullary canal of the proximal phalanx passing parallel to the longitudinal axis to the depth of the laser line. Next repeat the process in the intermediate phalanx. See clinical pearls for additional considerations related to optimal drill placement.

Next the appropriate IP tap is inserted and is buried to the laser line. Going beyond that point increases the risk of penetrating into the DIPJ. Attention is directed to the PP where tapping starts with the 2.7 mm tap, again buried to the laser line (Fig. 11.3). Based on the bite of the tap, the decision is either made to use the 2.7 mm PP implant or to thread with the 3.2 mm tap. Ultimately tapping should proceed in a sequential approach, gradually increasing size until the correct fit is achieved. Nonsequential tapping increases the risk of a stress riser particularly in osteoporotic bone. Our most common implant selection is a 4 mm IP with 2.7 mm PP implant with 10° of plantar flexion. Proceed next with implantation within each segment, inspecting each side for stress risers and stable implant seating (Fig. 11.4). Finally press fit the two components together until they are

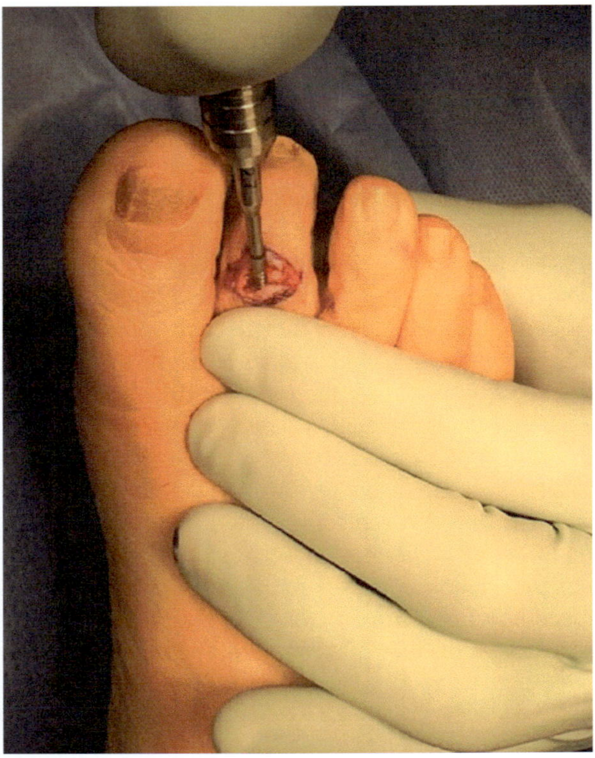

Fig. 11.3 Insertion of the proximal phalanx tap. The tap is inserted flush to the laser line and should be done in a sequential manner from the smallest tap to the desired tap size to ensure the best outcome

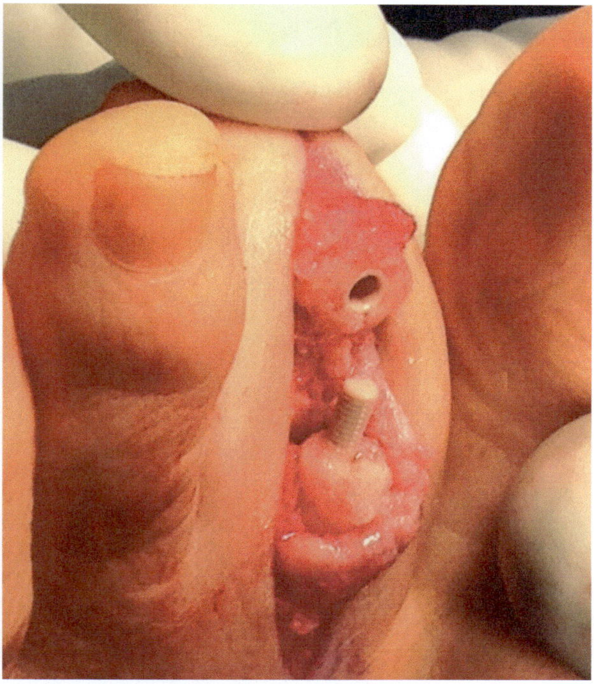

Fig. 11.4 Intraoperative image demonstrating that both components have been inserted in the appropriate position

flush, thus reducing the fusion site (Fig. 11.5). Proceed with deep and skin closure based on individual surgeon preference.

As detailed in other portions of this book, it is important to consider the biomechanics of the entire ray in selecting this treatment. In order to optimize outcomes, it is often necessary to perform concomitant realignment osteotomies and/or soft tissue rebalancing [4].

Outcomes

The benefits of PIPJ arthrodesis over arthroplasty are well known, with stable construct, superior propulsion, and enhanced digital purchase chief among them. With complication rates associated with K-wire fixated PIPJ arthrodeses between 16% and 31% [5, 6], more robust fixation devices such as PEEK implants have become ubiquitous. Current publications fail to delineate the successful outcomes of a two-component PEEK implant, but our own data is being reviewed at the time of this publication and will be presented in the near future. Although a stable pseudoarthrodesis is acceptable, complete osseous union is desirable. In our experience this technology has significantly enhanced our ability to optimize care.

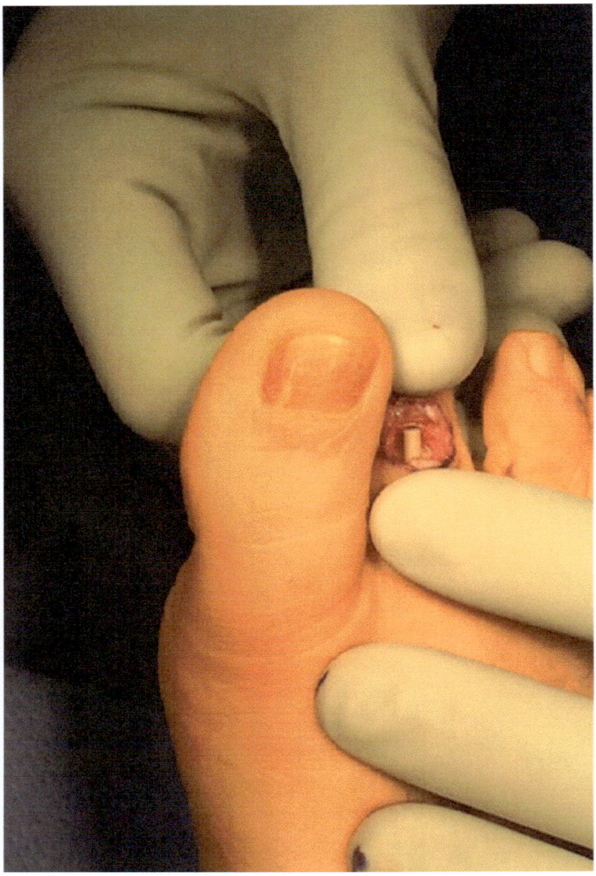

Fig. 11.5 Small ridges on the implant surface enable a press-fit design that will provide the necessary intraosseous stabilization

Clinical Pearls/Pitfalls

- Our preference is to raise a 2 mm subperiosteal flap along the dorsal aspect of the intermediate phalanx which will facilitate more robust suture closure that provides resistance against frontal plane rotation and acts as an additional point of fixation.
- Placement of the drill prior to tapping of the intermediate phalanx is important. Because of the differential height of the intermediate and proximal phalanx if the drill and implant are placed centrally in the sagittal plane, a dorsal step-off will become evident at the dorsal intermediate phalanx. Instead, if the intermediate phalangeal implant is placed ~2 mm above the center point, the dorsal cortical margins should be flush. The danger to this approach is that this places greater stress on the IP dorsal cortex and increases the risk of stress riser if the tap is inserted in a non-orthogonal manner. In patients with osteoporotic bone, we believe that the dorsal step-off is

acceptable in order to prioritize stable fusion. This issue is present with any two-component system for digital fusion.
- In the chronic setting, we frequently combine this with a MTPJ reconstruction and possible metatarsal osteotomy as well as addressing other deformities such as the first ray. This approach considers the entire mechanics of the ray which should limit recurrence and optimize outcomes.

References

1. Ramakrishna S, Mayer J, Wintermantel E, Leong KW. Biomedical applications of polymer-composite materials: a review. Compos Sci Technol. 2001;61(9):1189–224.
2. Kurtz SM, Devine JN. PEEK biomaterials in trauma, orthopedic, and spinal implants. Biomaterials. 2007;28:4845–69. https://doi.org/10.1016/j.biomaterials.2007.07.013.
3. Panayotov IV, Orti V, Cuisinier F, et al. Polyetheretherketone (PEEK) for medical applications. J Mater Sci Mater Med. 2016;27:118. https://doi.org/10.1007/s10856-016-5731-4.
4. Edwards WH, Beischer AD. Interphalangeal joint arthrodesis of the lesser toes. Foot Ankle Clin. 2002;7(1):43–8.
5. O'Kane C, Kilmartin T. Review of proximal interphalangeal joint excisional arthroplasty for the correction of second hammer toe deformity in 100 cases. Foot Ankle Int. 2005;26(4):320–5.
6. Kramer WC, Parman M, Marks RM. Hammertoe correction with K-wire fixation. Foot Ankle Int. 2015;36(5):494–502.

Chapter 12
PIPJ Arthrodesis with a Bioabsorbable Implant

Luke D. Cicchinelli

Presentation/History

Digital deformities are likely the single most common chief complaint of patients presenting to a foot and ankle specialists' office. The reasons for pain vary from drifting of the toes in all planes that cause painful callouses interdigitally to distal tip of toe corns and dorsal corns on the proximal or distal interphalangeal joints that are further irritated by closed shoe gear. In the failure of conservative and palliative measures, the goal of surgical intervention is a reliable lasting correction of the digital deformity at the apex or focal point of the deformity that eliminates any painful skin lesions and always a comfortable variety of closed shoe gear.

The purpose of this article is not an exhaustive review of the available techniques and science behind hammertoe/claw toe surgery nor a review of the existing literature on the topic. This already exists and is easily researchable. Specific to the use of 2.0 mm poly-L-lactic acid absorbable pin in hammertoe surgery, Konkel et al. published an excellent review of their clinical experience and their pertinent clinical and radiographic observations and results in Foot and Ankle International October 2011 [1]. Rather the author will in this article discuss his clinical approach to these so frequent digital deformities and the practical technique points that lead to reliable results. The Trim-it Drill pin has been and remains a mainstay of the author's approach to surgical correction of all levels of digital contractions since the first pin was implanted in November 2005. For appropriate complete disclosure and transparency, the author is the codeveloper of this device in conjunction with Arthrex, Inc. (Naples, Florida) and Dr. Gerard Bourke of Melbourne, Australia.

L. D. Cicchinelli (✉)
Private Practice, Centro Clinico Quirurgico, Vigo, Spain
e-mail: luke@cicchinelli.com

E. A. Cook, J. J. Cook (eds.), *Hammertoes*,
https://doi.org/10.1007/978-3-319-16552-3_12

Diagnosis/Assessment

A thorough preoperative assessment of the actual deformity to be managed is critical. It is still surprising to the author how many clinicians do not carefully evaluate the patient standing in the clinic. Every patient considering corrective surgery for a digital deformity must be evaluated carefully both seated and standing in the clinic. Frequently the nature of the reducibility of the deformity; its true deviation in the sagittal, coronal, or transverse plane; and the patient's actual chief complaint to be addressed are only ascertainable by a careful standing exam. The goal of the seated exam is primarily to assess whether the deformity is a fixed rigid deformity or passively reducible at the three pertinent articular levels. These levels are the distal interphalangeal joint, the proximal interphalangeal joint, and the metatarsophalangeal joint. In order to determine this effectively, the toes must be examined with the foot plantarflexed as well as dorsiflexed at the ankle level. A hammertoe that is passively reducible with the foot plantarflexed but not so with the foot dorsiflexed signifies the primary deforming or limiting anatomic structure as the long flexor tendon, flexor digitorum longus. This patient may benefit from a simple flexor tenotomy with no osseous work. If the hammertoe is not reduceable with the foot plantarflexed or dorsiflexed, this toe will require osseous work at some level for effective and lasting correction. The standing evaluation affords an opportunity to assess any contracture of hyperextension at the metatarsophalangeal joint level due to retrograde ground reactive force of full weightbearing on a contracted digit. Equally important is that it is only with the standing weightbearing exam that we can fully assess exactly where the chief complaint arises from, whether there are interdigital complaints as well and exactly how adjacent or multiple digits contribute to or do not to the overall symptom complex (Figs. 12.1 and 12.2).

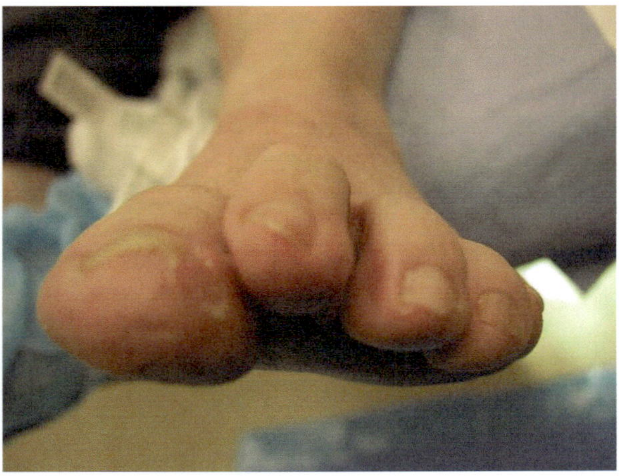

Fig. 12.1 Non-weightbearing view of a hammertoe deformity. This should also be evaluated in stance to appreciate fully the true deformity in all planes

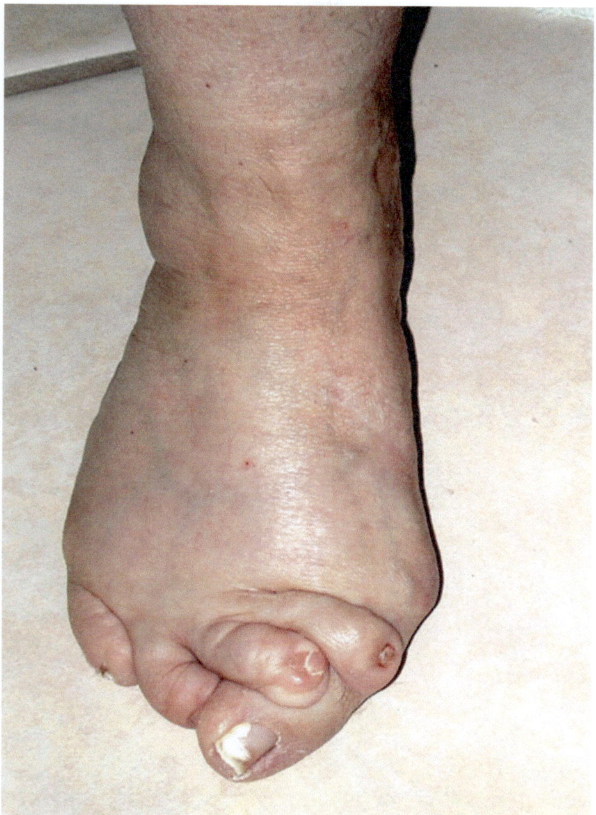

Fig. 12.2 Hammertoe deformity and transverse plane deviation of lesser toes

With a simple concise yet thorough exam, completed considerations of procedural selection may be undertaken. Specific to the use of the absorbable Trim-it Drill pin, again the motive of this requested article, the levels of correction to be entertained are the three articulations, the distal and proximal interphalangeal joints and the metatarsophalangeal joints. The surgical options for correction that involve absorbable pin stabilization are resection arthroplasty of either the distal or proximal phalangeal head with pinning or interphalangeal fusion of the proximal interphalangeal joint of stabilization with pinning of the distal interphalangeal joint. Additionally many surgeons consider stabilization across the metatarsophalangeal joint as well which brings special considerations in the use of an absorbable pin versus a metallic pin which will be discussed.

The Trim-it Drill pin device itself is available in sizes 1.5 mm and 2.0 mm and comes with a smooth metal predrill pin that is slightly undersized to the absorbable pin, and the 2.0 mm pin comes with a metal tip on one end and a tapered opposite end (Fig. 12.3) [2]. Both sizes come with a cannula and plunger system for effective and accurate countersinking of the absorbable pin at any place of insertion. The biomaterial is poly-L-lactate and is well tolerated in multiple locations and indica-

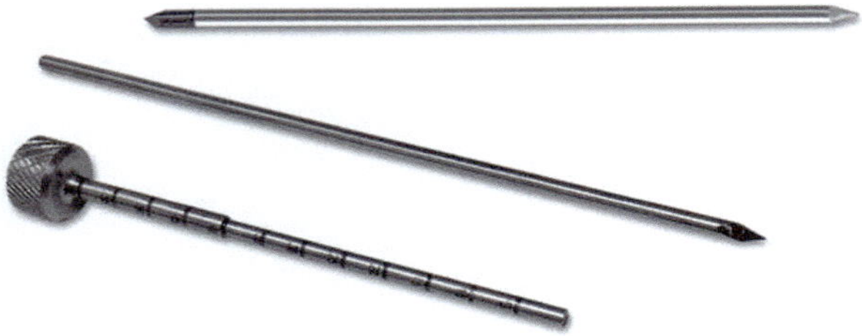

Fig. 12.3 The 2.0 mm polylactic acid pin, metal predrill pin, and tamp

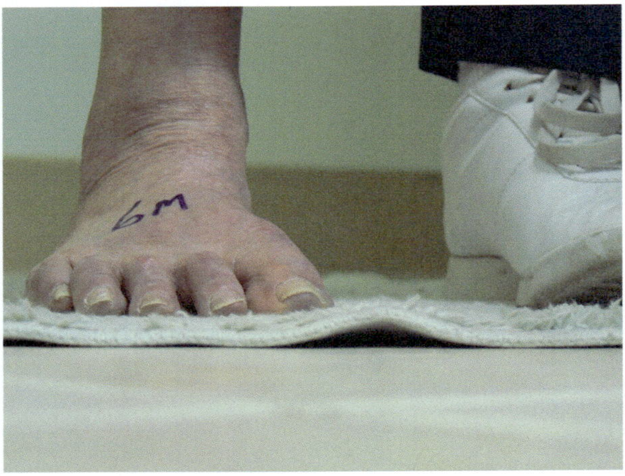

Fig. 12.4 A 6-month clinical photo of "flexed fusions" of the all lesser toes

tions in the entire body since its first use in absorbable screws in the late 1980s in Finland. The degradation process begins approximately 6 months post implantation and proceeds via hydrolysis and nonspecific enzymatic activity. The Konkel paper showed a gradual decrease in bone marrow edema on follow-up MRI between 10 and 19 months postoperatively, and by 34 months postoperatively, there was no residual bone marrow edema identified. The pin was conceived and designed to allow the exact implantation technique and instrumentation of a standard Kirschner wire yet make unnecessary the need for removal or externally protruding fixation in hammertoe surgery. The mechanical characteristics of the Trim-it Drill pin were designed to allow a memory or retention of an adjusted or molded position of the pin that facilitates the surgeon's ability to position the toe in any desired angle of correction prior to the placement of the initial surgical dressing. The most frequent application of this by the author is the achievement of a "flexed toe fusion" of approximately 15 degrees downward which simulates the resting flexion tension in the digits of the hand and affords a more functional and aesthetic result for patients undergoing hammertoe surgical correction (Figs. 12.4 and 12.5). In essence it allows a convenient and easy discouragement toward the not infrequent complaint of patients that postoperatively their toe is "too straight." This is particularly problematic for women in shoes with a heel that necessitate the equal amount of extension at the metatarsophalangeal joint as the amount of ankle flexion.

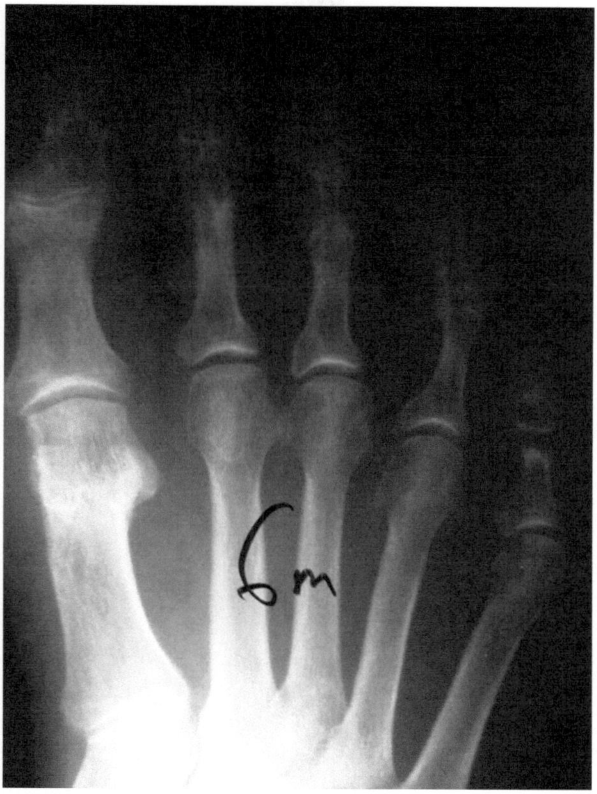

Fig. 12.5 The X-ray of Fig. 12.4 showing excellent osseous consolidation at the PIP joints

Treatment/Surgical Technique

The applications of the Trim-it Drill pin at each level of digital deformity will now be discussed starting distally. The true mallet toe contracture of a flexion deformity at the distal interphalangeal joint is readily corrected by a middle phalangeal head resection arthroplasty with or without a flexor tendon tenotomy. The correct use of the Trim-it Drill pin to stabilize this arthroplasty should the surgeon desire is to use the 1.5 mm pin metal predrill pin and create a pilot hole in the shaft of the middle phalanx and the distal phalanx. The absorbable pin is then drilled into the middle phalanx maximizing the length of the middle phalanx canal and cut to the appropriate length of the distal phalanx, and the distal phalanx is then "placed" over the pin affecting an "all-inside" technique. Alternatively the pin may be drilled out the pulp of the toe, retrograded out an additional 5–8 mm, cut flush at the skin level, and then tamped back into the distal phalanx with the cannula and plunger system.

Proximal interphalangeal joint contractures as in true hammertoe or claw toe deformities are ideally corrected with either phalangeal head resection arthroplasty and pin stabilization or interphalangeal fusion with pin stabilization. If the surgeon prefers a “soft” fusion or resection arthroplasty approach, the recommendation is to use the 2.0 mm pin in the toes 2 and usually 3 and most commonly the 1.5 mm pin in toes 4 and/or 5. The implantation technique options are the same as in the above description for the mallet toe correction. The recommended technique for a proximal interphalangeal joint fusion is either the “all-inside” technique or the use of the modified Trim-it Drill pin named the spin pin. The dissection and osseous resection of the head of the proximal phalanx and the base of the middle phalanx are per the surgeon’s preference. The “all-inside” technique is carried out by first creating pilot holes with the metallic predrill pin in the proximal phalanx and the middle phalanx. The predrill pin should be drilled to the base of the proximal phalanx, and the middle phalanx should be depth gauged using the laser mark measurement lines on the predrill pin. The maximal length of the absorbable pin may now be drilled into the medullary canal of the proximal phalanx. The pin is then cut sharply and obliquely to leave a point on the tip and the appropriate amount of pin extruding from the proximal phalanx based on the depth gauging length of the middle phalanx. The middle phalanx is then placed over the pin, and the joint is compressed closed. The soft tissues are closed per surgeon routine (Figs. 12.6, 12.7, 12.8, 12.9, 12.10, 12.11, and 12.12).

The modified Trim-it Drill pin called the spin pin has a fatigue mark or break away point designed into the pin that allows for exact sizing of every toe length based on appropriate depth gauging with the laser marked metal tip of the pin. This effectively allows for proximal interphalangeal joint fusion in each toe without any material traversing the distal interphalangeal joint. It is typically paired with a percutaneous flexor tenotomy to discourage late mallet toe contracture after a successful proximal interphalangeal joint fusion (Figs. 12.13, 12.14, 12.15, 12.16, 12.17, 12.18, 12.19, 12.20, 12.21, and 12.22).

In those cases where proximal interphalangeal joint fusion is desired and distal interphalangeal joint stabilization is sought as well, the Trim-it Drill pin may be drilled antegradely out the tip of the toe and then retrograded back into the base of

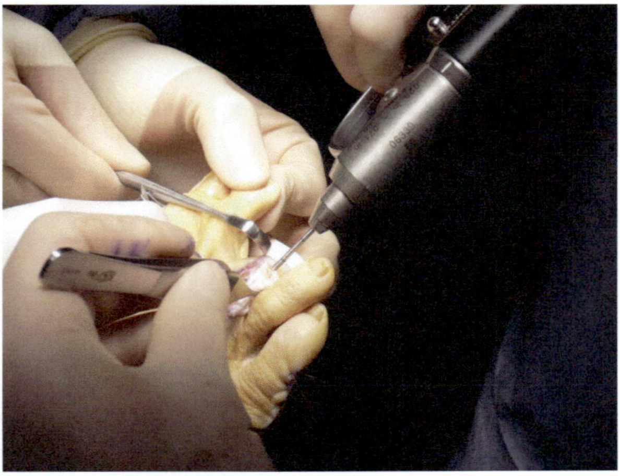

Fig. 12.6 Performing the pilot hole in the canal of the proximal phalanx with the metal drill pin

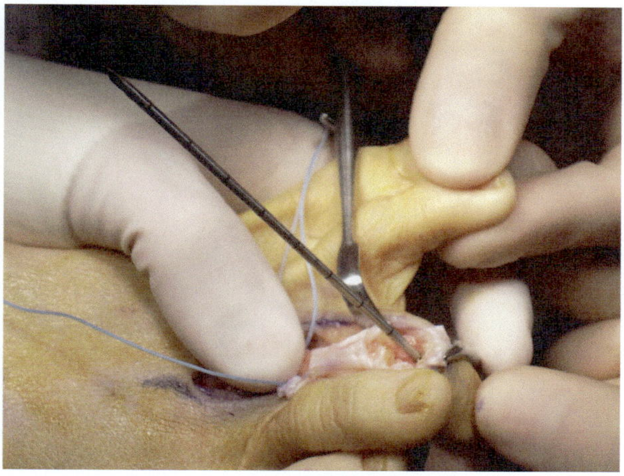

Fig. 12.7 Depth gauging and drilling of the pilot hole in the middle phalanx

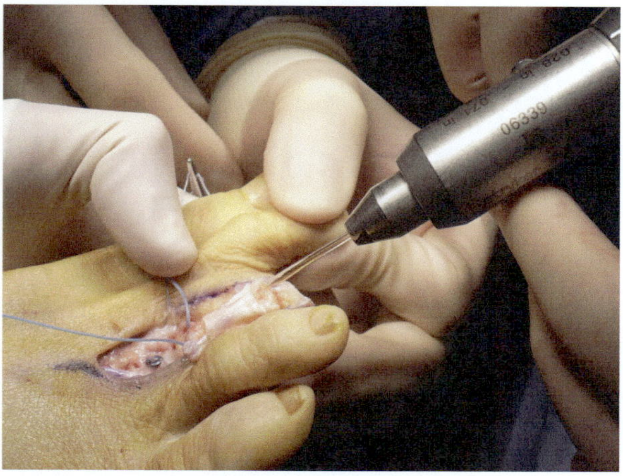

Fig. 12.8 Insertion of the 2.0 mm polylactic acid pin in the proximal phalanx

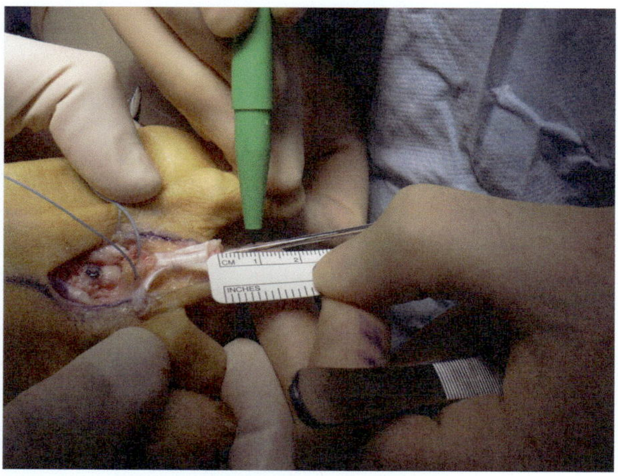

Fig. 12.9 Measuring of the correct length of absorbable pin to be implanted in the middle phalanx

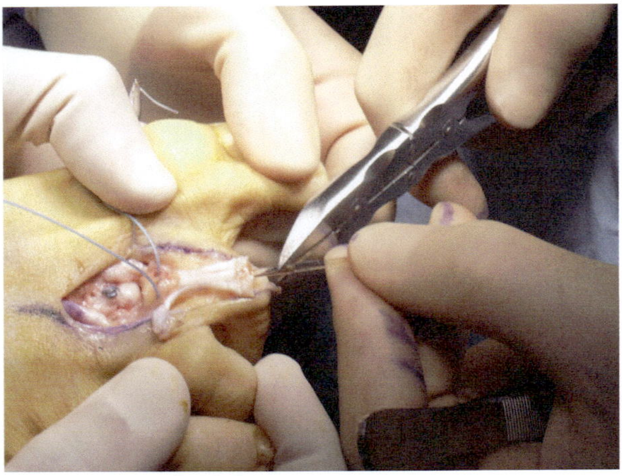

Fig. 12.10 The oblique trimming of the absorbable pin at the PIP joint

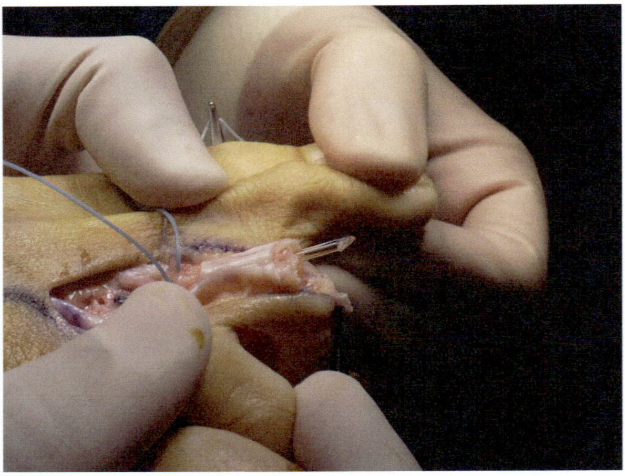

Fig. 12.11 The pin is prepared for engagement in the canal of the middle phalanx

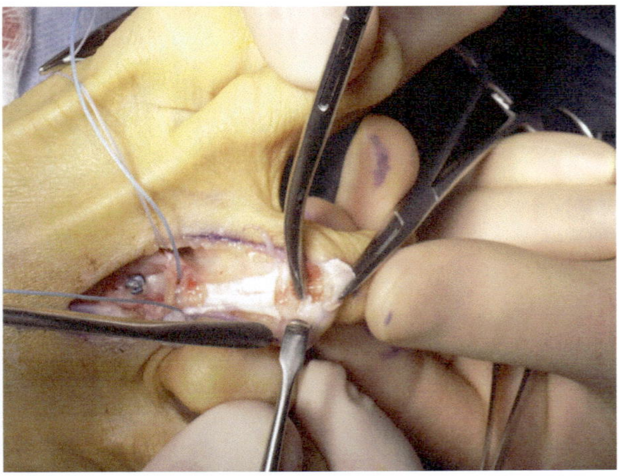

Fig. 12.12 The pin is bent slightly with a hemostat, and the middle phalanx is seated onto the pin

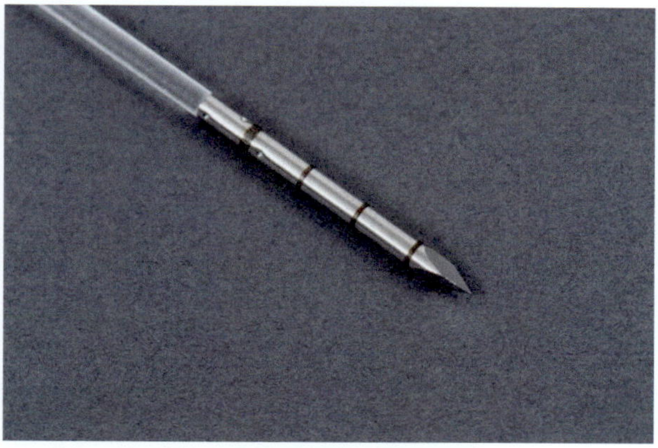

Fig. 12.13 Picture of the spin pin with the laser mark depth measurements

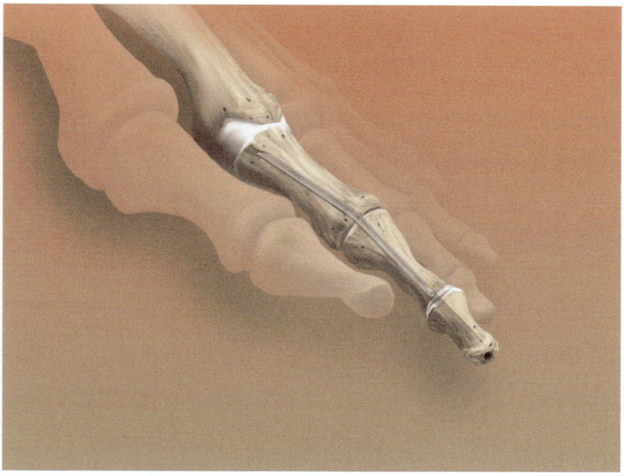

Fig. 12.14 Schematic of the spin pin measured exactly to the length of the proximal and middle phalanx

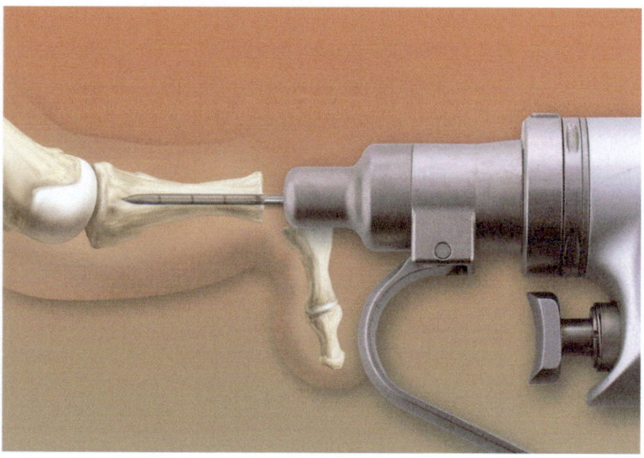

Fig. 12.15 The depth gauging of the proximal phalanx with the spin pin

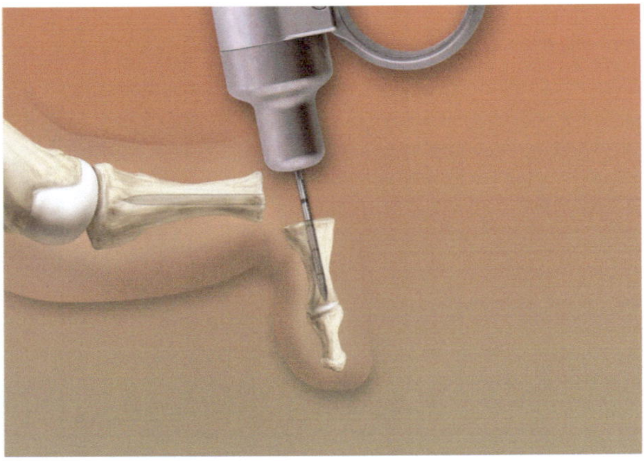

Fig. 12.16 The depth gauging of the middle phalanx with the spin pin

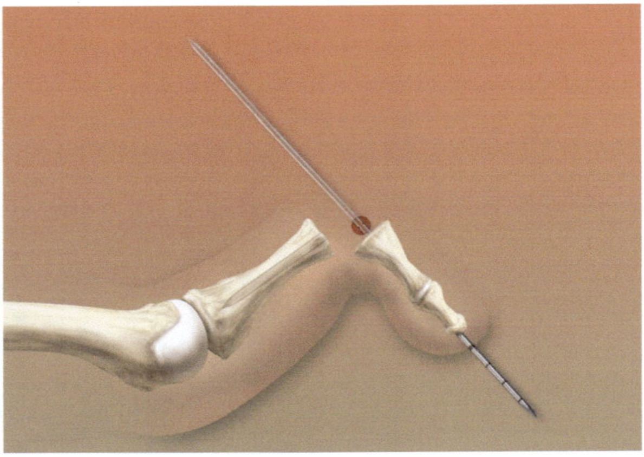

Fig. 12.17 The spin pin is advanced distally out the tip of the toe stopping when the breakaway fatigue mark is flushed with the base of the middle phalanx

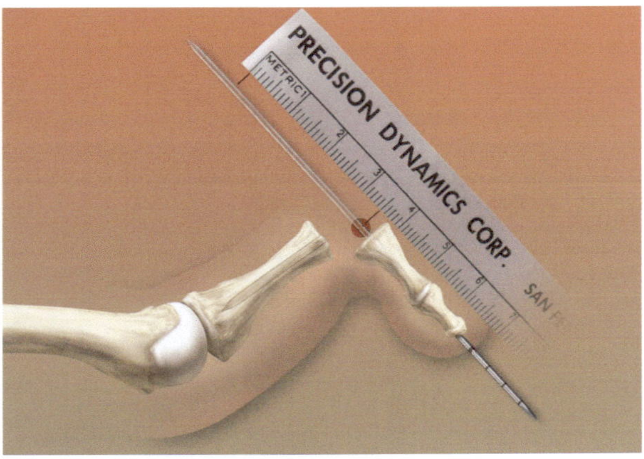

Fig. 12.18 The measurement of the pin to be implanted that equals the length of the proximal and middle phalanges

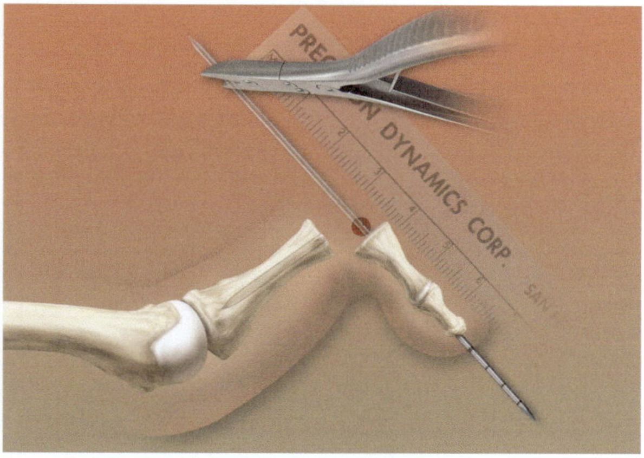

Fig. 12.19 The pin is snipped at the appropriate length

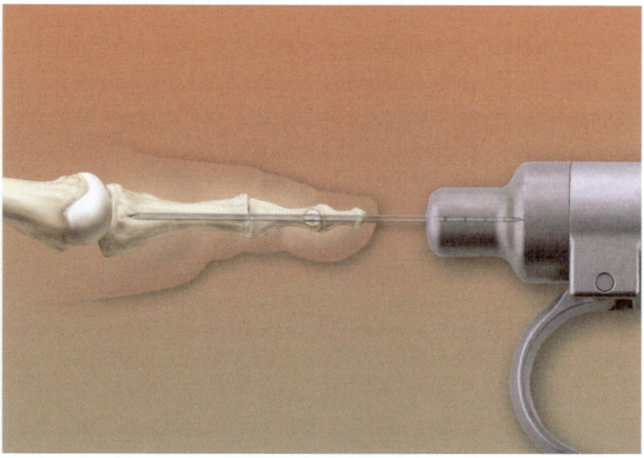

Fig. 12.20 The entire measured pin is now seated in the toe

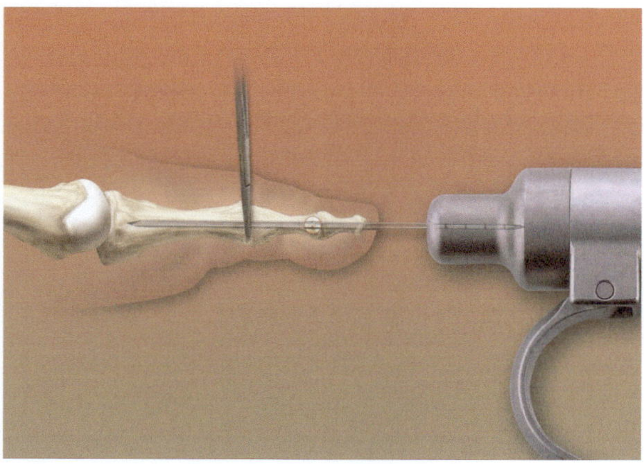

Fig. 12.21 A hemostat is used to grasp and immobilize the spin pin

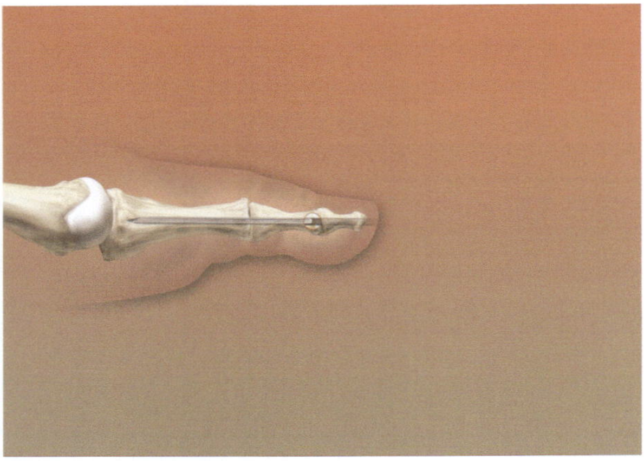

Fig. 12.22 The K-wire driver is then engaged and the pin "spins" off at the fatigue mark leaving the perfectly measured length of the proximal and middle phalanges implanted

the proximal phalanx. The procedure sequence is to predrill the canal of the proximal phalanx and middle and distal phalanges with the metallic predrill pin and then starting at the proximal interphalangeal joint drill out the tip of the toe. The absorbable pin is then retrogradely drilled to the base of the proximal phalanx, backed out 5–8 mm, and then cut flush with the skin and tamped back into so that all pin resides within the bone of the distal phalanx.

The last potential application of the Trim-it Drill pin is for stabilization of the metatarsophalangeal joint in those cases where extension deformity exists at this anatomic level in spite of complete hammertoe/claw toe reduction and pinning. The author routinely uses the 2.0 Trim-it Drill pin full length (100 mm) for digital stabilization in conjunction with panmetatarsal head resections and as an alternative to metallic Kirschner wire fixation with excellent and lasting results (Figs. 12.23, 12.24, 12.25, 12.26, and 12.27). In those cases where metatarsophalangeal stabilization is desired but the articular condition is healthy, the indications are less clear. In those cases of a dysfunctional MTP joint such as a subluxed proximal phalangeal base or substantial articular damage to the metatarsal head, the preference is for a 1.5 mm Trim-it Drill pin that traverses the joint and which will likely fatigue break or absorb in the first 18 months postoperatively while maintaining stable clinical correction in the sagittal plane. The 1.5 mm Trim it pin may also be considered for additional MTP joint stabilization in any case that involves a partial metatarsal head resection. Considerations for correction of transverse plane deformities such as medial or lateral drifting of toes or crossover toe are beyond the scope of this article.

In all the above clinical applications of the Trim-it Drill pin, the soft tissue closure is per surgeon preference. Prior to the placement of the initial intraoperative surgical dressing, the knee is bent on the operating room table, and the foot is loaded to simulate weightbearing. The final toe position is then adjusted via manipulation/bending of the toe to achieve the aforementioned flexed fusion that is more

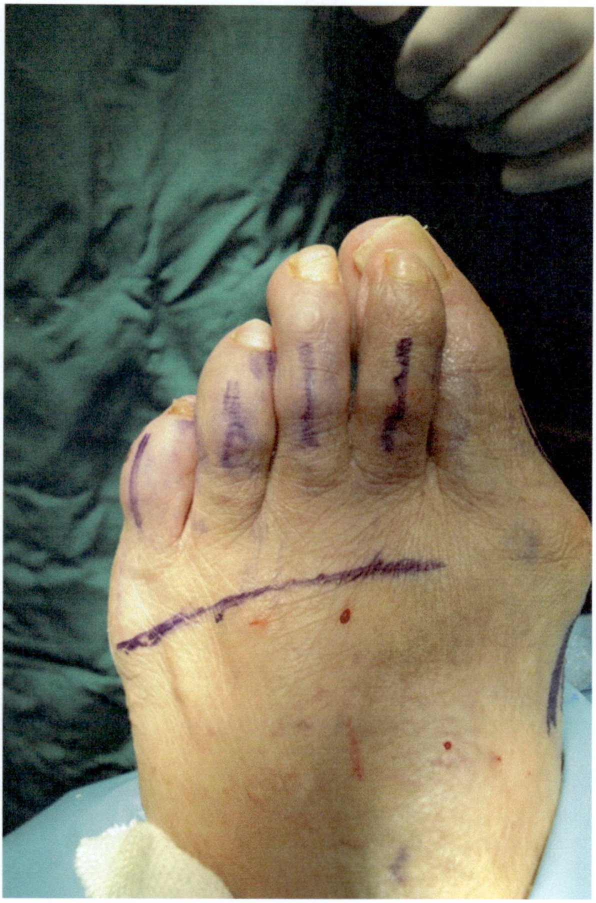

Fig. 12.23 Preoperative view of a case of panmetatarsal head resection

functional and aesthetic than a rigidly fused excessively straight toe. The final toe position may also be adjusted mildly in the transverse plane depending on the desired alignment with the adjacent toes. The clear advantage of the Trim-it Drill pin is that no pin is exiting the tip of the toe which allows a faster return to bathing and closed shoe gear. The author's preference is to change the surgical dressing at 1 week postoperatively and, if the incisions are stable, allow shower bathing and a return to closed shoe gear between 2 and 3 weeks postoperatively. In contrast to protruding metallic pins, this rapid return to closed shoe gear also reduces the amount of postoperative edema in the toes. The prolonged use of stable yet non-compressive surgical shoes and boots that is so common with protruding external Kirschner wire fixation of the toes post hammertoes allows the expected postoperative digital edema to persist longer than necessary.

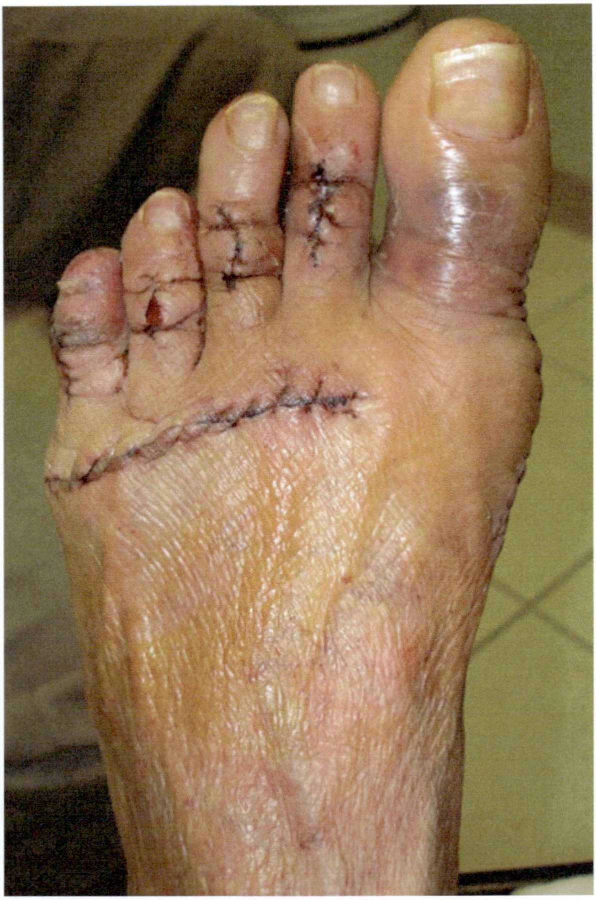

Fig. 12.24 One-week postoperative view of the patient in Fig. 12.23

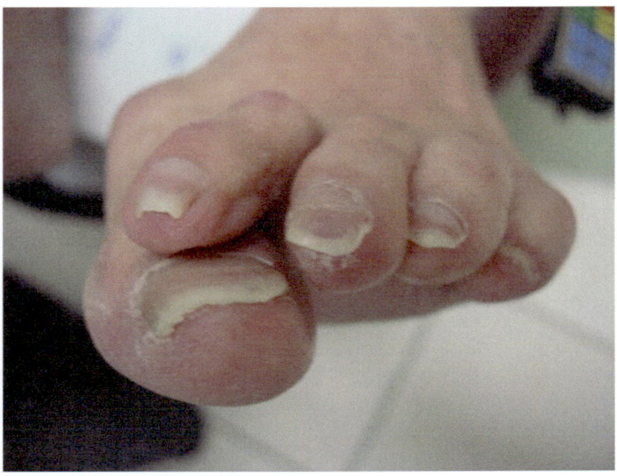

Fig. 12.25 Alternative view of the same patient preoperatively in Fig. 12.23

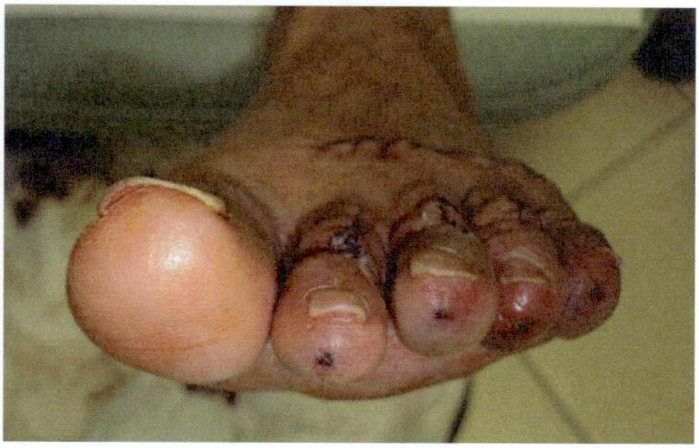

Fig. 12.26 The 1-week postoperative view of the patient in Fig. 12.23

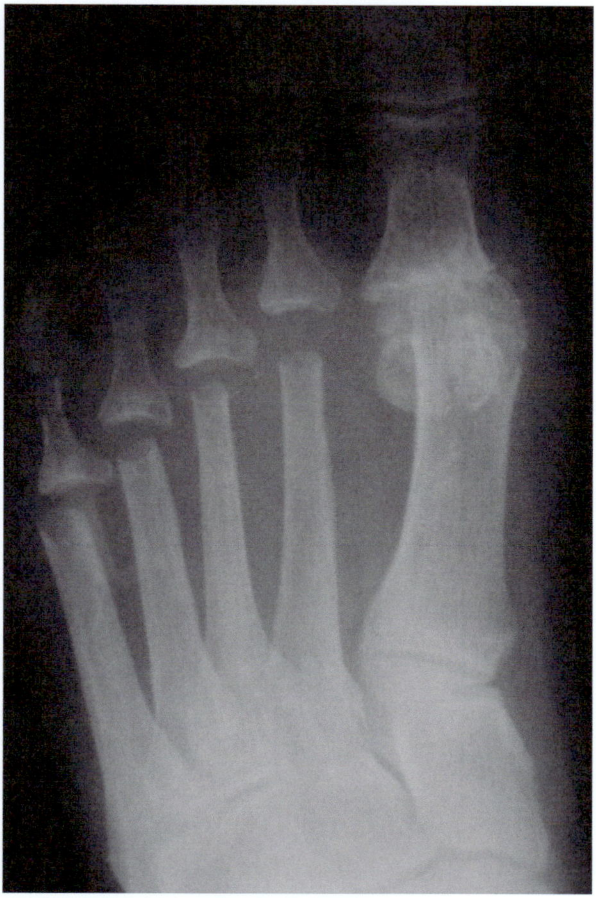

Fig. 12.27 Radiographs of the same patient with fixation of the panmetatarsal head resection with absorbable pins

Clinical Pearls/Pitfalls

- In the 7 years since the release and surgical application of the Trim-it Drill pin in hammertoes, some recurring questions have arisen from practicing surgeons. The most common questions entertained relate to digital edema, the occasional late extrusion of a pin from the tip of the toe, and an occasional radiographic appearance of osteolysis around the PIP joint fusion sites. The most common denominator in all these is deviation from the recommended and published surgical techniques. The absorbable pin does not even begin to hydrolyze for 6 months so any erythema and/or digital edema is not a reactive process to the poly-L-lactide pin. A frequent question is as to whether the pin may be causing a reactive soft tissue irritation and it is not. The last 30 plus years of worldwide experience with the biomaterial poly-L-lactide in all applications of orthopedic surgery for bone fixation shows the incidence of a true reaction to the material to be exceedingly low and in the tenths of 1%. The most common cause for soft tissue swelling and any persistent edema is residual movement or pistoning of the pin at the interphalangeal joint level. This creates a mini nonunion or pseudoarthrosis-type environment with the expected concomitant edema. The most common technique errors are not completely filling the entire length of the proximal phalanx with the Trim-it Drill pin during the "all-inside" technique and incomplete approximation of the PIP joint prior to closure of the skin. Regardless of the surgical technique variances, any pistoning or movement at the PIP joint will provoke continued movement, and resultant soft tissue edema and logically local erythema follow. This typically resolves with compression bandages and further controlled immobilization in surgical shoes and/or boots. The periodically noted osteolysis around the desired fusion sites is a further byproduct of any persistent micromotion in addition to the slow degradation profile of poly-L-lactic acid in an intramedullary location. There is no noted clinical consequence to this.
- The most common causes of the late extrusion of a Trim-it Drill pin from the tip of a toe are inadequate or errant tamping of the pin back into the distal phalanx. The available cannula and tamp system has largely reduced this complication, but there are still cases where the tamp skives or slips off the pin, and the sensation is that the tip of the pin is being retrograded back into the distal phalanx, but it is not. The pin in these cases may remain in the soft tissue pulp of the distal toe only to later cause some soft tissue irritation. The solution is simple; the pin is simply removed as if it was a standard metallic Kirschner wire under topical ethyl chloride anesthetic or in rare cases under local anesthetic (Figs. 12.28 and 12.29). The regular use of the "flexed fusion" technique also discourages any migration of the pin as the bend in the pin enhances its stability within the intramedullary canal and avoids and longitudinal shift or displacement.

- The Trim-it Drill pin is a well-accepted and reliable non-external fixation device for the reproduceable stabilization of the common hammertoe deformities so many patients suffer from. The absence of any protruding pin from the tip of the toe allows a faster return to closed shoe gear and a faster resumption of normal bathing which facilitate a quicker functional recovery for the patient and high patient acceptance. Strict adherence to the recommended surgical techniques is paramount to diminish any complications and to consistently achieve satisfactory surgical outcomes and satisfied patients.

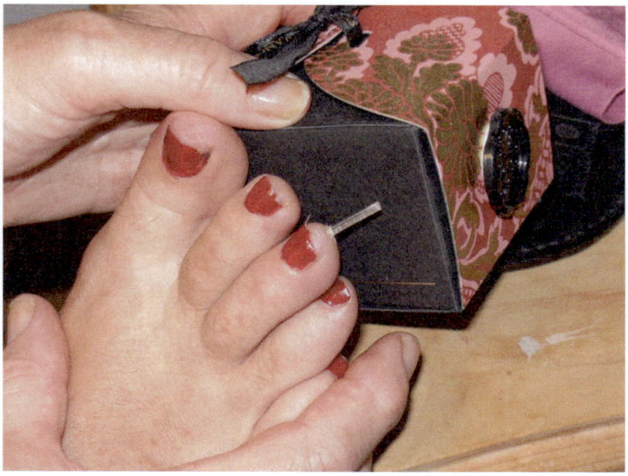

Fig. 12.28 Late migration of an absorbable pin out the tip of the toe

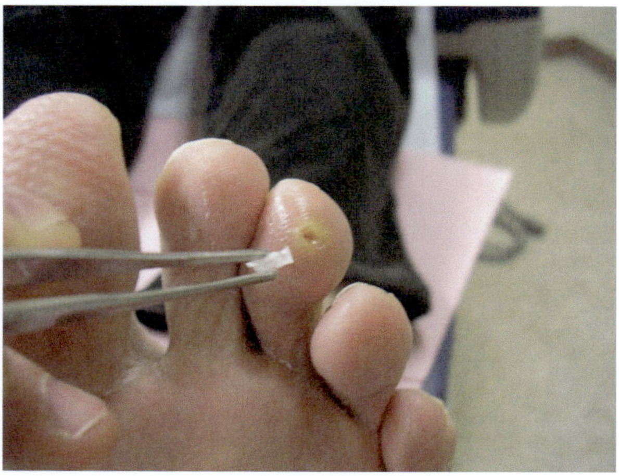

Fig. 12.29 The simple trimming and removal of the migrated pin from the tip of the toe

References

1. Konkel KF, et al. Hammertoe correction using an absorbable pin. Foot Ankle Int. 2011;32(10):973–8.
2. Cicchinelli LD. Hammertoe surgery and the Trim-it Drill pin. Foot Ankle Spec. 2013;6(4):296–302.

Chapter 13
Plastic Surgery Procedures for Hammertoe Correction

Peter Blume, Beau Vesely, and Rene Hymel

Case #1 Bilobed Flap Presentation

A 52-year-old female presents with the concern of an occasionally painful lesion on the dorsal lateral aspect of her left second digit (Fig. 13.1). She notes that it has drained clear gelatinous material and reduces in size but often returns within a month or two. Shoe modification and intralesional injection, with cortisone or 4% alcohol sclerosing solution, are often attempted for conservative therapy.

Diagnosis

Digital mucoid cysts present as a solitary, round or oval, clear to flesh-colored nodular lesions on the dorsal aspect of the fingers and toes. They are uncommon in the younger population and occur in a greater frequency in females (3:1 ratio) [1]. The pathophysiology is poorly understood, but they are often located at the level of the distal interphalangeal joint and are attributed to osteoarthritic changes caused most commonly by a mallet toe deformity. The patient's symptoms result from increased pressure and shoe gear irritation. Conservative therapy often fails, requiring surgical excision [2].

P. Blume (✉)
Yale School of Medicine, New Haven, CT, USA

B. Vesely
Krohn Clinic, Black River Falls, WI, USA

R. Hymel
Baton Rouge General Hospital, Hammond, LA, USA

E. A. Cook, J. J. Cook (eds.), *Hammertoes*,
https://doi.org/10.1007/978-3-319-16552-3_13

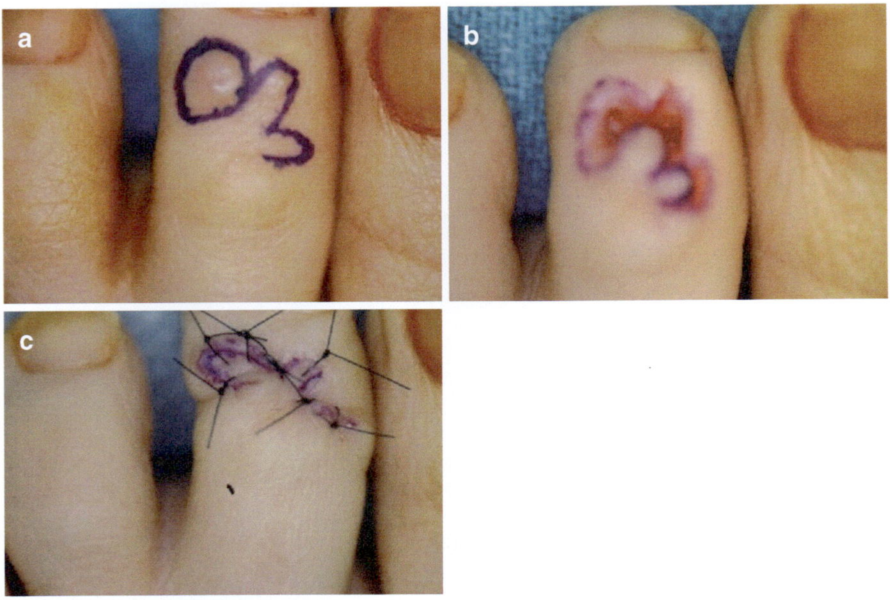

Fig. 13.1 (**a**) Small lesion noted to lateral second DIPJ. (**b**) Resection of lesion with planning of double-lobe flap outlined with skin marker. (**c**) Flap following transposition and closure with simple interrupted suturing technique

Surgical Technique and Pearls

The bilobed flap was designed to move additional skin over a larger distance than what is available with a single-lobe flap. This flap does not typically require additional skin grafting and allows for primary closure [3]. The bilobed transpositional flap extends beyond the excised lesion and utilizes adjacent donor sites for closure of the defect. This allows for redistribution and redirection of skin tension, allowing for primary closure of the soft tissue defect [4].

The two flaps that are separated by an angle share a common pedicle and encompass the epidermis, dermis, and subcutaneous tissue. The vascular supply is composed of a source artery and its associated vein from the local subdermal plexus that perforates the subcutaneous tissue.

Careful dissection, delicate soft tissue handling, and hemostasis are imperative for preservation of blood supply and tissue integrity.

The technique for creating a bilobed flap includes an initial full-thickness excision through the subcutaneous tissue of the lesion. Following excision of the lesion, assess the lines of maximal extensibility and RSTL. The pinch test can help determine how supple the adjacent tissue is and determine the axis of rotation for flap planning. Variations of the bilobed flap design exist, but the most common configuration is a 90-degree angle [5]. The rotation of this flap consists of a 360-degree circle for rotation on an axis point [6]. A design is constructed with the adjacent lobe with 75% of the size of the original defect and the secondary lobe approximately 50% of the original defect [7]. Outlining the plan with a fine tip surgical marker works best when working on small digital areas. Full-thickness incisions perpendicular to the skin, avoiding skiving, and atraumatic technique with single-prong skin hooks can help prevent complications such as scar formation, wound edge, and flap necrosis. The flap can be elevated from deeper connective tissue, with care to include subcutaneous adipose tissue to remain within the flap. The local tissue surrounding the donor site should be carefully undermined with dissection scissors. Undermining, however, should be limited with only enough to produce laxity, thus increasing the extensibility of local skin and decreasing tension on the flap during closure. The larger adjacent flap can be rotated into the primary defect and then the second lobe into the primary flap donor site. Careful closure avoiding strangulating the soft tissue and avoiding suturing the acute angles of the flap can prevent necrosis and dehiscence at the surgical site. Closure should be performed with simple interrupted technique and with suture no larger than 4-0 nylon to avoid suture-induced ischemia. Subcutaneous sutures are rarely necessary and should be avoided to prevent tissue reactivity. Any dog ears created from excess skin should not be removed, as they will resolve spontaneously over 2–3 weeks.

Outcomes

Excision of a lesion with the adjunctive bilobed flap closure has been demonstrated to be highly curative with successful results and low complication rates as adjunctive treatment of digital mucoid cysts [8]. A retrospective review completed by this author found that there were zero recurrences, flap failures, or significant complications in a cohort of 15 patients with an average follow up of 4.6 years. This flap does not typically require additional skin grafting and allows for primary closure. The long-term reproducibility and functional outcome of the bilobed flap are quite predictable. With appropriate application and incisional planning, it can make an excellent tool for the podiatric surgeon.

Case #2 V-to-Y Advancement Flap

Presentation/History

A 46-year-old female returns to the clinic with continued frustration and pain of her left fifth toe. The toe has caused her discomfort for a number of years. Conservative offloading and padding have been unsuccessful. On exam, there is tenderness of the digit with noted soft tissue contracture of the fifth digit, without an overlying skin lesion.

Diagnosis/Assessment

Congenital overlapping fifth toe

Surgical Technique

The V-to-Y advancement type flap moves in a single direction, without any lateral or rotational components. One can only expect approximately 20% skin lengthening with the use of a V-to-Y technique [9]. The length of the V arms can vary on the degree of contracture present. The length of each individual arm should be equal. The acuity of the angle and arm length determines the lengthening achieved. The apex of the V should bisect the axis or orientation of the contracture. Undermining the surrounding tissue should be minimally performed, releasing enough tension to allow closure with 4-0 or smaller suture as undermining can violate the local vascular supply. Reapproximation of skin edges is planned with the toe held in its corrected position. It can be helpful to mark this level with a hash mark as to where the apex of the flap should be sutured to its adjacent skin edge. An apical stitch can then be thrown followed by simple interrupted closure of the remaining portion of the newly formed Y. The remaining closure can be performed with simple interrupted suturing technique (Fig. 13.2).

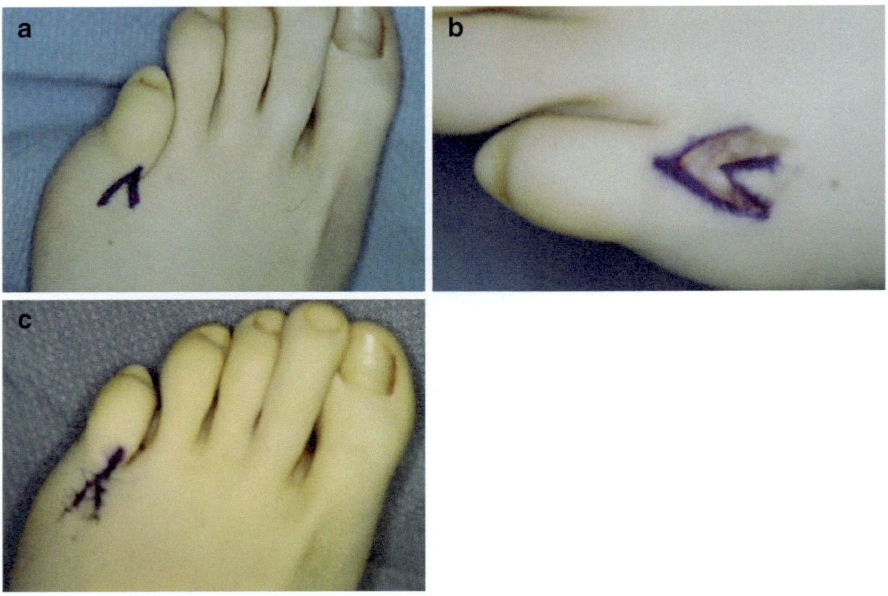

Fig. 13.2 (**a**) Congenital deformity noted at the left fifth toe with planned incision outlined with skin marker (**b**) Incision made and ready for advancement. (**c**) Closed with simple suturing technique being sure to not overly tighten sutures

Outcomes

Hand surgeons have routinely used V-to-Y flaps for digital reconstruction following traumatically amputated terminal phalanges [10], and their long-term viability has been proven.

Pearls

The V-Y advancement flap, commonly used in fingertip injuries, when indicated and carefully performed, gives excellent contour and padding. This advancement flap maintains toe length and provides good cosmesis for digital surgery [10].

Case #3 Combined Advancement Flap (Butler Procedure)

Presentation/History

A 67-year-old woman who previously underwent corrective surgery of her overlapping fifth toe was referred for a second opinion. The patient reports a history of increasing deformity and pain. She had poor results with conservative therapy consisting of padding and careful shoe gear selection. She was not pleased with her previous surgical result (Fig. 13.3). On exam, her deformity was reducible with pain on palpation to the lateral and dorsal fifth toe.

Diagnosis/Assessment

Recurrent cock up deformity of the fifth digit following hammertoe correction surgery

Surgical Technique

A modification of the Butler procedure incorporates the use of the V-to-Y and a Y-to-V to correct the deformity and was used in this revision.

The Y-to-V plasty is the opposite of the V-Y flap by increasing tension in line with the Y-to-V and releasing tension perpendicular to the flap. The incisions of the Y-V plasty are carried deep into the subcutaneous tissue layer with gentle undermining of the surrounding tissue. The subcutaneous tip of the flap should be gently

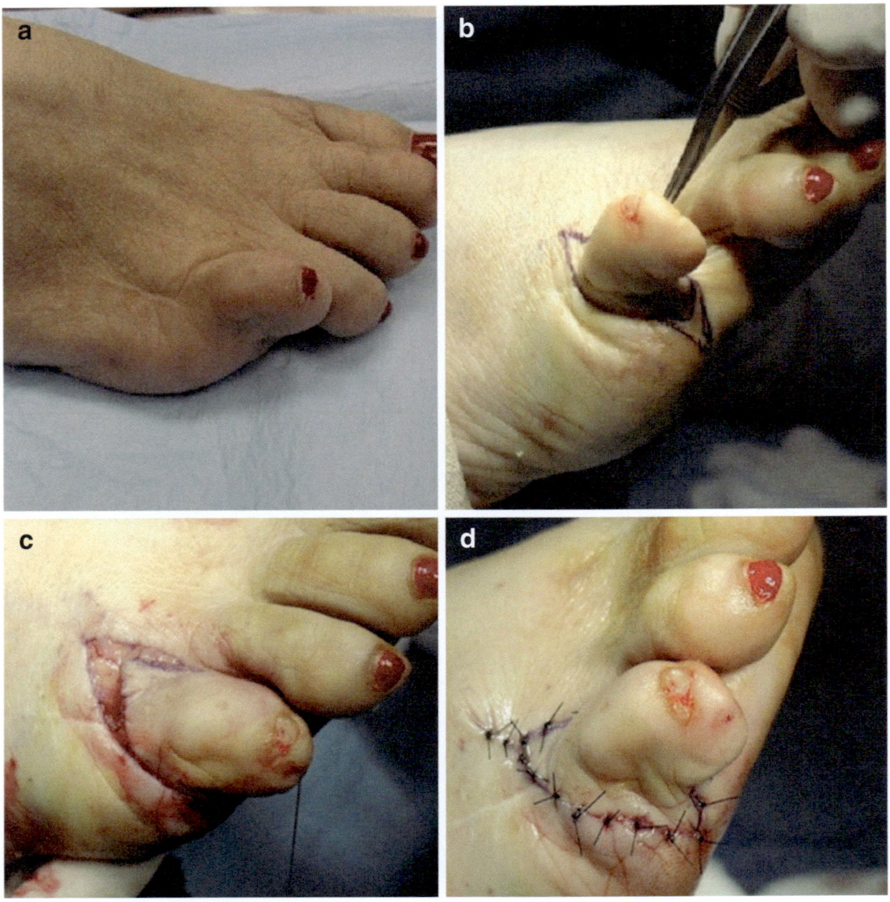

Fig. 13.3 (**a**) Recurrence of overlapping fifth toe deformity with minor scar contracture noted (**b**) Incision planned (**c**) Incision made with delicate soft tissue handling (**d**) Closed with simple interrupted suture technique

held in position with a skin hook with care taken not to damage the skin layer of the tip. Dorsally the V incision is created for planned lengthening. After the incision is made, the digit should be manually reduced, held, and marked for length of the stem of the Y. Next, the Y-to-V portion of the incision is outlined plantarly for planned excision of redundant tissue. The Y-to-V should be checked to ensure enough tissue has been resected. Once pleased with the tailoring of the final skin plasty, any adjunctive procedures can be performed as needed. The surgical incision can be closed primarily with an assistant holding the toe in a corrected position. Again, a focus on delicate tissue handling while placing apical stitches and closing the incision is imperative. It is advocated that the toe be bandaged to help hold the toe in the desired position for several weeks while healing.

Outcomes

The patient was pleased with her result and had excellent deformity correction with significant pain relief. In 1993 DeBoeck published a retrospective study of 23 cases of overriding of the fifth toe treated by Butler's arthroplasty. Satisfactory results were obtained in all but one patient, and all could wear normal shoe gear [11].

Pearls

The use of the V-Y and V-to-Y/Y-to-V combination tools is helpful in the correction of revisional surgery, as well as the congenital overlapping fifth toe. They can both provide soft tissue lengthening and have excellent exposure for adjunctive osseous and capsulotendon procedures in digital correction.

These flaps can be done in series to release a contracture over the dorsum of the forefoot, in areas of burn scar contracture or applied to contracted digits.

Case #4 Z-Plasty Presentation

A 64-year-old male presents with a recurrence of a second digit contracture of his left foot. He complains of pain at the distal tip of the toe and as a diabetic is concerned about possible ulceration. He would like to have the toe corrected to prevent a future ulceration and possible infection (Fig. 13.4).

Diagnosis

Complications including scar contracture following digital arthroplasty are not uncommon [12]. Scar formation and contracture in digital correction can produce a reducible deformity at the surgical site, thus the need for revisional surgery with soft tissue correction.

Surgical Technique

To design the z-plasty, the central limb is placed parallel to the contracture axis or along the direction of the desired length increase. The extending limbs should be of equal length with all angles created equal and parallel to the RSTL. Keeping the

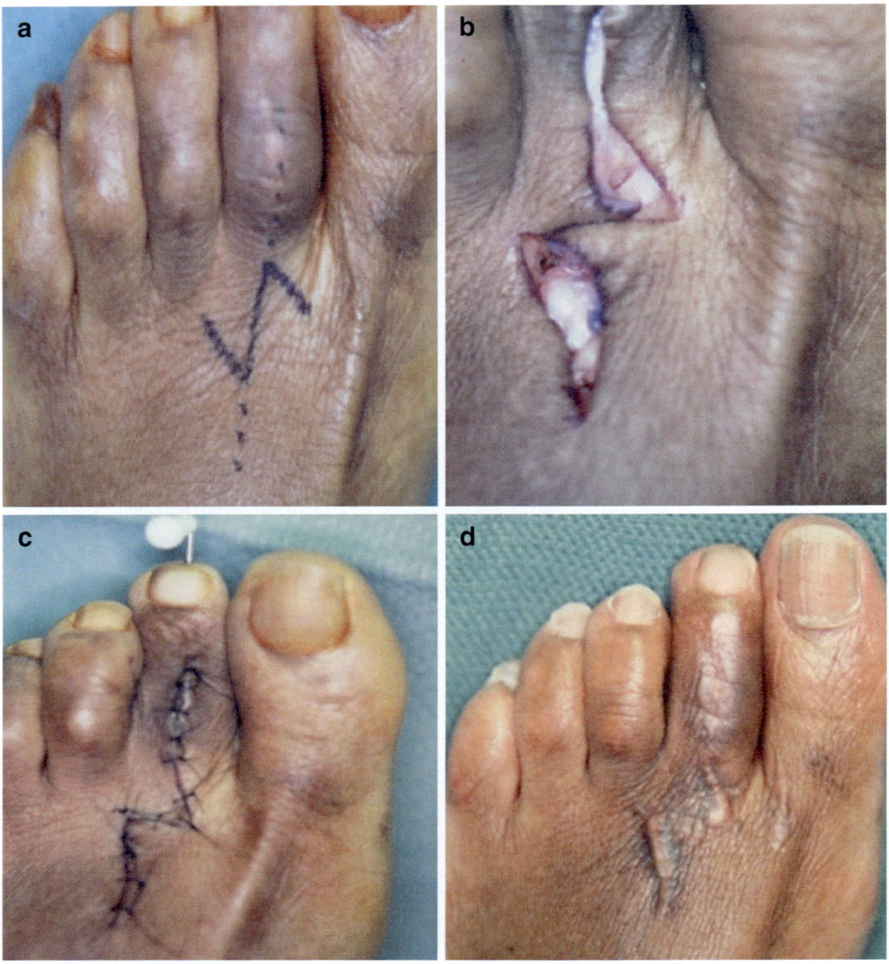

Fig. 13.4 (**a**) Long arm of Z parallel to scar contracture (**b**) Incision made with delicate tissue handling (**c**) Arthrodesis of the proximal interphalangeal joint with primary closure (**d**) Incision is healed with additional length provided by Z-plasty

length and angle of each flap precisely equal is key to avoid mismatched flaps that may be difficult to close [13]. Z-plasties designed with 90° angles can create dog ears that are also difficult to excise and close primarily [14]. On the other hand, angles created too acutely can lead to necrosis of the flap tip [15]. The flaps should be fully elevated to slightly beyond their bases to allow for ease of rotation; however, care must be taken to avoid undermining the tip of the flaps. An imaginary line connecting the two noncentral incisions becomes the new central line or diagonal of the final Z after the flaps have been transposed. Careful closure is imperative to prevent dehiscence at the surgical site. Closure should be performed with simple interrupted technique and with suture no larger than 4-0 nylon to avoid suture-induced ischemia.

The first stitch should first be placed in the midpoint of the newly formed central arm. The base of the flaps should then be reapproximated followed by oblique sutures to advance the tip of each Z-flap. Finally an apical or Gillies' corner stitch can be applied to the tip of each flap for final closure.

Clinical Pearls/Pitfalls

Tissue lengthening procedure such as the Z-plasty, with or without tendon and osseous work, is a useful technique for the correction of digital deformities. It is especially useful in the correction of revisional digital procures via lengthening a linear scar contracture, dispersal of a scar tissue, and realigning a scar within the RSTL [16]. A Z-plasty should only be considered if there is sufficient skin laxity perpendicular to the direction of the skin to be lengthened, as length is gained at the expense of width [13]. The Z-plasty should also not be used if the original scar lies within the RSTL, as the newly formed central arm wound lies perpendicular to the RSTL [17]. The amount of length achieved is determined by both the arm length and angle. The basic Z-plasty (typically 60° arm angles) can be modified by varying arm length and angle [9]. Z-plasty is a useful technique in revisional digital surgery and can lengthen a scar by up to 75% and reorient the direction by 90 degrees [18–20].

Atraumatic technique with delicate tissue handling is critical for success. This involves the use of the use of skin hooks and fine-toothed forceps for tissue handling. Care should be taken to avoid compromising the flap's blood supply by traumatizing the base or twisting or kinking the base during advancement. Hemostasis is also crucial as hematoma formation can have devastating effects on flap survivability and can be performed with bipolar cautery. Hematoma increases the risk of tissue necrosis, infection, and subsequent flap failure. Nonreactive sutures are preferred for closure, and deep absorbable sutures should be avoided when possible.

Possible complications of z-plasty include flap necrosis, hematoma formation under the flaps, wound infection, trapdoor effect, and sloughing of the flap caused by high wound tension. These can be avoided by careful design planning with correct patient selection, meticulous dissection and tissue handling, appropriate hemostasis, and closing the incisions under minimal tension.

Case #5 Double Z-Plasty Presentation

A 64-year-old African American male who suffered extensive third-degree burns to the left lower extremity from a campfire accident >10 years ago presents for evaluation. He relates pain to the distal dorsal second toe from rubbing in shoe gear and difficulty in wearing steel-toed boots required for his work. He has failed all conservative measures of tapping and padding and would like to pursue surgical correction.

Diagnosis/Assessment

Ridged elevated second digit secondary to scar contracture from third-degree burns to the left foot

Surgical Technique

A double Z-plasty, a modified version of the single Z-plasty, can be used when there is insufficient laxity of adjacent soft tissues in an area that does not permit the use of a large single Z-plasty. Two Z-plasties are designed so that their central incision or diagonal stem of the Z is parallel (Fig. 13.5b). The initial incision, which will become the diagonal line of the Z, is made longitudinally along the length of the scar or along the direction to be lengthened. The other incisions are then made off of this central line at 45°–60° angles and should parallel the RSTL. The limbs of the Z-shaped incision should be of equal length. The flaps are then elevated and transposed in a manner similar to the single Z-plasty reviewed in the previous case.

Outcomes

Three cases of necrosis of tip of Z-plasty flaps occurred which were under 3 mm and resolved gradually in a cohort of 23 patients who underwent double Z-plasties for burn contractors of the hand [21]. In three contractures, the release was inadequate, and an additional procedure under local anesthesia was performed to achieve deformity correction [21].

Pearls

The repair of postburn deformities must prioritize function over form, must be based on careful assessment of the patient's goals and desires, and should respect the timing and duration of physiologic scar maturation [22]. Achauer noted that the optimum timing of reconstructive surgery from a biological standpoint is diametrically

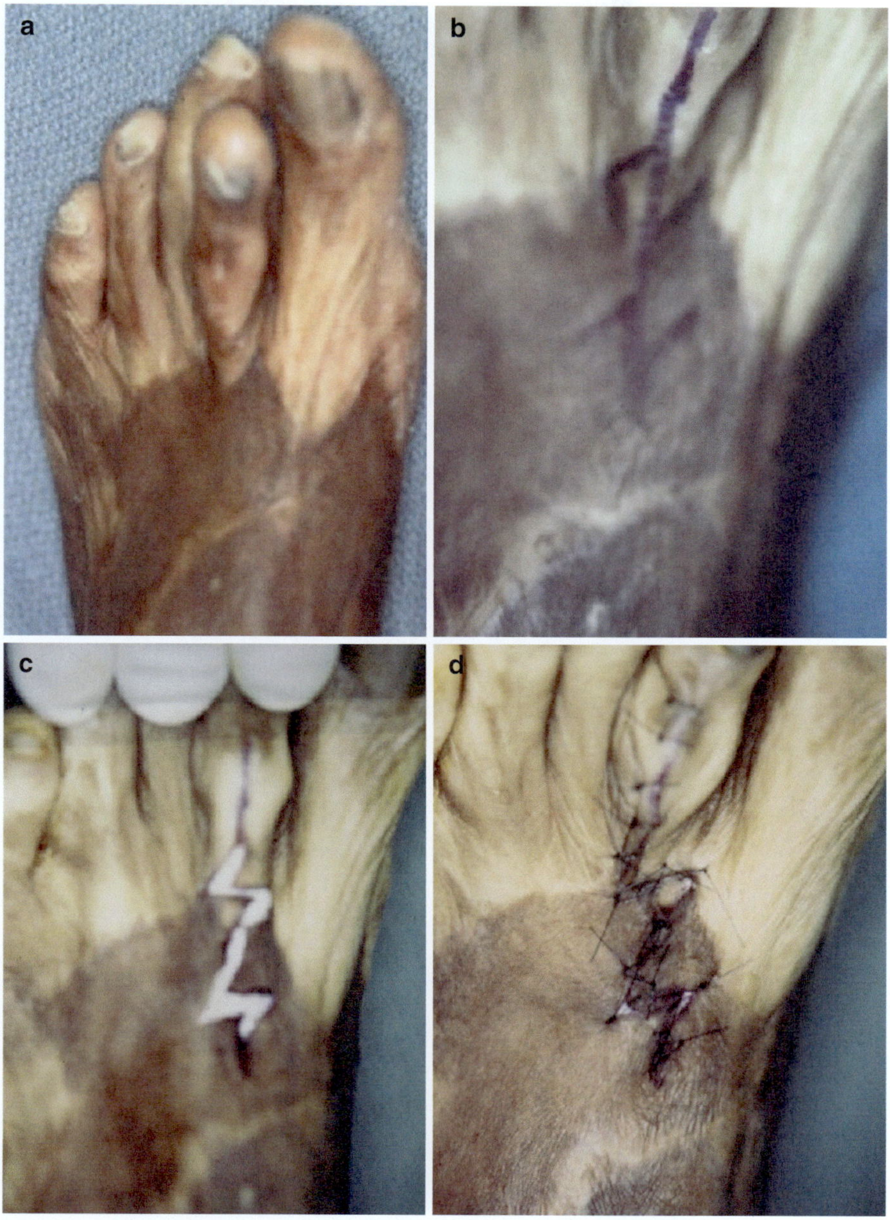

Fig. 13.5 (**a**) Significant scaring present from full-thickness burns (**b**) Incision outlined with skin marker (**c**) Incision made full thickness (**d**) Incision reapproximated in improved position

opposed to the optimum timing from the standpoint of rehabilitation and the patient's mental well-being [23]. Scar maturation usually occurs around 12 months post burn, and therefore most corrective procedures should be delayed at least this long. Others advocate waiting up to 2 years for full scar maturation before proceeding with reconstructive surgery [24]. Surgical manipulation of an active, red, immature scar is not only technically more difficult but also may be associated with renewed and more aggressive scar formation postoperatively. Furthermore, many hypertrophic scars tend to involute over time [22].

Clinical Pearls/Pitfalls

The successful incorporation of a tissue transfer for digital reconstruction should include several steps. A surgeon must identify the goals of the flap which ultimately provide landmarks for design, orientation, and anatomic application. This will allow for correct incision planning. The general health assessment of the patient, the source of blood flow to the flap, donor site and recipient site selection, and the optimum positioning and design of the flap are paramount to its success. The viability of the flap is directly and proportionally affected by the level of atraumatic technique used and the reduction in undermining peripherally to the flap. Hemostasis must remain a priority because hematoma formation can have devastating effects on flap survivability. Hematoma increases the risk of tissue necrosis, infection, and subsequent flap loss. The donor site must be evaluated for tissue mobility and elasticity in order to reduce tension after transposition. The manual pinch test is very useful for this indication. One should always have a backup plan when considering flap elevation and division due to the possibility of the flap failure. The adverse outcome can leave the patient with a large tissue deficit and impact healing and function. The intraoperative care of the flap does play a direct role in the success of the flap. Atraumatic dissection and careful handling of the flap are highly recommended. This involves the use of bipolar cautery, sharp dissection rather than cautery dissection, the use of skin hooks or fine-toothed forceps to handle tissue, and delicate handling of the flap. Care should be taken to avoid compromising the flap's blood supply by traumatizing the base or twisting or kinking the base during movement. Nonreactive sutures are preferred for closure, and deep absorbable sutures should be avoided when possible.

Advancement flaps should be placed so as to benefit from the elasticity of the surrounding skin while bearing in mind the regional blood supply. They should be perpendicular to the RSTL and advance in a movement parallel to the LME. Although advancement flaps allow for closure of the donor and defect simultaneously, their use can be limited in the foot, due to mobility restrictions and the need for broad exposure to underlying osseous pathology.

Summary

The bilobed flap, V-Y skin plasty, and Z-plasty are extremely useful adjunctive procedures for correction of digital deformities. Multiple geometric constructs have been described, and each has its own unique principles which can be adapted to certain locations and conditions. The versatility, reproducibility, and long-term functional outcomes that these flaps provide are well known and should be utilized where appropriate by today's foot and ankle surgeon.

References

1. Dockery G, Crawford M. Textbook –lower extremity soft tissue and cutaneous plastic surgery. Edinburgh/New York: Saunders; 2006. p. 314–5.
2. Jager T, Vogels J, Dautel G. The Zitelli design for bilobed flap applied on skin defects after digital mucous cyst excision. A review of 9 cases. Tech Hand Up Extrem Surg. 2012;16(3):124–6.
3. Sahin C, et al. Bilobed flap for web reconstruction in adult syndactyly release: a new technique that can avoid the use of skin graft. J Plast Reconstr Aesthet Surg. 2014;67:815–21.
4. Hallock GG. The sacred heart Bilobed flap: a simple method for closing small scalp defects. Plast Reconstr Surg. 2015;136:286e.
5. Bouche RT, Christensen JC, Hale DS. Unilobed and bilobed skin flaps. Detailed surgical technique for plantar lesions. J Am Podiatr Med Assoc. 1995;85(1):41–8.
6. Jelinek NJ, Cordova KB. Bilobed flap for reconstruction of small alar rim defects. Dermatol Surg. 2013;39(4):649–52.
7. Sanchez-Conejo-Mir J, Buneo Montes J, Moreno Giminez JC, Camacho-Martinez F. The bilobed flap in sole surgery. J Dermatol Surg Oncol. 1985;11(9):913–7.
8. Blume PA, Moore JC, Novicki DC. Digital mucoid cyst excision by using the bilobed flap technique and arthroplastic resection. J Foot Ankle Surg. 2005;44(1):44–8.
9. Dockery G, Crawford M. Textbook –lower extremity soft tissue and cutaneous plastic surgery. p. 151–2.
10. Bharathi RR, Jerome TJ, Kalson NS. V-Y advancement flap coverage of toe-tip injuries. J Foot Ankle Surg. 2009;48(3):368–71.
11. DeBoeck H. Butler's operation for congenital overlapping of the fifth toe. Acta Orthop Scand. 1993;64(3):343–4.
12. Femino JE, Mueller K. Complications of lesser toe surgery. Clin Orthop Relat Res. 2001;391:72–88.
13. Lesavoy MA. Local incisions and flap coverage. In: Plastic surgery. Philadelphia: W.B. Saunders Company; 1990. p. 1441–58.
14. Bark SE, Keplinger LM, Meyr AJ. Precise intraoperative 60° skin Z-plasty. J Foot Ankle Surg. 2010;49:191–3.
15. Thordarson DB. Congenital crossover fifth toe correction with soft tissue release and cutaneous Z-plasty. Foot Ankle Int. 2001;22(6):511–2.
16. Crawford ME, Dockery GL. Use of Z-skin plasty in scar revisions and skin contractures of the lower extremity. J Am Podiatr Med Assoc. 1995;85(l):28–35.
17. Hove CR, Williams EF III, Rodgers BJ. Z-Plasty: a concise review. Facial Plast Surg. 2001;17(4):289–94.
18. Miguel DA. Elongation through Z-Plasty: an experimental study comparing 11 Z-Plasty variations on nonbiologic tissue. Plast Reconstr Surg. 2012;129(5):890–2.
19. Myerson MS, Fortin P, Gilard P. Use of skin Z-plasty for management of extension contracture in recurrent claw and hammertoe deformity. Foot Ankle Int. 1994;15(4):209–12.

20. Barreiros H, Goulao J. Z-Plasty: useful uses in dermatologic surgery. An Bras Dermatol. 2014;89(1):187–8.
21. Davami B. V-M plasty and double Z-Plasty, two versatile flaps for treatment of post burn syndactyly. Tech Hand Up Extrem Surg. 2009;13(3):124–9.
22. Cartotto R, Cicuto BJ, Kiwanuka HN. Common postburn deformities and their management. Surg Clin N Am. 2014;94:817–37.
23. Achauer BM. Burn reconstruction. New York: Thieme Medical Publishers Inc.; 1991.
24. Huang T. Overview of burn reconstruction. In: Herndon DN, editor. Total burn care. 3rd ed. Philadelphia: Saunders Elsevier; 2007. p. 674–86.

Suggested Reading

Gillies HD. The design of direct pedicle flaps. Br Med J. 1932;2(3752):1008.
Zimany A. The bi-lobed flap. Plast Reconstr Surg (1946). 1953;11(6):424–34.

Chapter 14
Tendon Lengthening Procedures

Mark Gilheany

Introduction

Tendon lengthening procedures are a common component of surgical algorithms utilised in the reduction of lesser toe deformity [1–6]. These algorithms most commonly involve bone and joint surgery with decompression and/or balancing of soft tissues which may include the skin, ligament, joint capsule and/or tendon. Patient factors such as age, co-morbidities, stage and extent of presenting deformity, flexibility of presenting deformity and expectations of both the patient and the surgeon all impact upon decision-making in respect to these algorithms.

In addition to acting as a component of a procedure, isolated or multiple tendon procedures of both the short and long flexors and extensors can be performed as independent procedures to reduce or correct deformity in appropriate circumstances.

Isolated tendon procedures are generally considered not suitable for patients where the deformity is so significant that skin plasty, ligament release and/or osseous procedures are required concurrently to address non-reducible or multiple plane deformity. In these later circumstances, the tendon procedures are executed as a component of an algorithm which may include procedures to the above tissues. In addition to further soft tissue procedures, osseous procedures may include arthroplasty, arthrodesis or osteotomy at the phalanx and metatarsal level.

Underpinning the use of tendon lengthening procedures in the lesser toes is the concept of decompression and/or balancing of soft tissues about an abnormal joint flexion which has a component of sagittal plane imbalance. Despite widespread use [7] and support [8], the evidence base for the performance of tendon lengthening procedures as a stand-alone procedure is equivocal, principally due to a lack of well-designed prospective trials [9]. This does not imply that such procedures are

M. Gilheany (✉)
Foot Ankle Specialists, Traralgon, VIC, Australia
e-mail: admin@fasa.net.au; www.footanklespecialists.com.au

E. A. Cook, J. J. Cook (eds.), *Hammertoes*,
https://doi.org/10.1007/978-3-319-16552-3_14

not appropriate; simply that further outcome studies are warranted. This concept is highlighted by more recent level 3 and 4 evidence reporting promising results in the treatment of pre-ulcerative and ulcerative lesions in the neuropathic foot using isolated flexor tenotomy [10–12].

In this chapter tendon lengthening procedures to the lesser toes are discussed specifically relating to considerations in lengthening of flexor digitorum longus (FDL), flexor digitorum brevis (FDB), extensor digitorum longus (EDL) and extensor digitorum brevis (EDB). There is an emphasis placed on the potential for adverse outcomes if a functional surgical approach is not pursued when executing what can be sometimes viewed as routine or simplistic procedures.

Presentation

Any sagittal plane deformity of the lesser toes may benefit from extensor or flexor tendon lengthening procedures. This most commonly relates to the various presentations of an underlying muscle imbalance which has led to sagittal plane toe deformity affecting multiple digits. It has been suggested that the definitions associated with lesser toe deformity, claw, hammer and mallet toes, are often confused by clinicians, and on this basis the various forms of the deformity are best described as a functional continuum [13, 14] or by plane of deformity [15] (Fig. 14.1). This anatomic approach to understanding the deforming forces also provides a basis for planning rational and functional surgical approaches.

A functional approach to surgical planning must also acknowledge that the causes of imbalance can be varied and multifactorial [3, 4, 16] and that surgical approaches will by necessity reflect this variability [8, 17, 18].

Additionally there are specific clinical circumstances where isolated toe pathology is amenable to isolated flexor and extensor tendon balancing. These

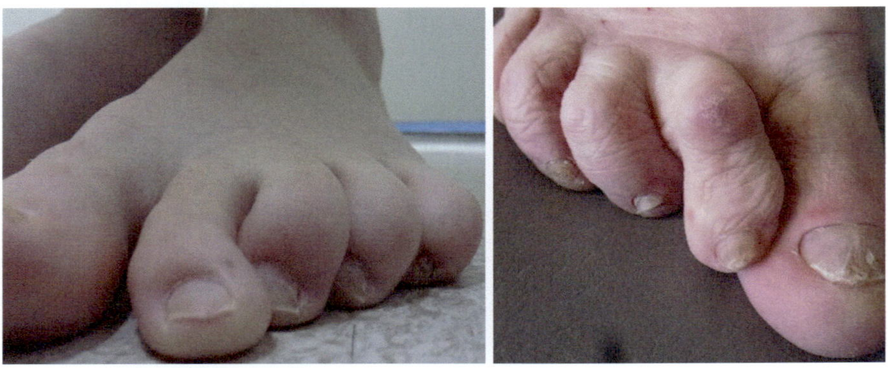

Fig. 14.1 Lesser toe deformities can be viewed as a functional progression of imbalance at the interphalangeal joints which leads ultimately to rigid deformity over time. The extent and location of joint adaptation will relate to underlying functional adaptation

include pressure lesions affecting the apex of toes or about the interphalangeal joints of toes (Fig. 14.2) and curly toe deformity in the paediatric population (Fig. 14.3).

Sagittal plane soft tissue imbalance will over time result in contracture and adaptation of joint structure and function. It is accepted that both extensor overpowering and flexor overpowering can result in sagittal plane deformity [4]. At a clinical level, however, it can be deceptively difficult to determine whether it is the flexors or extensors which are the overpowering deforming force.

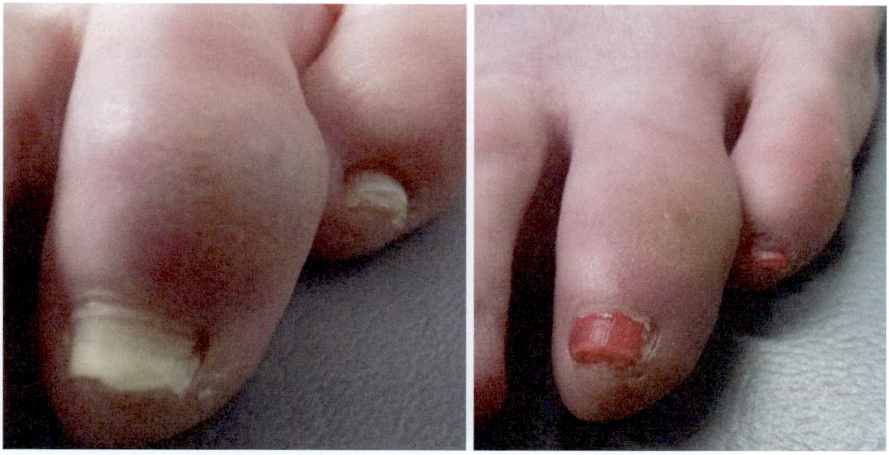

Fig. 14.2 Excessive tendon tension resulting in curled toe and lesion. Pre-flexor tendon (FDL) and post-flexor tendon (2 weeks) release. The hyperkeratotic lesion resolved by the eighth post-operative week

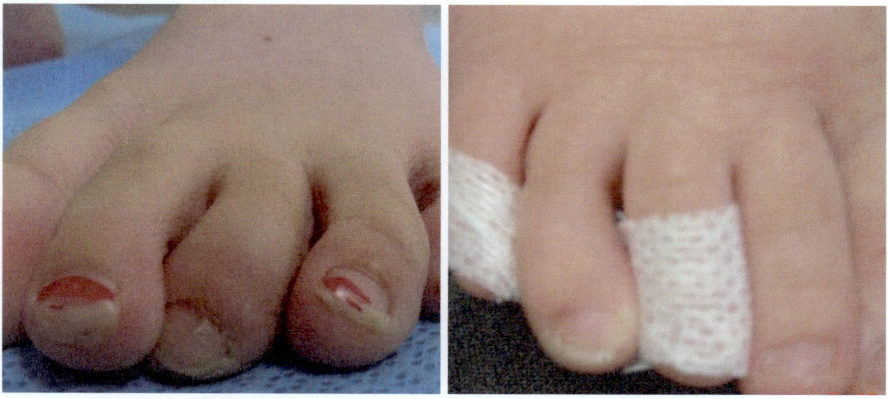

Fig. 14.3 Paediatric curly toe syndrome secondary to congenitally tight FDL. An example of a simple splinting technique which can be used both preoperatively and postoperatively (to maintain correction) is pictured

Diagnostic Assessment

Surgical reduction of toe deformity relies upon tendon lengthening within sequential dissection and release protocols as a means to neutralise deforming force about the digit. This can be achieved by selectively lengthening either extensor or flexor tendons in isolation or concurrently. Postoperative splinting is used in various forms to maintain the digital alignment in a neutral position with repair of the tendons to a neutral functional outcome or selective lengthening of extensor or flexor tendons based upon assessment of functional imbalance. This neutralising effect can also be achieved by the secondary decompression effect of osseous procedures such as joint fusion or arthroplasty.

The surgical algorithms generally report surgical techniques which rely on intraoperative assessment and decision-making using sequential releases. This approach does not necessarily recognise the importance of understanding the dynamic nature of digital deformity. A diagnostic and subsequent procedural alternative is to identify the primary deforming force based upon clinical assessment and understanding of foot function preoperatively. Understanding the foot type including adaptive function on the deforming muscle tendon unit is an imperative element of surgical planning.

A simplistic example can be used to demonstrate this point. The unstable hyperpronated foot will exhibit excessive flexor contracture as a stabilising mechanism. The cavus foot will tend to exhibit excessive extensor activity during gait. Both these circumstances although due to inherently differing foot types can produce clinically similar sagittal plane contracture of the lesser digits.

To assist the assessment muscle imbalance and/or dominanance, a simple functional test (the digital balance test) is used by the author to assist in determining which tendon group requires lengthening and potentially which tendon group should not be lengthened.

To perform the digital balance test, the patient should be in a relaxed standing position. The clinician notes the severity and anatomic location of the contracture.

Then the patient is asked to purposefully contract the toe flexors; the clinician notes whether the deformity increases with this action. Then the patient is asked to actively contract the toe extensors; again the clinician notes whether this either reduces or exacerbates the sagittal plane toe deformity. Worsening deformity with either extension or flexion provides guidance as to which muscle group is the overpowering force. This in turn guides the soft tissue rebalancing required to reduce toe deformity (Fig. 14.4).

When electing to consider tendon lengthening procedures, it is important to consider these elements of functional anatomy not just from a surgical planning perspective but also both from a non-surgical and post-surgical perspective. For example: Would the patient benefit from targeted splint or exercise therapy to address the imbalance? Is there a role for ortho-mechanical or ergonomic modification to address the imbalance?

Another important element of clinical presentation is the common origin of the lesser extensor and flexor tendons. This means that consideration to multiple tendon

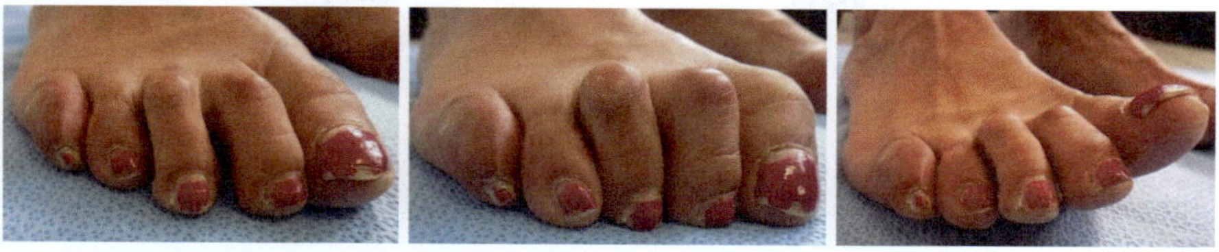

Fig. 14.4 Weight-bearing digital balance test. Note that gripping the ground increases the deformity whilst extending the toes decreases deformity. This indicates that the flexor tendons are overpowering the extensors. In this scenario strengthening the extensor muscles may reduce the need for surgical lengthening of the flexors. If surgery is required, then flexor lengthening is indicted not extensor. The reverse is applied if worsening deformity is noted with extensor contraction

lengthenings must always be given before proceeding with an isolated tendon lengthening. Isolated tendon lengthening provides the potential for muscle tendon imbalance which can result in further deformity affecting other digits.

Surgical Techniques

As reviewed above, the goal of tendon lengthening is to decompress a flexed or extended joint via appropriate tendon relaxation. Surgically this can be achieved via complete tenotomy (sharp release of the tendon) or tendon lengthening procedures. Both of these options can be performed via open or percutaneous technique.

Open techniques provide direct visualisation of the structure to be lengthened and allow protection of neurovascular structures. Open techniques are more commonly utilised in combination with osseous procedures such as digital arthrodesis or arthroplasty.

Percutaneous techniques require accurate understanding of surface anatomy as the procedure is performed without direct visualisation of neurovascular structures and target tissue. Percutaneous procedures in isolation provide advantages such as suitability for performance in office-based settings under local anaesthesia whilst also resulting in less risk of deep fascia scarring and adhesions.

When planning tendon lengthening procedures either open or percutaneously performed, the location of release will have an impact not just reduction and balance of deformity but capacity for healing of the flexor or extensor complex uneventfully. The complex arrangements of the extensor apparatus and the flexor vincula [19] provide a stable construct against which functional healing can occur (Fig. 14.5). Tendon lengthening performed outside of these zones relies on open, accurate and stable repair of the lengthened tendon or permanent loss of tendon function, and associated gait complications may result.

Percutaneous procedures can also be performed in combination with percutaneous osteotomies.

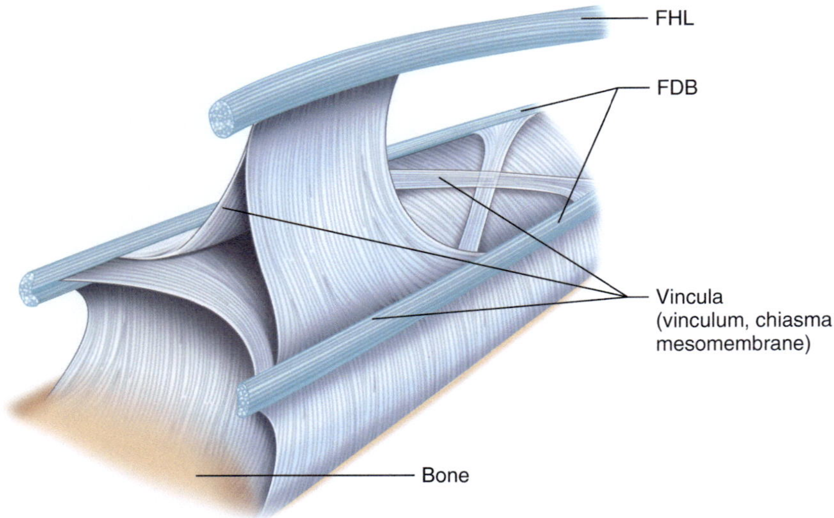

Fig. 14.5 Diagrammatic representation of the flexor vincula. These facial attachments demonstrate the close functional relationship between the short and long flexors of the toes. This anatomical relationship is an important consideration from a functional and surgical perspective when performing tendon lengthening procedures. (Adapted from Sarrafian)

Key points to remember when planning tendon lengthening:

- Tendon lengthening is a powerful surgical tool for a broad range of conditions and patient groups.
- Tendon lengthening procedures decompress joint tension.
- Reduction in tendon tension acts to weaken the muscle tendon unit.
- This weakening affect should be planned to establish balance about the joint.
- The extensor and flexor tendons of the lesser toes originate from common muscles; changing tension in one tendon will affect tension in the other tendons.
- Tendon lengthening procedures are often a component of more extensive procedure(s).
- Excessive tendon lengthening procedures can result in temporary or permanent weakness.
- Inappropriate or excessive tendon lengthening procedures can contribute to joint instability or deformity.
- Consider the complex arrangement of the flexor vincula and extensor apparatus when planning incision sites.

Open Tendon Lengthening

The classical description of open tendon lengthening involves a Z-plasty focused upon the EDL tendon. As an isolated procedure, it is generally described as undertaken proximal to the extensor hood of the metatarsophalangeal joints. This proximal placement means that stable open repair of the lengthened tendon should be performed. Percutaneous tenotomy at this level is not appropriate. A short incision with blunt dissection to expose the paratenon is utilised. The paratenon is reflected, the tendon is lengthened and sutured in its new physiologic length using either absorbable or non-absorbable sutures depending on surgeon preference, and the paratenon repaired prior to skin closure (Fig. 14.6).

If additional soft tissue release and/or osseous procedures are planned at the metatarsophalangeal joint level, a tendon Z-plasty can be undertaken as a component of comprehensive sequential release.

Flexor lengthening is not generally described as an open procedure unless as a component of a flexor tendon transfer. Technically it is unlikely that an open Z-plasty on the plantar aspect of the toes can be performed without resulting in extensive scar contracture and significant disturbance of flexor vincula.

An alternative to the Z-plasty proximally performed is to reflect the hood ligament at the level of the metatarsophalangeal joint and perform Z lengthening at this level. This approach is more generally applied when more extensive dissection is required for correction of toe deformity involving osseous and joint capsular structures. During this technique the opportunity to evaluate the tension of extensor digitorum brevis is possible, with release or lengthening as appropriate. This sequential

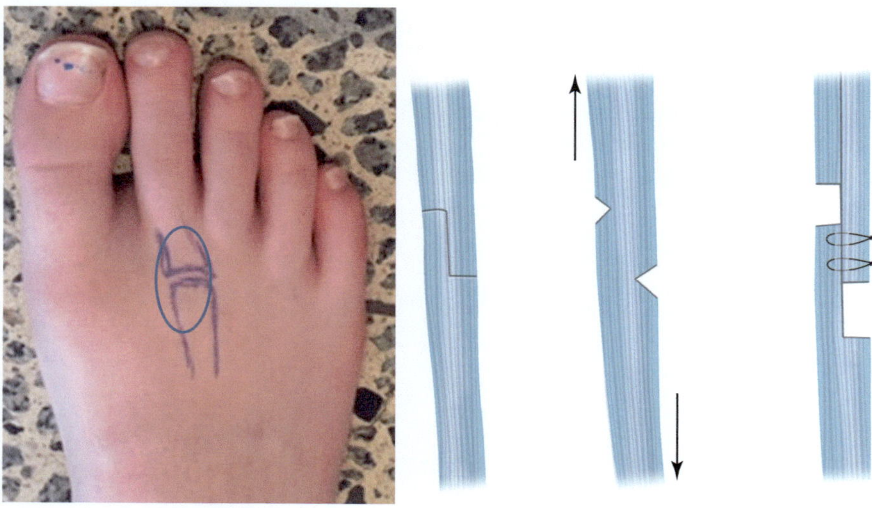

Fig. 14.6 Diagrammatic representation of the technique and positioning of traditional Z lengthening performed at or proximal to the extensor apparatus

loading to determine effective reduction of contracture is well described and not the focus of this chapter.

A further option is the use of multiple "Zs" or partial tendon release performed at intervals on alternating sides of the tendon followed by a manual stretch to lengthen fibres without complete release at any point. When using this technique, suture repair of the tendon is not necessary, and the paratenon does not have to be reflected (Fig. 14.7).

Percutaneous Tendon Lengthening

Percutaneous techniques have also been extensively described in the literature. Percutaneous tenotomies are ideally performed utilising either a minimally invasive (MIS) scalpel blade or utilising a sharp 18 or 19 gauge needle. If a small portal is utilised, there is generally no need for suturing of the skin. In the author's experience, using an 18 or 19 gauge needle results in return to function in a faster timeframe than when using a scalpel, but the technique is less reliable in inexperienced hands. The author reserves a 67 MIS blade for use when the contracture is significant and capsular structures need to be released (Fig. 14.8).

Technical illustrations of percutaneous lengethening, generally describe tenotomy via a medial approach with a rotation of the blade to allow release of the tendon as the toe is placed into flexion or extension [6] (Fig. 14.9). In the author's view, this approach provides potential for neurovascular and/or skin injury without careful control of the blade.

An alternative is to approach medial or lateral to the tendon from a dorsal portal for extensor and plantar portal for flexor (Fig. 14.10). Orientation of the blade towards the underlying phalanx protects the patient from inadvertent skin laceration. It is important to be aware that without primary repair of lengthened tendon, failure of the tenotomised ends of the tendon to heal may be a complication. Placing the percutaneous lengthening within the hood ligament dorsally and within the flexor vincula plantarly reduces this potential.

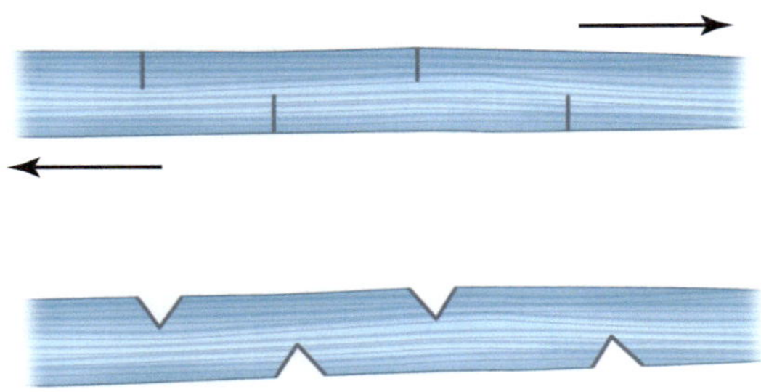

Fig. 14.7 Diagrammatic impression of multiple Z lengthening technique

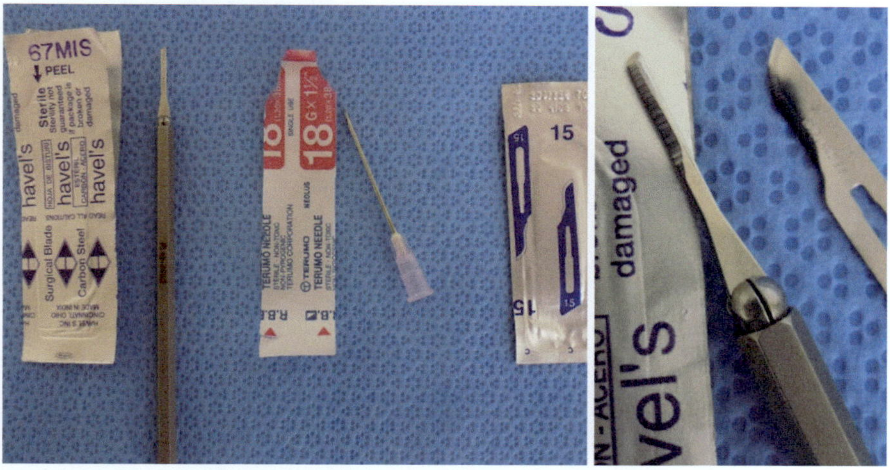

Fig. 14.8 Examples of instruments that can be used for percutaneous tendon lengthening. Note contrast between a standard 15 blade and a mini 67 blade

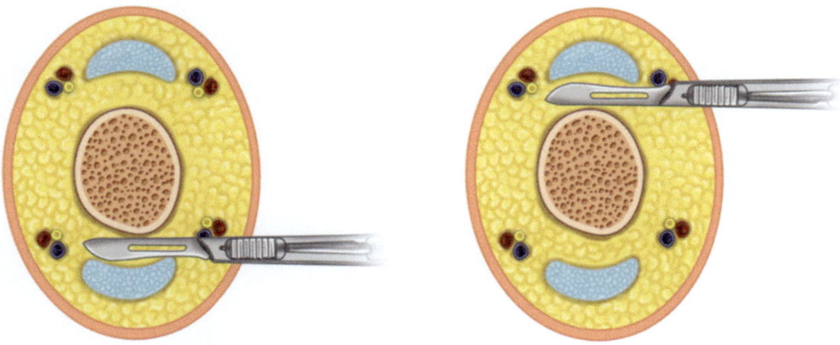

Fig. 14.9 Traditional approaches describe the blade has been rotated to allow release of the tendon. Potential neurovascular injury is a potential concern

Percutaneous approaches also allow for release or lengthening of the short flexors in addition to the long flexor/extensors selectively as required (Fig. 14.11).

Post-operative Care

In all cases of isolated tendon lengthening and/or tenotomy, meticulous attention to post-operative splinting is required for a minimum of 4 weeks. Initially, operative dressings should be applied to achieve this goal followed by low-allergenic tape or

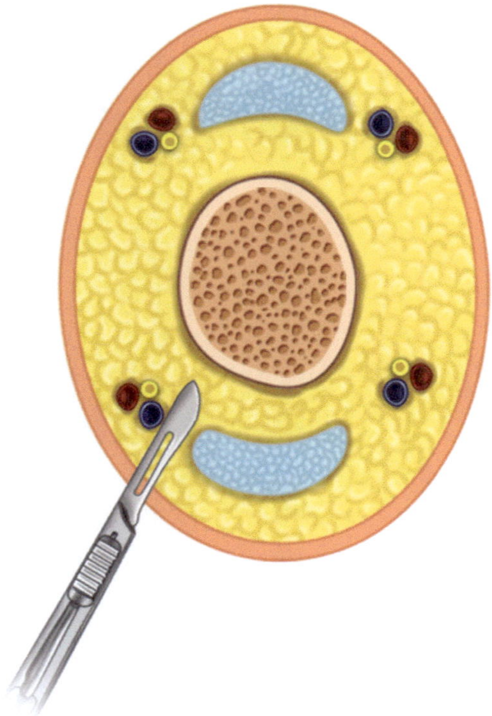

Fig. 14.10 An alternative approach involves approaching the tendon more directly and angling the blade towards the bone. Using this technique the surgeon can also approach the tendon via both medial and lateral incisions

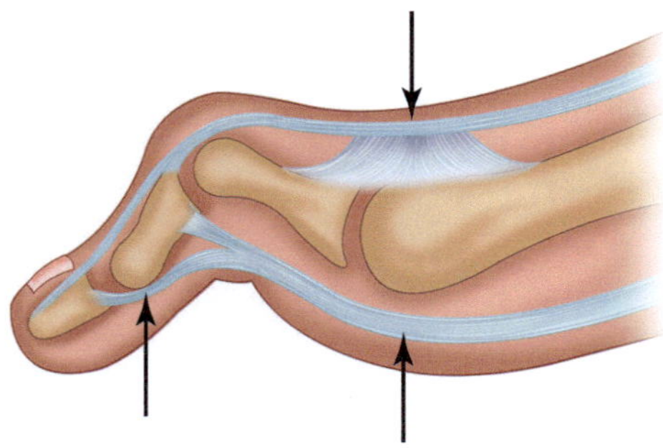

Fig. 14.11 The above diagram illustrates the locations of portal entry to effect release for the various tendon contractures encountered with toe imbalance. Note that each entry point is within either the flexor or extensor expansion

Steri-Strips. Taping can be followed with individually prepared silicon splints (Fig. 14.12).

Such splinting may require regular changing by a trained therapist to ensure that the correction is not lost. To augment this splinting, author preference is to utilise a solid-sole post-operative sandal for 2–3 weeks post tendon lengthening procedures

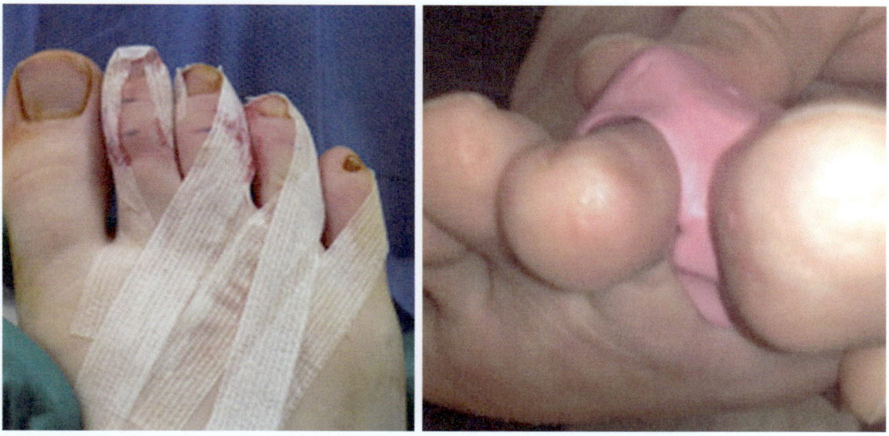

Fig. 14.12 Examples of post-operative splinting. Immediate post-tendon lengthening using Steri-Strips. Taping using nonallergenic tape should continue for the first 4 weeks. This can be followed by the use of silicon splints

even if the procedure is performed in isolation of osseous procedures. This maintenance of digital position is required to reduce potential for inappropriate loss of flexor or extensor power to one of all the digits as a complication of tendon lengthening.

Outcomes

Tendon lengthening although technically considered relatively simple to perform requires skill in assessment, operative planning and meticulous post-operative care. Adverse outcomes may occur if these principles are not adhered to.

Adverse outcomes include iatrogenic deformity in the form of variations of swan neck deformity [18, 20] or loss of muscle function to one or more digits with associated instability. Complete loss of function although a potential risk post tendon lengthening of the toes has not been reported broadly in the literature and can be regarded as a low risk assuming appropriate perioperative care is undertaken. Management of expectations from both a clinician and patient perspective is key to address concerns in respect of over- or under-correction which may be seen with tendon lengthening in isolation.

However, the outcomes are generally considered acceptable when appropriate techniques are used providing significant improvement in digital deformity even where a deformity appears semi-rigid (Fig. 14.13).

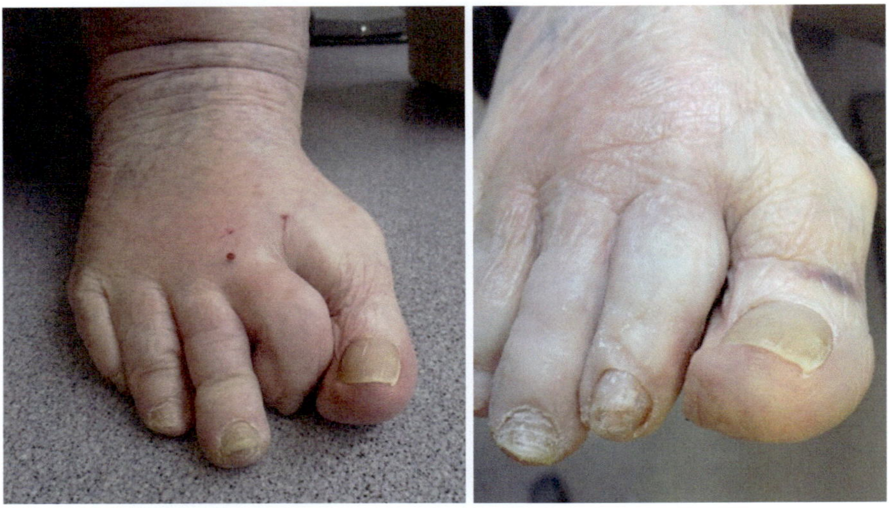

Fig. 14.13 Significant semi-rigid deformity with apical lesion in a patient not fit for osseous procedures. One month post ambulatory percutaneous flexors release (longus and brevis) with release of proximal interphalangeal joint capsule. The extensor structures were preserved

Swan Neck Deformity: A Unique Complication of Flexor Tendon Lengthening

Swan neck deformity has been described as a hyperextension deformity arising from rupture of the plantar plate of flexor tendons of the toes and fingers described originally as associated with rheumatoid arthritis [20] (Fig. 14.14). The condition can affect either the distal or proximal interphalangeal joints. This can be an iatrogenic complication of tendon lengthening most particularly when FDL is tenotomised in isolation. This is more of a risk if excessive tension in FDB is not addressed or the plantar ligamentous/capsular structures of the distal interphalangeal joint are inadvertently released (Figs. 14.13 and 14.14).

Joint hypermobility can also be a precursor to this deformity if tendon lengthening is performed without assessment of inherent joint stability (Fig. 14.15).

To avoid the formation of swan neck deformity when performing flexor lengthening procedures, the surgeon should consider what the effect of releasing FDL on the stability of the proximal and distal interphalangeal joints will be. Consideration to concurrent lengthening of FDB is essential. However, when performing complete resection of both flexors, the potential for instability and/or loss of function should be discussed [21].

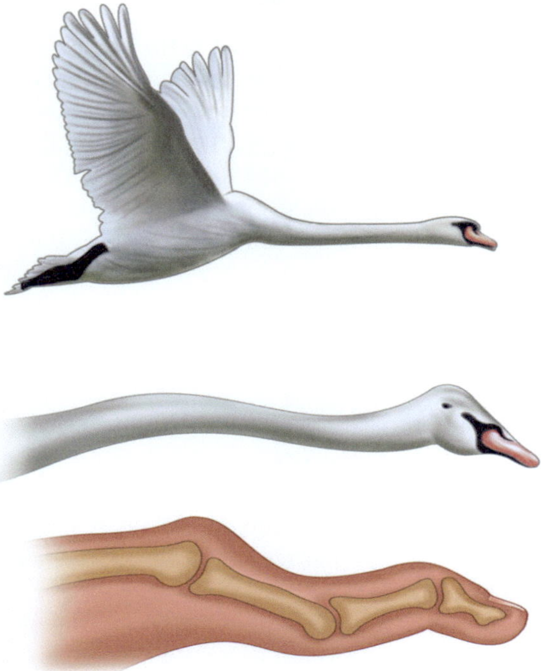

Fig. 14.14 Swan neck deformity. (Adapted from Dreyfus)

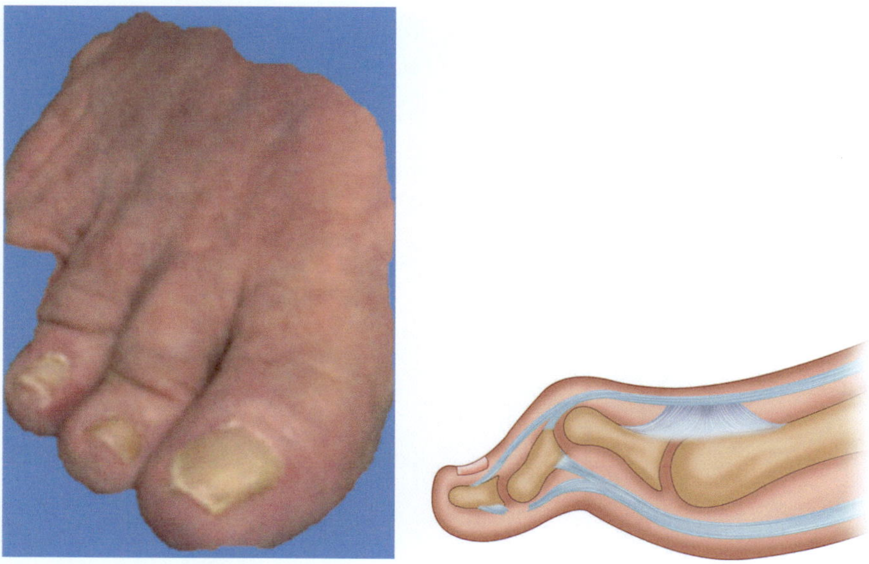

Fig. 14.15 Distal interphalangeal (DIP) joint swan neck deformity post FDL lengthening without lengthening of FDB

Clinical Pearls for Tendon Lengthening

Percutaneous isolated tendon lengthening is ideally suited to an ambulatory environment under local anaesthetic. This also allows the patient to assist by contracting the flexor or extensor during the procedure which provides the surgeon real-time feedback as to the degree of lengthening achieved.

After all tendon lengthening procedures, post-operative splinting utilising either internal splints such as K-wire or external splints such as a bandage or taping is critical to maintaining the tendon at its desired length.

Splinting should be utilised for 4 weeks as a minimum.

Capsulotomy and ligament release or balance are often required to reduce persistent contracture. This can also be performed percutaneously and concurrently to tendon lengthening.

Care is required when performing plantar capsulotomy at the DIP or PIP to avoid potential swan neck deformity.

Healing of the tendon with return to function is an expectation post tendon lengthening. Lack of appropriate splinting may allow healing of the tendon in a persistent contracted state. Similarly inappropriate lengthening and splinting may result in dysfunction (Fig. 14.16).

Positioning of the portal to enable lengthening procedure and choice of blade will influence recovery (Fig. 14.17).

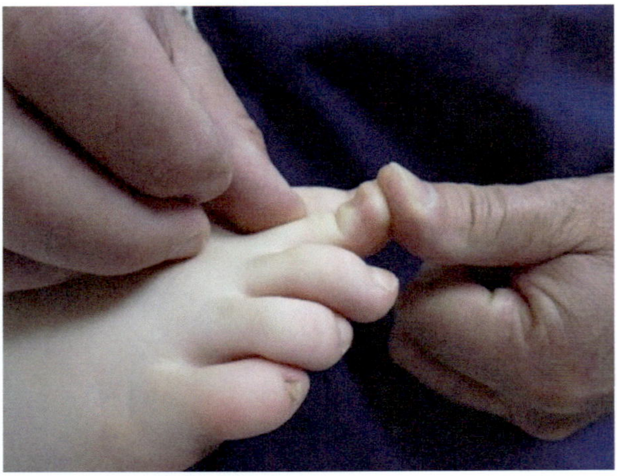

Fig. 14.16 DIP joint hypermobility. Care to preserve plantar ligament structures when performing flexor lengthening is paramount in this circumstance

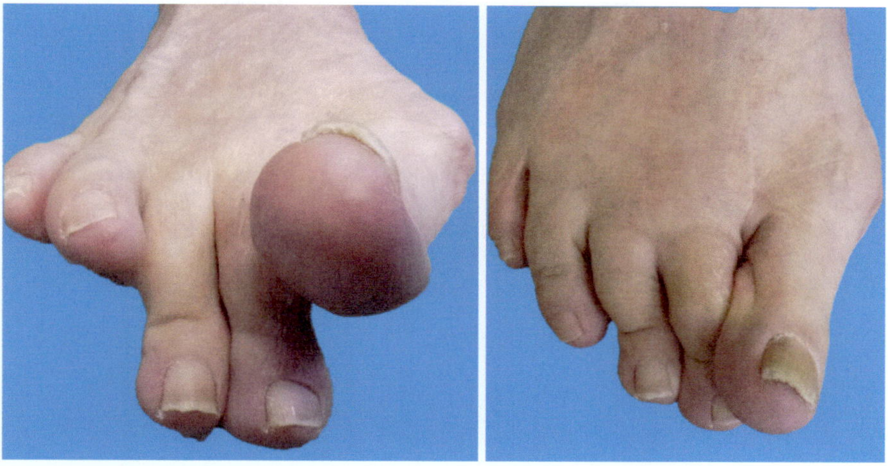

Fig. 14.17 Painful second and third overload during weight bearing post excessive and inappropriate lengthening/release of EDL to the second and third toes. The picture on the left is non-weight bearing and on the right is weight bearing

References

1. Ellington K. Hammertoes and clawtoes: proximal interphalangeal joint correction. Foot Ankle Clin. 2011;16:547–58.
2. Thomas JL, et al. Diagnosis and treatment of forefoot disorders. Section 1: digital deformities. J Foot Ankle Surg. 2009;48(2):230–8.
3. Coughlin M. Chapter 7: Lesser toe deformities. In: Coughlin M, Saltzman MR, editors. Surgery of the foot and ankle. 8th ed. Philadelphia: Mosby; 2007.
4. McGlamry ED, et al. Chapter 9: Lesser ray deformities. In: Banks A, Downey M, Martin D, Miller S, editors. Foot and ankle surgery. 3rd ed. Philadelphia: Lippincott; 2001.
5. Isham S, Nunez O. Isham hammertoe procedures for the correction of lesser digital deformities. In: Maffuli N, Easly M, editors. Minimally invasive surgery of the foot and ankle. London/Dordrecht/Heidelberg/New York: Springer; 2011. p. 171–83.
6. Dockery G. Chap. 25: Digital procedures. In: Dockery G, Crawford M, editors. Lower extremity soft tissue & cutaneous plastic surgery: Saunders. ISBN: 9780702049514.
7. Molloy A, Shariff R. Mallet toe deformity. Foot Ankle Clin. 2011;16:537–46.
8. Solan MC, Davies MS. Revision surgery of the lesser toes. Foot Ankle Clin. 2011;16:621–45.
9. Roukis TS, Schade VL. Percutaneous flexor tenotomy for treatment of neuropathic toe ulceration secondary to toe contracture in persons with diabetes: a systematic review. J Foot Ankle Surg. 2009;48(6):684–9.
10. Kearney TP, Hunt NA, Lavery LA. Safety and effectiveness of flexor tenotomies to heal toe ulcers in persons with diabetes. Diabetes Res Clin Pract. 2010;89:224–6.
11. van Netten JJ, Bril A, van Baal JG. The effect of flexor tenotomy on healing and prevention of neuropathic diabetic foot ulcers on the distal end of the toe. J Foot Ankle Res. 2013;6(1):3.
12. Tamir E, Vigler M, Avisar E, Finestone AS. Percutaneous tenotomy for the treatment of diabetic toe ulcers. Foot Ankle Int. 2014;35(1):38–43.
13. Joost CM, Schrier JCM, Verheyen C, Louwerens JW. Definitions of hammer toe and claw toe. an evaluation of the literature. J Am Podiatr Med Assoc. 2009;99(3):194–7.
14. Schrier JC, Louwerens JW, Verheyen CC. Opinions on lesser toe deformities among Dutch orthopaedic departments. Foot Ankle Int. 2007;28(12):1265–70.

15. Barakat MJ, Gargan MJ. Deformities of the lesser toes – how should we describe them? The Foot. 2006;16:16–8.
16. Caselli MA, George DH. Foot deformities: biomechanical and pathomechanical changes associated with aging, Part I. Clin Podiatr Med Surg. 2003;20(3):487–509.
17. Coughlin MJ. Operative treatment of the mallet toe deformity. Foot Ankle Int. 1995;16(3):109–16.
18. Myerson MS, Jung HG. The role of toe flexor-to-extensor transfer in correcting metatarsophalangeal joint instability of the second toe. Foot Ankle Int. 2005;26:675–9.
19. Sarrafian SK. Anatomy of the foot and ankle. Descriptive topographic functional. 2nd ed. Philadelphia: Lippincott; 1993. p. 283–03 & 551–8.
20. Dreyfus JN, Schnitzer TJ. Pathogenesis and differential diagnosis of the swan-neck deformity. Semin Arthritis Rheum. 1983;13(2):200–11.
21. Bauer T. Percutaneous forefoot surgery. Orthop Traumatol Surg Res. 2014;100:191–204.

Chapter 15
Flexor to Extensor Tendon Transfers

Kris DiNucci and Kenneth Hegewald

Presentation/History

Hammertoe deformity in the presence of deformity at the metatarsophalangeal joint can be a challenging clinical entity for foot and ankle surgeons. The progressive nature of hammertoe deformities can lead to subtle subluxation, instability, and possible digital dislocation across the metatarsophalangeal joint. As the deformity progresses, worsening in sagittal plane and transverse plane alignment is typical.

Patients will often seek treatment options when the dorsal aspect of the lesser digits begins to encroach on shoe gear causing pain and inflammation. As the deformity progresses, patients may complain of more diffuse pain across the forefoot. Obtaining a comprehensive history is important in identifying and differentiating plantar plate injuries as this separate entity may need additional surgical attention. Patients may complain of lack of digital purchase, which should raise concern to integrity of the plantar plate. Key elements in the history include patient activity level and duration of symptoms. Chronic hammertoe deformities are typically more recalcitrant to common surgical approaches and may require adjunctive procedures to stabilize digital contracture while correcting deformity. When dorsal subluxation persists despite a stepwise approach to hammertoe deformity correction, the flexor digitorum longus to extensor tendon transfer is an excellent surgical adjunctive procedure [1–9].

K. DiNucci (✉)
Foot and Ankle Center of Arizona, Scottsdale, AZ, USA

K. Hegewald
Cascade Orthopedics and Sports Medicine Center, Hood River, OR, USA

E. A. Cook, J. J. Cook (eds.), *Hammertoes*,
https://doi.org/10.1007/978-3-319-16552-3_15

Diagnosis/Assessment

After obtaining a comprehensive history with a judicious physical examination is important with special attention to key areas. Reducibility of the deformity should be assessed, as this will require additional ancillary procedures. Fixed deformities will often require arthroplasty or arthrodesis to obtain deformity correction, while more supple deformities may be amenable to soft tissue balancing and reconstruction. A full weight-bearing examination should be performed to assess deformity when the foot is loaded (Fig. 15.1). A gait evaluation will show a non-weight-bearing deformity through the swing phase of gait and expose extensor substitution and can further give clues on etiology and appropriate treatment options.

After assessing flexibility of the digit, special attention should be given to evaluate stability across the metatarsophalangeal joint. A vertical stress test has been previously described to assess stability across the metatarsophalangeal joint [10]. Variations in this technique have also been described. Evaluation of the plantar plate integrity can be evaluated clinically by grasping the proximal phalanx and applying a dorsiflexion translocation drawer stress with the other hand grasping the metatarsal neck (Fig. 15.2). Gross instability across the metatarsophalangeal joint is suspicious for plantar plate insufficiency, and surgical treatments to address this pathology may be necessary.

Further diagnostic workup includes weight-bearing radiographs of the foot to assess and isolate deformity in all three planes. Weight-bearing AP, lateral, and oblique views are the standard protocol for assessment. Advanced imaging techniques are rarely indicated unless there is further suspicion for the presence of plantar plate pathology. In these instances, the authors prefer metatarsophalangeal arthrogram, which can be easily performed with a radio opaque contrast agent and access to a fluoroscopy unit. Contrast dye is injected under live fluoroscopic imaging.

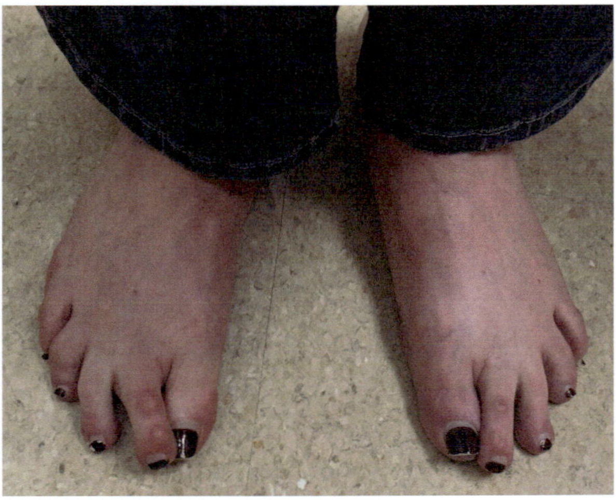

Fig. 15.1 Weight-bearing evaluation, showing accentuation of transverse plane deformity

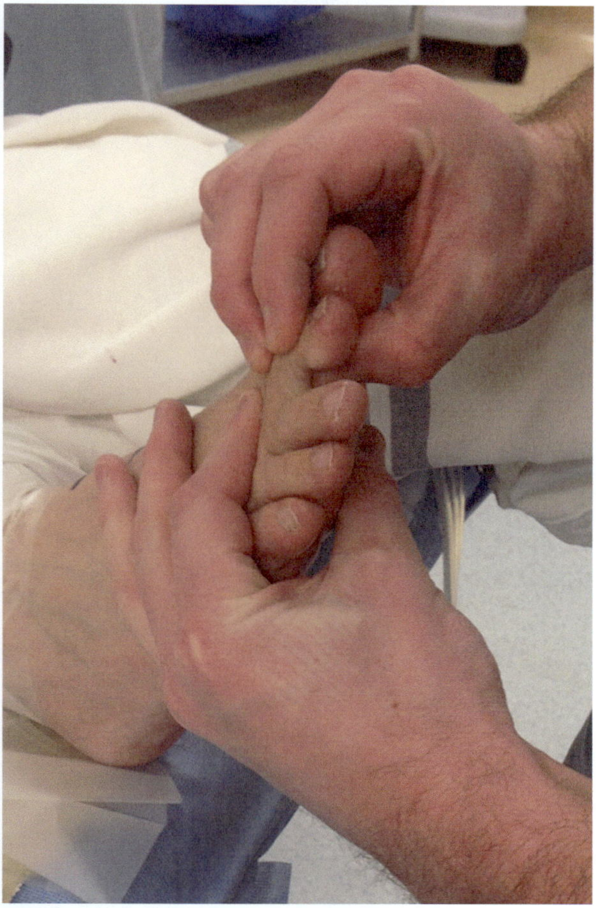

Fig. 15.2 Vertical stress test of metatarsophalangeal joint

Extravasation of the dye beyond the capsular lining suggests tear of the plantar plate (Fig. 15.3). Further diagnostic modalities to assess plantar plate integrity include ultrasound and magnetic resonance imaging [11]. While imaging can be helpful in isolation of deformity and pathology, a thorough physical examination and history are key for a complete presurgical evaluation.

Surgical Technique

Several surgical techniques have been described for flexor to extensor tendon transfers [1–9]. Techniques vary based on tendon harvest point, tendon routing, and fixation methods. Three surgical techniques will be described.

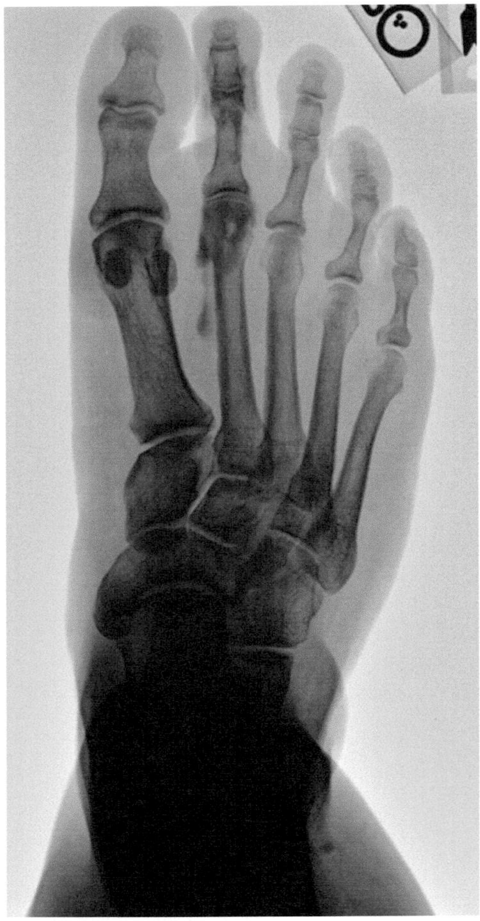

Fig. 15.3 Extravasation of contrast dye after capsular injection

Technique One: Split Flexor Digitorum Longus

A standard dorsal incision is performed over the digit. Incision should allow full visualization of middle and proximal phalanx while avoiding excessive skin tension during retraction. The long extensor tendon is transected at the level of the proximal interphalangeal joint. Arthrotomy is performed of the proximal interphalangeal joint. Medial and lateral collateral ligaments should be sharply released from the proximal phalangeal head and middle phalangeal base to allow full visualization. A standard arthroplasty is performed and the head of the proximal phalanx is removed. If performing interphalangeal arthrodesis, the articular cartilage at the base of the middle phalanx is removed or the joint is prepared by the surgeon's preference. A longitudinal incision is performed though the interphalangeal fibrous plate. Depth control is important to avoid damage to underlying flexor tendons. At this point a hemostat can be utilized to split the medial and lateral flexor digitorum brevis tendon slips. After separating the medial and lateral tendon slips of the short flexor, the long flexor tendon is seen centrally. The long flexor is grasped utilizing hemostat or right angle. The digit is then placed in maximal plantarflexion to obtain maximum length. The tendon is then cut as distally as possible while keeping brevis tendon slips intact. The long flexor tendon is split longitudinally at midline and separated. Approximately 1.0–1.5 cm of the tendon is split. The medial and lateral aspects of the tendon are brought dorsally (Fig. 15.4). If IPJ arthrodesis is to be performed, fixation is employed at this time. The paratenon of the tendon is removed to allow for appropriate tenodesis. The digit is plantarflexed to appropriate level, and the flexor tendon is the sewn into place at the dorsal aspect of the proximal phalanx. It is important the foot is placed in a simulated weight-bearing position to assure of appropriate physiologic tension across the transfer site. The long extensor tendon is then repaired. The transfer is completed by securing the flexor tendon to the extensor tendon via suture methods at surgeon's preference. This step is important to avoid proximal migration of the tendon transfer on the proximal phalanx and a resultant loss of correction.

Technique Two: Transfer via Osseous Tunnel

Dissection is performed as described above. The long extensor tendon is transected and retracted proximally to the level of the metatarsophalangeal joint to allow full exposure of the base of the proximal phalanx. Release of the long flexor tendon is performed as described above. Alternatively, the long flexor can be released through small stab incision at the central aspect of the plantar interphalangeal joint. The DIP is dorsiflexed to allow sharp release of the long flexor tendon. A dorsal to plantar osseous tunnel is then created at the base of the proximal phalanx. Sequential

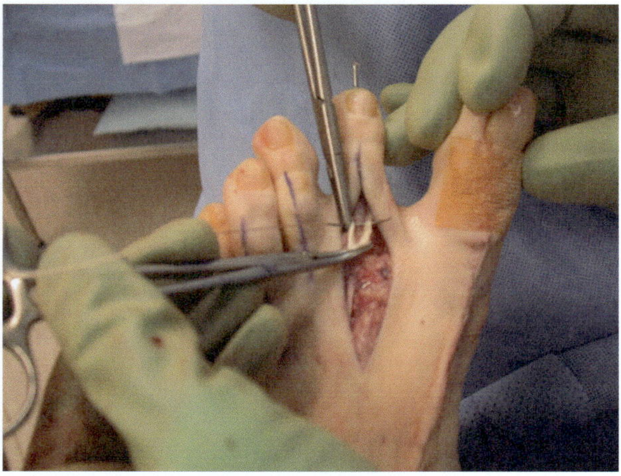

Fig. 15.4 Split long flexor tendon being sutured over dorsal aspect of proximal phalanx

drillings are performed from 2.0–3.5 mm taking care to avoid destruction of the medial and lateral cortex. Modifications in drill size may be necessary depending on size of the digit. Drilling is performed in the metaphyseal portion of the base distal enough to avoid destruction of the subchondral plate, preserving the articular integrity of phalangeal base. The long flexor tendon is then routed dorsally through the osseous tunnel (Fig. 15.5). This can be performed by creating a suture lasso with 21 gauge wire or similar tendon passing instruments (Fig. 15.6). The digit is plantarflexed to reduce deformity and correction is held with use of a hemostat. The transfer is completed after repair of the extensor tendon, by suturing the long flexor tendon into the long extensor tendon.

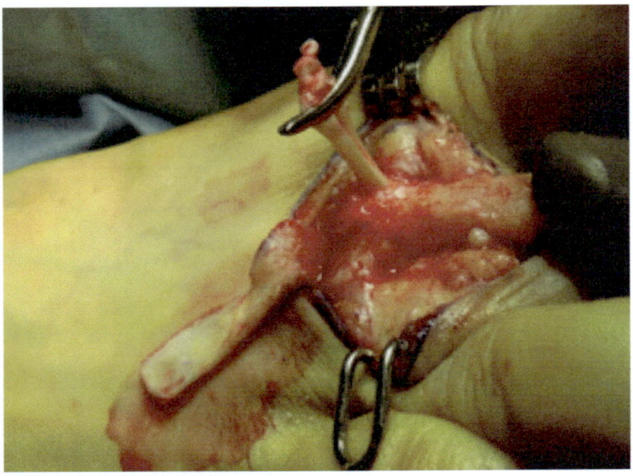

Fig. 15.5 Routing the long flexor tendon through osseous tunnel

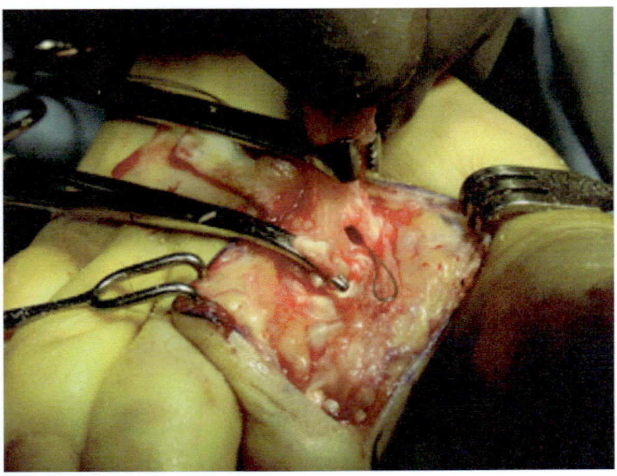

Fig. 15.6 Lasso technique for tendon transfer

Technique Three: Medial/Lateral Transfer

This technique can be performed without long extensor tenotomy, and proximal interphalangeal joint arthrotomy is not necessary. Incision is carried along the medial or lateral aspect of the digit taking care to avoid underlying neurovascular damage (Fig. 15.7). Subperiosteal dissection is performed along the medial or lateral aspect of the proximal phalanx. The authors find this method preferred when concomitant transverse plane deformity is present. For instance, if adduction deformity is noted, a lateral approach will allow transverse plane deformity correction when transfer is completed.

Dissection is carried plantarly in subperiosteal fashion to the flexor tendons. The brevis is split to allow access to the long flexor tendon as described above. The long flexor is cut after maximal plantarflexion of the digit. The long flexor is brought dorsally along the proximal phalanx (Fig. 15.8). The digit is plantarflexed, and the long flexor tendon is sewn into the long extensor tendon to complete the transfer (Fig. 15.9). Subtle transverse plane correction should be anticipated.

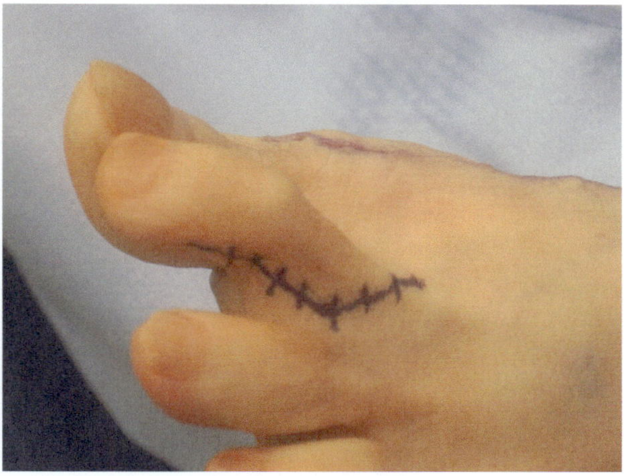

Fig. 15.7 Incision placement for lateral approach to long flexor tendon

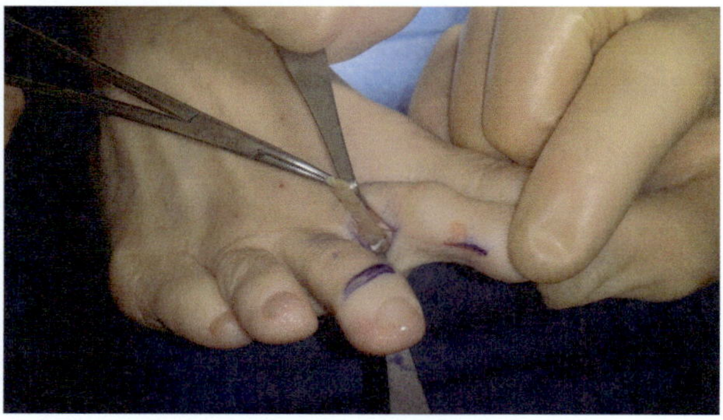

Fig. 15.8 Flexor tendon brought dorsally through lateral approach

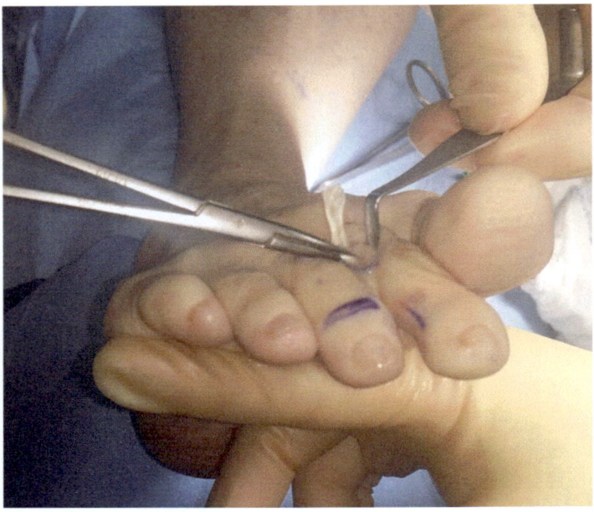

Fig. 15.9 Completion of tendon transfer with tenodesis to long extensor tendon

Outcome/Case Resolution

When performed correctly the flexor to extensor tendon transfer is a powerful and efficacious augmentation in digital deformity correction. Several studies have demonstrated the usefulness and long-term efficacy of this procedure [6–9]. The procedure allows for immediate weight-bearing and range of motion in a protective postoperative shoe. It is not uncommon for edema to persist for several months after the procedure, and occasionally patients will notice extra tissue along the dorsal aspect of the transfer site. When meticulous dissection and soft tissue handling are performed, the procedure allows for low complication rates. Fracture of the digit postoperatively after flexor digitorum longus transfer has been described [12]. Furthermore, surgeons should be cautious of large deformity correction and potential vascular embarrassment, which can lead to tissue necrosis and gangrene. To circumvent these complications, meticulous dissection is important as well as appropriate preoperative work up to ensure adequate vascular perfusion.

Clinical Pearls/Pitfalls

- Extensive dissection should be avoided to prevent potential neurovascular damage and vascular embarrassment to the digit.
- Care should be taken to preserve the extensor digitorum brevis tendon slips thereby preserving function when performing an arthrodesis of the interphalangeal joint.
- Use of a hemostat for temporary fixation of flexor tendon allows for evaluation of appropriate tension prior to tenodesis with extensor tendon.
- Debridement of the tendon slips to remove the paratenon is important to allow for appropriate tenodesis.

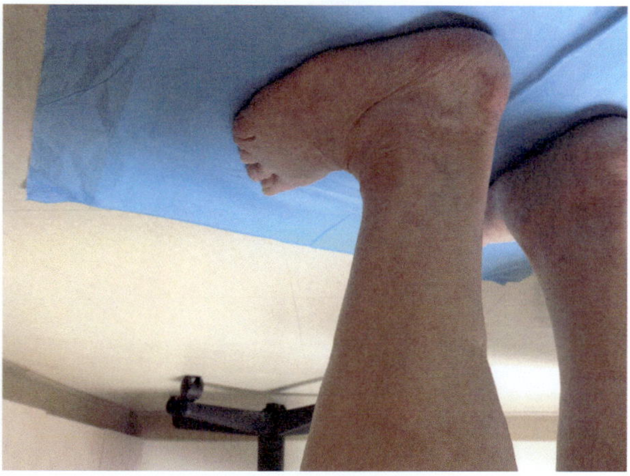

Fig. 15.10 Pre-operative hammertoe presentation

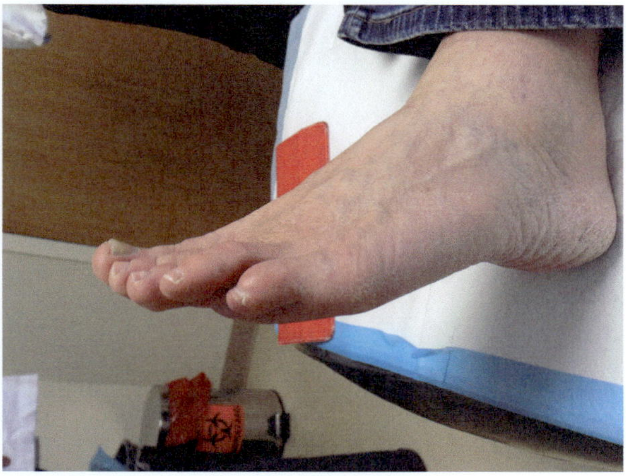

Fig. 15.11 Post-operative hammertoe correction

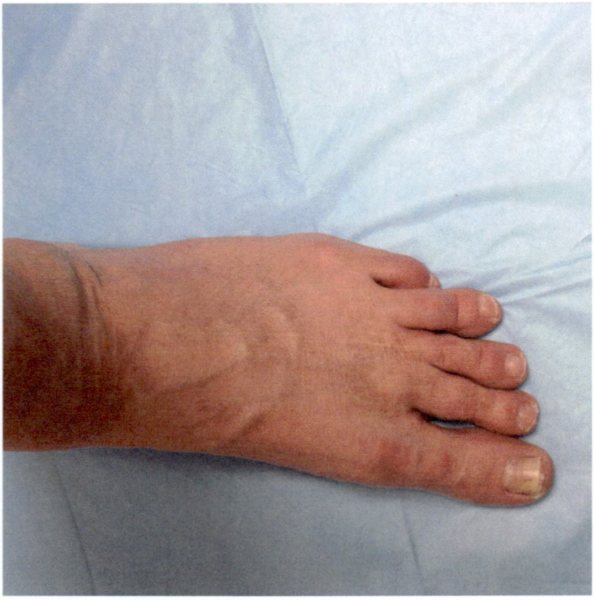

Fig. 15.12 Post-operative hammertoe correction

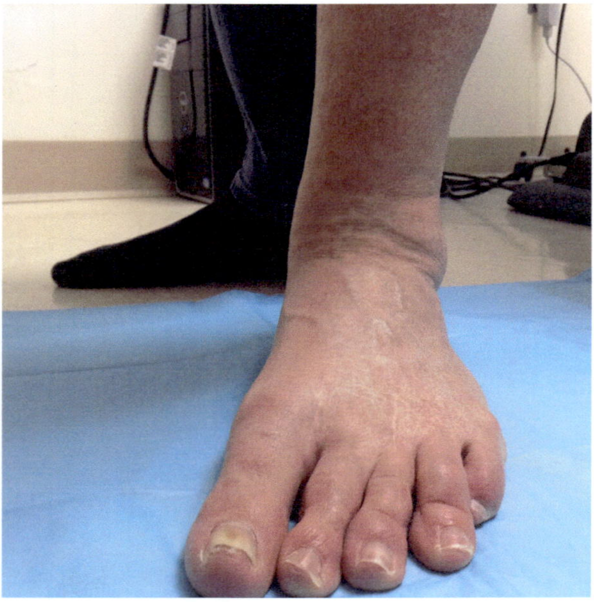

Fig. 15.13 Post-operative hammertoe correction

References

1. Taylor RG. The treatment of claw toes by multiple transfers of flexor into extensor tendons. J Bone Joint Surg. 1951;33:539–42.
2. Sgarlato TE. Transplantation of the flexor digitorum longus muscle tendon in hammertoes. J Am Podiatry Assoc. 1970;60(10):383–8.
3. Kuwada GT. A retrospective analysis of modification of the flexor tendon transfer for correction of hammer toe. J Foot Surg. 1988;27(1):57–9.
4. Thompson FM, Deland JT. Flexor tendon transfer for metatarsophalangeal instability of the second toe. Foot Ankle. 1993;14(7):385–8.
5. Schuberth JM, Jensen R. Flexor digitorum longus transfer for second metatarsophalangeal joint dislocation/subluxation. In: Reconstructive surgery of the foot and leg. Update '97. Tucker: The Podiatry Institute; 1997. p. 11–4.
6. Myerson MS, Jung HG. The role of toe flexor-to-extensor transfer in correcting metatarsophalangeal joint instability of the second toe. Foot Ankle Int. 2005;26(9):675–9.
7. Boyer ML, DeOrio JK. Transfer of the flexor digitorum longus for the correction of lesser-toe deformities. Foot Ankle Int. 2007;28(4):422–30.
8. Barbari SG, Brevig K. Correction of clawtoes by the Girdlestone-Taylor flexor-extensor transfer procedure. Foot Ankle. 1984;5(2):67–73.
9. Bouche RT, Heit EJ. Combined plantar plate and hammertoe repair with flexor digitorum longus tendon transfer for chronic, severe sagittal plane instability of the lesser metatarsophalangeal joints: preliminary observations. J Foot Ankle Surg. 2008;47(2):125–37.
10. Thompson FM, Hamilton WG. Problems of the second metatarsophalangeal joint. Orthopedics. 1987;10:83–7.
11. Klein EE, Weil L Jr, Weil LS, Knight J. Magnetic resonance imaging versus musculoskeletal ultrasound for identification and localization of plantar plate tears. Foot Ankle Spec. 2012;5(6):359–65.
12. Fishco WD, Roth BJ. Digital fracture after a flexor tendon transfer for hammertoe repair: a case report. J Foot Ankle Surg. 2010;49:179–81.

Chapter 16
Tendon Transfers for Digital Deformities and Hammertoes

Lawrence A. DiDomenico, Frank A. Luckino III, and Danielle N. Butto

Presentation/History

Digital deformities may present in a variety of forms. Mallet toe, hammertoe, claw toe, and curly toe deformities have all been described [1]. Shoe gear, genetics, neuromuscular imbalances, inflammatory arthritis, and trauma have all been shown to be potential causes [1–3]. Though most of the literature would point to a biomechanical imbalance between the extrinsic and intrinsic musculature, three categories have been described for classification of digital deformities: flexor stabilization, flexor substitution, and extensor substitution [4].

Mallet toe is a flexion contracture in the sagittal plane of the distal phalanx on the middle phalanx at the distal interphalangeal joint (DIPJ). The deformities are usually fixed; however, they can present as flexible or semirigid too. Pain is caused due to repetitive trauma of the distal toe hitting the ground or the irritation to the dorm of distal interphalangeal joint. This trauma can cause a distal toe callus and/or ulceration with an associated bursitis to the interphalangeal joint. Correction of a mallet toe is achieved by removal of the deforming flexor digitorum longus tendon force [5] and releasing the interphalangeal contracture if needed.

L. A. DiDomenico (✉)
Department of Surgery, St. Elizabeth Health Center, Youngstown, OH, USA

Northside Medical Center, Youngstown, OH, USA

F. A. Luckino III
Northeast Ohio Foot and Ankle Specialists, Canton, OH, USA

Mercy Medical Center, Canton, OH, USA

D. N. Butto
Trinity Health of New England Medical Group, Hartford, CT, USA

Saint Francis Hospital, Hartford, CT, USA

E. A. Cook, J. J. Cook (eds.), *Hammertoes*,
https://doi.org/10.1007/978-3-319-16552-3_16

A hammertoe is a deformity which is typically associated with a contracture in the sagittal plane at the proximal interphalangeal joint (PIPJ). This deformity can have a component of transverse and frontal plane deformity too. The middle phalanx is plantarflexed on the proximal phalanx. The deformity sometimes involves a dorsal contracture at the metatarsophalangeal joint. The distal interphalangeal joint is in either a flexed, extended, or neutral position [6]. A dorsal, painful callus or ulceration is often present over the PIPJ.

A curly toe is characterized by a flexion contracture, internal rotation, and varus deformity of the interphalangeal joints of the affected toes. Curly toe deformities are often seen in pediatric patients [7]. On the other hand, an adductovarus deformity occurs at the proximal interphalangeal joint in the frontal and sagittal planes. The deformity commonly occurs with a pronated foot type. The quadratus plantae loses its normal vector pull. The direction of pull is shifted medially, therefore creating a varus and adductus pull on the digit [8].

The crossover hammertoe presents with pain and swelling at the plantar aspect of the metatarsophalangeal joint capsule. As the deformity progresses, the proximal phalanx hyperextends and deviates in a coronal or sagittal plane and usually crosses over the great toe. The second digit is the most common digit affected [9]. The plantar plate is often ruptured in this deformity.

A heloma dura can be present at either the proximal interphalangeal joint or distal interphalangeal joint. When present on the lateral nail fold, the lesion is called a Lister's corn. An interdigital heloma molle develops because of the malalignment of the toes associated with deformity resulting in increased pressure between the lateral aspect of the base of the fourth digit proximal phalanx and the medial aspect of the head of the fifth digit proximal phalanx. The etiology is secondary to malalignment of an enlarged or deformed distal, middle, or proximal phalanx [8].

A claw toe is characterized by hyperextension of the MTP joint and flexion of the PIP and DIP joint. With a claw toe, there may be an associated callosity beneath the involved head of the metatarsal, overlying the PIP joint, and even at the tip of the toe [10].

Each of the types of hammertoes can be associated with pain, soft tissue irritation, and callus formation than can lead to ulceration. In addition, when a hammertoe deformity is present and there is a dorsal contracture at the metatarsalphalangeal joint causing retrograde pressure, there is a significant increase in plantar pressure present at the metatarsal head and a distal displacement in the fat pad which can lead to pain, soft tissue changes, callus formation, and ulceration [11].

It is important to identify the underlying cause of the hammertoe deformity. Flexor stabilization typically occurs in a pronated foot type. As the foot pronates, the flexor digitorum longus fires earlier in the gait cycle gaining a mechanical advantage over the interossei muscles. An adductovarus rotation of the fourth and/or fifth digit is typically present [12, 13]. Flexor substitution is often associated with a weak triceps surae. The deep posterior group musculature overpowers to accommodate for the weak triceps surae. The flexors gain an advantage over the interossei [12].

Extensor substitution occurs in the swing phase of gait with the long extensors gaining a mechanical advantage over the lumbricals [12]. Generally there is contracture at the metatarsalphalangeal joint level with bowstringing of the extensor tendons [13]. Neuromuscular disorders such as Charcot-Marie-Tooth (CMT), poliomyelitis, muscular dystrophies, and lumbar disc disease may lead to contractures at the metatarsophalangeal and interphalangeal joints (IPJ) of the lesser digits [2] manifesting most commonly as a claw toe deformity. A high-arched, cavus foot type is often exhibited with this type of deformity as well [14]. Hibbs originally termed this foot type a "claw foot" where there are high arch, plantar calluses, and prominent metatarsal heads secondary to the digital deformities [15]. Though this type of digital contracture is typically seen in patients with neuromuscular disease [16], it can be seen in a flatfoot deformity, as well as rheumatoid and diabetic patients [4].

A thorough history from the patient is crucial. Patients may relate a positive family history of a high-arched foot type with neuropathic type symptoms. Muscle weakness with complaints of a foot drop with tripping or instability with gait may be present [17]. A patient may describe difficulty with shoe gear secondary to prominences at the dorsal and proximal IPJs. Callus formation secondary to prominent metatarsal heads leads to metatarsalgia as a common complaint [14, 16].

Diagnosis/Assessment

A thorough weight-bearing and non-weight-bearing exam, as well as gait analysis, should be performed on all patients. One should employ the Silfverskiold test to assess for underlying equinus deformity. Next, the overall foot type should be classified, and attention is then drawn to the digital deformity or deformities. The involved toes should be evaluated in the sagittal, transverse, and frontal plane. One should determine whether the deformity is flexible, semirigid, or rigid. A push-up test as described by Kelikian with plantar pressure applied at the metatarsalphalangeal joint (MTPJ) will allow one to determine the flexibility of the deformity [14]. Long-standing deformities may lead to dislocation at the level of the MTPJ. The Lachman test can be employed to assess for pathology at the metatarsalphalangeal joint. With the metatarsal immobilized and proximal phalanx held in 20–25° of dorsiflexion, the proximal phalanx is translated vertically. A positive test is greater than 2 mm of dorsal displacement or 50% subluxation to the vertical height of the metatarsal head [18].

Standard, three-view radiographs should be evaluated. The anterior-posterior projection is utilized to assess transverse and sagittal plane deformity [13]. The "gun-barrel sign" is a hallmark of sagittal plane deformity as one visualizes the medullary canal of the middle phalanx [13, 14]. The lateral view clearly demonstrates sagittal plane pathology.

In deformities where pathology of the plantar plate is in question, an MRI can be ordered for further evaluation. On T1-weighted images, the plantar plate is seen as a continuous low-signal structure. On gradient-echo images, the plantar plate is slightly hyperintense from the flexor tendons. In plantar plate rupture, the signal is higher in intensity and more widespread, extending beyond the immediate area of the plate attachment on the proximal phalangeal base. Proximal-to-distal continuity of the plate is lost and the rupture is isointense with synovium and joint fluid. Associated findings include MTPJ synovitis and synovitis or effusion in the flexor tendon sheath [19].

In order to understand the disease process, one must have a sound understanding of the anatomy. The MTPJ, PIPJ, and DIPJ are stabilized by collateral ligaments obliquely on either side of the joint. Plantar stability is provided by the plantar plate, a thick fibrocartilaginous structure that prevents dorsal subluxation of the digit at the MTPJ level [13]. The extensor digitorum longus tendon acts as a dorsiflexor of the ankle through the swing phase of gait. The tendon splits once it passes the ankle into four separate slips which insert on the dorsal aspect of the middle and distal phalanges of digits 2–5. The extensor digitorum brevis tendon has three separate slips to digits 2, 3, and 4 and inserts at the extensor expansion of the corresponding EDL tendon. The extensor expansion has attachments plantarly with the capsule, plantar plate, and flexor tendon sheath at the level of the MTPJ. Therefore, the pull of EDL and EDB causes significant dorsiflexory power at the level of the MTPJs and minimal at the IPJs. The flexor digitorum brevis originates at the medial calcaneal tuberosity. It courses distally and splits into two slips that attach to the plantar aspect of middle phalanx. The flexor digitorum longus originates in the posterior compartment of the leg and courses to the digits through the split in FDB tendon to insert on the distal phalanx.

When non-weight-bearing, the long flexor flexes the MTPJ and IPJ. During weight-bearing, the long flexor tendon will pull the distal phalanx proximally, buckling the toe. In a weight-bearing situation, firing of the long flexor alone will produce a claw toe, while pull of the long and short flexors will recreate a true hammertoe [13].

With extensor substitution typically presenting in a neuromuscular disease patient, such as CMT or polio/post-polio, a thorough neuromuscular exam is paramount. The pathomechanics of CMT is well documented; however, this may not correlate with nonprogressive causes for the cavus foot type. Typically in the CMT population, the disease process begins with atrophy of the intrinsic musculature. With loss of stability of the lumbricales at the level of the MTPJ, there is unopposed pull of the long extensor tendons and the long flexor tendons. This causes extension at the MTPJ and flexion of the phalanges. Subsequently, there is a generalized weakness of the tibialis anterior tendon as well as the peroneus brevis tendon. The muscle strength to the long flexors and peroneus longus is preserved. The weakness in the anterior compartment requires the extensor digitorum longus (EDL) tendon to compensate for the lack of dorsiflexion at the level of the ankle. This further exacerbates the hyperextension, hammertoe contracture [20].

DM and RA Foot Types Similar to CMT

The long extensor to the hallux will cause a similar deformity at the great toe as seen in the lesser digits [20]. In Hibbs' original description, he felt there were two concerns that needed to be addressed surgically. First, correction of what he called an "exaggerated arch" and secondly removal of the extensor overpowering to the digits. The former could be corrected through a Steindler stripping and latter correction achieved by the release of the long extensor tendons and transfer of the proximal portion to the lateral cuneiform [15].

Before surgery is being considered for any type of digital contracture, vascular status must always be assessed. Should there be a concern, noninvasive vascular studies with digital pressures and/or toe-brachial indices (TBIs) can be ordered. Further neurologic workup may include an electromyographic (EMG) or a nerve conduction velocity (NCV) study. If the foot deformities have been progressive versus static, this should prompt a more in-depth workup by a neurologist [21].

In preparing the patient for surgery, the surgeon should educate the patient that the digital deformity is a chronic soft tissue pathologic process that has occurred because of tendon imbalance and secondary soft tissue contractures at each segment of the involved joint/joints of the proximal, middle, and distal phalanx. Although the digit as an entity may present as a deformity, each separate segment (proximal, middle, and distal phalanx) does not exhibit any bony pathology. The goal for a successful outcome is to balance the toe and "weaken" the overpowering tendon and "strengthen" the weaker tendon pull to balance the toe. Essentially, the surgeon is removing the deforming soft tissue attachments from the toe, placing the toe in the desired position and then rebuilding the attachments to the toe with tendon transfers under physiologic tension to improve digital alignment and function. The end result should provide a stabile, neutrally placed toe with some weakening in one part of the toe and some strengthening in another part of the toe.

Treatment/Surgical Technique

The Modified Girdlestone–Taylor Procedure (Flexor Digitorum Longus Transfer)

The modified Girdlestone-Taylor procedure is used to treat flexion contractures of the distal interphalangeal joint and/or proximal interphalangeal joint. One can perform the procedure through a midline incision approach on the lateral aspect of the hallux and the medial or lateral aspect of the second, third, and fourth toes and the medial aspect of the fifth toes. By placing the incision on the lateral aspect of the hallux and the medial aspect of the fifth toe, this provides a good location for cosmetic purposes.

It is recommended that one use fine double skin hooks for retraction in order to avoid soft tissue compromise. Deepen the incisions in the same plane being careful to avoid the neurovascular bundles. The dissection is carried to the plantar aspect of the soft tissues of the respective toe. Identify the flexor digitorum longus and trace it distally to its attachment to the distal phalanx. Detach the distal aspect of the flexor digitorum longus, clamp with an Allis clamp, and retrieve proximally within the wound to the web space.

Next, attention is directed to the flexor digitorum brevis tendon. Detach (both the medial and lateral slips) of the tendon from the base of the middle phalanx. A capsulotomy at the interphalangeal joint (for a flexion contracture of the proximal interphalangeal joint) and/or the distal interphalangeal joint is performed allowing the contracture to be reduced.

A K-wire (preferably 0.062 inches) is inserted from the distal tip of the distal phalanx to the base of the proximal phalanx. It has been the authors' experience to be cautious not to overcorrect the flexion contracture by placing the distal interphalangeal joint and the proximal interphalangeal joint into a neutral or extended position and to place it into a neutral to slight plantar flexion position. If an isolated flexor digitorum longus tendon transfer is being performed, there should not be a contracture at the metatarsalphalangeal joint; therefore, there is no need to pin across the metatarsalphalangeal joint with the K-wire. Next, while the toe is held in anatomical alignment and held into the desired position, the flexor digitorum longus tendon is transferred and sutured into the extensor soft tissue (extensor hood) of the proximal phalanx under physiologic tension. The excess tendon of the flexor digitorum longus is resected and the skin is lightly re-approximated with typical skin closure.

Advantages: With the scars located on the lateral aspect of the hallux and the medial or lateral aspect of the second, third, and fourth toes and the medial aspect of the fifth toe, the procedure leaves a much more cosmetic pleasing result. Additionally, by performing the flexor digitorum longus transfer, this removes the pathologic sagittal plane force as well as any additional pathological pull in the frontal and transverse plane allowing the toe to be placed in a neutral position. Postoperatively, there is a much more natural clinical look in terms of the length of the toe. The digits retain stability in the transverse and frontal plane as the medial and lateral collateral ligaments are left intact. The toe is not shortened as there is no bone resection. There is minimal postoperative edema since all the directions consist of soft tissue only and there is no bony involvement which often occurs with bony procedures. Any resulting bursa, hyperkeratosis, and ulceration eventually dissipate as the deforming forces are removed and relieve the pressures.

Since there is no surgery on the bony structures, there is no rotation, shifting, malalignment, or shortening of the digits. The tendon transfer treats the underlying pathology, the dynamic/static deforming force of the tendon, therefore, eliminating the need to disturb the natural osseous structures of the three phalanxes. Postoperatively, the K-wire is removed at approximately 7–10 days based on the patients' preoperative deformity. Lastly, if a problem would occur postoperatively, one could always perform a bony procedure if necessary.

Disadvantages: In terms of disadvantages, this is a more technically challenging surgical procedure in terms of dissection. The approach makes for a difficult space to work between toes. While possible complications are similar to those with any other digital surgery, more unique complications to this procedure consist of overcorrection or hyperextension leading to a recurvatum deformity of the corrected joints, maceration, and wound issues of the incision sites secondary to interdigital contact.

The Modified Hibbs Procedure (Extensor Tendon Transfers)

The modified Hibbs procedure is indicated for patients who exhibit extensor substitution/recruitment. Dorsal subluxations/dislocations at the metatarsalphalangeal joints are frequently linked with claw toes and hammertoes. These deformities typically result with the recruitment of a tight extensor digitorum longus (extensor substitution/recruitment) to support dorsiflexion against a tight posterior muscle group (equinus contracture).

For treating hammertoes 2–5, beginning at the second metatarsalphalangeal joint, make an oblique dorsal incision proximal to the base of the fourth metatarsal. Deepen this incision in the same plane and avoid all neurovascular structures. Be sure to avoid and preserve the superficial nerves in the subcutaneous tissues as these will be running longitudinally. Great care of the soft tissue is essential, and fine double skin hooks are recommended for retraction in order to avoid soft tissue compromise. Identify the extensor tendons (extensor digitorum longus and brevis) and separate only these tendons from the subcutaneous tissues. There is no need to dissect any other tissues other than separating the soft tissues from the extensor digitorum longus and brevis tendon. The extensor digitorum longus and brevis tendons lie deep to the superficial nerves. The surgeon should separate and track the extensor tendons longitudinally. Isolate the second, third, and fourth extensor digitorum longus tendons, respectively, and cut these tendons as far proximal within the incision site. Clamp each one of the most distal aspect of the proximal portion of the cut extensor digitorum longus with a small mosquito hemostat. Clamp the most proximal aspect of the distal cut portion of the extensor digitorum longus tendon with an Allis clamp. The distal cut portions of the extensor digitorum longus tendons are then reflected from the remaining soft tissues as far distally within the incision site and retracted out of the way. The distal portion of the second extensor digitorum longus tendon is reflected distally and temporarily placed in the first web space of the foot. The third extensor digitorum longus tendon is placed similarly in the second web space, and the fourth extensor digitorum longus tendon is placed in third web space. The fifth extensor digitorum longus tendon is identified, and a Z-lengthening procedure is performed allowing the tension and contracture to be released from the fifth extensor digitorum longus tendon.

Attention is directed to the second, third, and fourth metatarsalphalangeal joints as far distal in the incision site. The second, third, and fourth extensor digitorum brevis tendon is traced as far distal within the incision site, and a tenotomy is performed as far distal as possible. An Allis clamp is applied to most proximal portion of the cut second, third, and fourth extensor digitorum brevis tendons, and these tendons are retracted proximal. At this time, complete exposure of the metatarsalphalangeal joint is achieved. A capsulotomy at the second, third, fourth, and fifth metatarsalphalangeal joints is completed. This facilitates release of all contractures via sharp and blunt dissection and/or the use of a McGlamry elevator. Following this release, the surgeon should realize that all the soft tissue deforming forces have now been removed and the digits should naturally revert to a "neutral position."

In most scenarios, when a digit involves the extension contracture, there is also a flexion component in the deformity. In deformities which exhibit both flexion and extension deformities, additional soft tissue procedures need to be performed to address flexion contractures of the second, third, fourth, and fifth digits (flexor tendon transfers). The flexor tendon transfer is then performed at each toe. Once this is accomplished, insert a 0.062 K-wire from the distal aspect of the toes through the distal interphalangeal joint, the proximal interphalangeal joint, and the metatarsophalangeal joint to the base of the second, third, fourth, and fifth metatarsals. Ensure there is good anatomical alignment of the toe relative to the metatarsal. Be sure the distal interphalangeal joint, the proximal interphalangeal joint, and the metatarsophalangeal joints are maintained and the toe is in the desired position.

Next, proceed to back to the dorm of the foot and perform a tendon transfer (a weave graft) of the distal stump of the proximal extensor digitorum brevis into the most proximal portion of the distal extensor digitorum longus stump of digits 2, 3, and 4 under physiologic tension. This tendon transfer will essentially weaken the extensor pull of the respected toes. Suture the Z-lengthened fifth extensor digitorum longus with physiologic tension while maintaining good anatomic alignment. Next, pass the distal stumps of the proximal portion of the second and third extensor digitorum longus tendons deep to the soft tissue structure (to avoid pressure on the neurovascular structures)with the fourth extensor digitorum longus. Suture together the distal stumps of the proximal portion (we typically use 0 Vicryl) of the second, third, and fourth extensor digitorum longus tendons, and transfer them into the peroneus tertius or the periosteum of the intermediate cuneiform with the surgical assistant loading the ankle at 90° relative to the leg. Again, this tendon transfer should be executed under physiologic tension. This method facilitates a mechanical gain in dorsiflexion. We typically close the deep subcutaneous tissues with 4-0 Monocryl. Be sure to avoid the superficial neurovascular structures. Close the skin using 4-0 Prolene. Following K-wire removal, one should emphasize physical therapy for the patient in order to help resolve any edema and soften the postoperative fibrosis and scar tissue formation. Emphasize active and passive manipulation of the joints that underwent surgery. Typically one instructs patients about home exercise programs they can use to maintain plantarflexion and dorsiflexion at the surgical sites.

In scenarios that involve the great toe individually or in combination, the same decision and principle should be maintained.

A key component to performing tendon transfer for the correction of digital deformities is identifying which procedure to perform for the given pathology. Most digit deformities are associated with an abnormal pull and biomechanics of the short and long flexors and extensors that have caused the toe or multiple toes to deform. The goal of the surgery must balance the flexors and extensors in order to prevent recurrence or continued progression of the deformity. Once the surgeon removes the deforming force, a recurrence should not occur. If the surgeon appropriately addresses the multiplanar digital deformity, he or she should be able to correct the toe in all planes.

A modified Girdlestone-Taylor procedure can transfer the flexor digitorum longus tendon to the extensor hood of the proximal phalanx. The modified Hibbs procedure can decrease the extensor tendon retrograde buckling on the respected metatarsal in the sagittal plane. Furthermore, this release will assist the surgeon to mobilize the respected toes out of frontal and transverse plane deformities while providing excellent exposure to the metatarsophalangeal joint.

Making a sound decision in which procedure or combination of surgical procedures (flexor tendon transfer and/or extensor tendon transfer) to perform is paramount. The foot and ankle surgeon must be able to identify the appropriate pathological process in order to perform the proper surgical procedure to address given underlying pathology. Digital deformities present in many ways. The pathology can present to an isolated joint of a toe, multiple joints of a toe, a single toe, and multiple toes, bilaterally, and can also involve other components of pathology such as an equinus contracture; metatarsals deformities; systemic diseases such as rheumatoid arthritis, diabetes mellitus, polio, and Charcot-Marie-Tooth disease; and other neuromuscular diseases.

For example, a patient may present with heloma dura at the lateral aspect of proximal interphalangeal joint of the fifth toe (often referred to as a "HD5"). Often times, this deformity can present with a flexion contracture at the proximal interphalangeal joint and/or distal interphalangeal joint. In addition, a varus rotation and a transverse pull medially can be involved. In presentations such as this, there is no extensor pathological process involved; therefore, the surgeon would need to make the decision to address this three-plane deformity involving only the flexion contracture. In a scenario such as this, the surgeon would proceed with a flexor digitorum longus tendon transfer to the extensor hood of the proximal phalanx. This will remove the deforming force of the flexion contracture plantarly, the medial and transverse pull, as well as the frontal plane rotation. The flexor digitorum brevis (both the medial and lateral) insertion is removed from the base of the middle phalanx; a capsulotomy is performed at the contracted joints (DIPJ and/or PIPJ) essentially removing the remaining sagittal plane (flexion) deforming forces. This allows each segment of the toe to realign into a neutral position. Next a K-wire is used to stabilize the DIPJ and PIPJ. The surgeon should attempt to insert the K-wire from the distal tip of the distal phalanx to the base of the proximal aspect of the proximal phalanx keeping the joints in a neutral to slight plantar flexion. Once the toe is fixated and positioned in the desired position, the tendon transfer should be completed under physiological tension.

In another scenario, a patient may present with an isolated second digit crossover hammertoe and plantar plate tear. Typically this involves a three-plane deformity involving both the extensor and flexor tendons along with associated soft tissue contractures at the metatarsalphalangeal joint, at the proximal interphalangeal joint, and possibly at the distal interphalangeal joint. The surgeon would address this case with an isolated extensor tendon transfer, a complete metatarsalphalangeal joint capsulotomy, and flexion tendon transfer. By completing this, all deforming forces are removed from the respected deformed toe, and the toe should be able to be placed in the neutral position. Remember, there is no bony pathology to any segment of the proximal, middle, and distal phalanx in digital deformities – the digits are deformed because of the soft tissue contractures and malalignment that occur secondary to chronic abnormal biomechanical pull from the tendon imbalance. Once the surgeon has adequately reduced the deforming forces, the toe should be able to retain a neutral position. A K-wire is inserted from the distal aspect of the distal phalanx across the DIPJ, PIPJ (maintaining a neutral-slight plantar flexion position) across the metatarsalphalangeal joint and into the base of the metatarsal. Once the surgeon identifies the "new neutral desired position," then the appropriate tendon transfers are performed under physiologic tension so that the new insertion of the tendons on the toes provides adequate function to each component of the toe.

When performing a modified Hibbs procedure for an isolated crossover hammertoe, one can make an incision that is approximately 2–3 cm. Begin the incision at the second metatarsalphalangeal joint, and direct it proximal and lateral parallel to the long extensor tendon. Deepen the incision in the same plane to the level of the extensor digitorum longus tendon. Lateral to the extensor digitorum longus tendon lies the smaller extensor digitorum brevis tendon. Transect the extensor digitorum longus as far as proximal in the incision site, and transect the extensor digitorum brevis as far as distal in the incision site. At this time, one can appreciate fantastic exposure to the second metatarsalphalangeal joint. The exposure of the metatarsalphalangeal joint will allow the surgeon to perform a complete release of the contracted and fibrous/deformed capsular tissue, essentially removing all deforming forces of the metatarsalphalangeal joint. This facilitates the release of all contractures via sharp and a blunt dissection using a McGlamry elevator, which allows for anatomic restoration of the metatarsalphalangeal joint. At this time, the toe should be relaxed into a neutral "limp position" as all the deforming forces of the second metatarsalphalangeal joint are gone.

Next, attention is directed to the medial aspect of the second digit where one can perform a modified Girdlestone-Taylor procedure. Use a midline incision approach on the medial aspect of the toe. We recommend that the surgeon use fine double-prong skin hooks for retraction in order to avoid soft tissue compromise. Then deepen the incision in the same plane, taking care to avoid the neurovascular bundles. Carry the incision deep to identify the flexor digitorum longus and trace it distally to its insertion of the distal phalanx. Detach the distal insertion of the flexor digitorum longus from the distal phalanx and direct it proximal to the web space. Proceed to direct the attention to the flexor digitorum brevis tendon where a release (both the medial and lateral slips) of the flexor digitorum brevis from the base of the middle phalanx and capsulotomy at the interphalangeal joint (for a flexion contracture of the proximal interphalangeal joint) is done. If the distal interphalangeal joint is contracted, perform a capsulotomy there as well. At this time, the deforming forces are removed from the appropriate joints. The surgeon can place the second toe into the desired anatomic position and insert a 0.062-inch Kirschner wire to stabilize and align the digit in the corrected position. Insert the K-wire from the distal tip of the distal phalanx to the base of the second metatarsal. With all the deforming forces gone and the digit in the desired anatomic position (in relation to the metatarsal), suture the flexor digitorum longus to the extensor hood under physiologic tension. It is imperative to suture this under physiologic tension as this tendon transfer will assist the lumbricales with plantarflexion and allow the toe to purchase the ground postoperatively.

Direct attention back to the dorsum of the second metatarsalphalangeal joint, and transfer the distal stump of the proximal end of the extensor digitorum brevis tendon into the proximal end of the distal stump of the extensor digitorum longus tendon via a weave graft under physiologic tension. Again, it is important to do this under physiologic tension in order to allow for the extensor digitorum brevis to dorsiflex the toe. Essentially, the modified Hibbs procedure allows the patient to maintain dorsiflexion of the toe but essentially "weakens" the dorsiflexor of the second digit. The modified Hibbs procedure is indicated for patients who exhibit isolated extensor substitution/ recruitment or global extensor substitution/recruitment to the forefoot. Dorsal subluxations/dislocations at the metatarsalphalangeal joint are frequently linked with claw toes and hammertoes, including the crossover toe variety.

In scenarios when patients present with global deformities of all toes, the respected procedures can be done for each involved segment. Again, these procedures can be performed on isolated individual toes or multiple toes. Each segment of each toe needs to be appropriately assessed.

Outcomes/Case Resolutions

The flexor tendon transfer is reported as the most consistent and successful treatment in eliminating pain and normal function of the MTPJ [18]. Flexor tendon transfers were first described in the literature by Taylor in 1940 and Girdlestone in 1947. The objective of the procedure is to allow the long flexor to substitute for intrinsic muscle weakness and provide plantarflexion of the digit along with releasing the plantar contracture at the distal digit allowing extension of the IPJ [22].

Bhatia et al. validated the flexor tendons ability to stabilize the digit at the MTPJ level in their biomechanical study [18, 23].

In a caderveric study by Ford et al. in 1998, it was found that transfer of the FDL stabilized the second MPJ similarly to a primary plantar plate repair. In addition, this stabilization was found to be similar to the stability provided by an intact plantar plate [18].

A finite element analysis of the FDL transfer revealed that the tendon transfer achieves a strong and sufficient reduction in the dorsal placement proximal phalanx [24].

Boyer and DeOrio treated both flexible and rigid hammertoe deformities utilizing the flexor tendon transfer with K-wire fixation. They reported an 89% success rate with no postoperative floating toe [25].

Gadzag and Cracchiolo reported success with the flexor tendon transfer is treating instability of the second metatarsophalangeal joint in 11/18 patients. All of their patients achieved postoperative stability and had complete relief of pain [26].

It has been almost 100 years since Hibbs' original description, which involved release of all soft tissue structures from the plantar heel and release of the long extensors with transfer to the lateral cuneiform. Hibbs reported no complications with the 25 operations that were performed [15]. This was a common procedure in the 1970s; however, it fell out of favor secondary to postoperative complications. According to Ruch, complications included flail lesser digits and flexor contractures at the distal IPJ. There was also little improvement in forefoot equinus visualized following the procedure [27, 28]. There have been some modifications of the procedure since that time [12].

Brody and Grumbine reported on 30 patients over a 3.5 year period that were treated with a combination of extensor transfers and peroneus tertius reconstruction for flexible claw toe deformities. Good to excellent results were reported in 28/30 patients, or 93.3%. Complications reported included pain, swelling, numbness, infection, and scarring [29].

Boffeli et al. recently reported on early minimally invasive techniques for CMT disease. In contrast to our technique, Boffeli describes the long extensor transfer being performed through a separate 3 cm longitudinal incision. The EDL tendons were bundled together and then transferred to the lateral cuneiform with an interference screw. It was noted for hammertoe correction that tenotomy of the long extensor tendons and capsulotomy at the level of the MTPJ may be adequate in early stages of the disease process when the deformity is still flexible. A plantar IPJ capsulotomy and flexor tenotomy may be needed for additional correction. They added that an IPJ fusion of the hallux, PIPJ fusions of digits 2–4, and arthroplasty of digit 5 may be employed as well [30].

Clinical Pearls/Pitfalls

- In terms of advantages with this proposed approach, the scars with the flexor tendon transfer procedure are located on the medial or lateral aspect of the respected digit or digits so the procedure leaves a much more cosmetically pleasing result. There is also a much more natural appearance to the digits postoperatively. Additionally, no shortening occurs, and the medial and lateral collateral ligaments remain intact so no frontal plane or transverse plane complications can occur. The cubic volume of bone is not altered so instability and shortening cannot occur. Because one limits dissection to soft tissue only, the postoperative edema is minimal in relation to bony procedures. Of note, any resulting bursa, hyperkeratosis, and ulceration eventually dissipate without specifically addressing them surgically. This is because the surgeon has corrected the deforming forces and relieved the abnormal pressures.
- It has been the authors experience when addressing patients who suffer from plantar plate tears that keeping the treatment simple and direct is best. The suggested treatment consists of a modified Hibbs procedure to the specific joint coupled with a flexor tendon transfer. The modified Hibbs procedure removes the deforming force by releasing the long and short extensor tendon. This provided excellent exposure to the metatarsalphalangeal joint. This should remove all dorsal and transverse and/or frontal plane deformity from the toe on the metatarsal. The flexor tendon transfer then will release the flexion contracture of the toe and correct all planes of deformity. Once this is accomplished, and the tendon transfers are done, the toe will maintain its position.
- Oftentimes, the authors will be questioned, does the plantar plate need to be directly repaired? Our experience is no. Once the deforming forces are

removed and the tendon transfer and balancing of the joint are complete, the deformity should not occur and the plantar plate will heal itself given the deformity and the abnormal pressures and position are no longer causing a pathologic process.

- With the incision placement with these particular procedures, neurovascular bundles will be readily visible, so gentle retraction with fine skin hook retractors is vital to prevent complications with wound healing.
- Since there is no work actually performed on the bone itself, there is typically minimal swelling localized to the digit, postoperatively.
- With the incision of the FDL transfer being placed either medial or laterally, the scars are well hidden and allow for excellent cosmesis.
- Since there is no osseous involvement, there is no shortening, translation, or rotation of a toe.
- Because the collateral ligaments are not invaded with an FDL transfer, this eliminates the concern of transverse and rotational malalignment.
- With respect to the modified Hibbs procedure, upon skin closure one needs to pay attention to detail in order to avoid significant scar tissue formation to the dorm of the foot and aggravation to superficial nerves. Typically the dorsum of the foot has a thin soft tissue envelope; therefore, the surgeon must take caution with retraction to protect the dorsal tissues in order to prevent wound issues.
- Following a Hibbs procedure, patients will have weakness with dorsiflexion power of their digits as well as limited range of motion with dorsiflexion to the involved toes. Following an FDL transfer, the patient will have increased plantar flexion power to the involved toe at the MTP and decreased power and limited range of motion of the PIPJ and DIPJ. These consequences should be discussed preoperatively with the patient.
- As pins are being placed for stabilization in the digits, slightly plantarflexing the digit at the PIPJ will help reduce chances for a recurvatum deformity.
- One must remember to dorsiflex the ankle as the long extensor tendon is being transferred to the dorsolateral aspect of the midfoot or peroneal tertius tendon under physiologic tension, so it will continue to aid with dorsiflexion at the level of the ankle.
- A recurvatum deformity at the level of the PIPJ can be a complication seen with the FDL tendon transfer procedure. Slight plantar flexion at the PIPJ when fixated should help reduce the potential complication.
- Patients with progressive, neuromuscular disease may show a recurrence of the contracture when an isolated arthroplasty procedure is performed; however, once a tendon transfer is complete, a recurrence should not be possible as the deforming force is removed.
- By avoiding osseous procedures on the phalanges such as an arthroplasty, one can avoid instability from decreasing the cubic volume of bone that is removed. This loss of cubic volume of bone can cause destabilization to

the respective joint. In addition, the secondary skin changes and edema can be diminished and potentially avoided.
- By not performing arthrodesis of the IPJ, one can avoid shortening, as well as malalignment of the transverse, sagittal, and frontal plane. Additionally, the long-term sequela of secondary skin changes and postoperative edema can be minimized and/or avoided.
- The authors suggest using an Allis clamp and small mosquito hemostats on the tendons. The Allis clamps are used to coordinate the extensor digitorum brevis tendonsinto the distal portion of the extensor digitorum longus tendon with the transfer. The mosquito hemostat is used to coordinate the proximal portion of the extensor digitorum longus tendon into the peroneal tertius or midfoot. Additionally, the use of the two distinct clamps assists in keeping the tendons organized throughout the dissection and transfer.
- Lastly, if complications with a tendon transfer do occur, the surgeon always has the ability to proceed with a bony procedure if needed.

Case 1

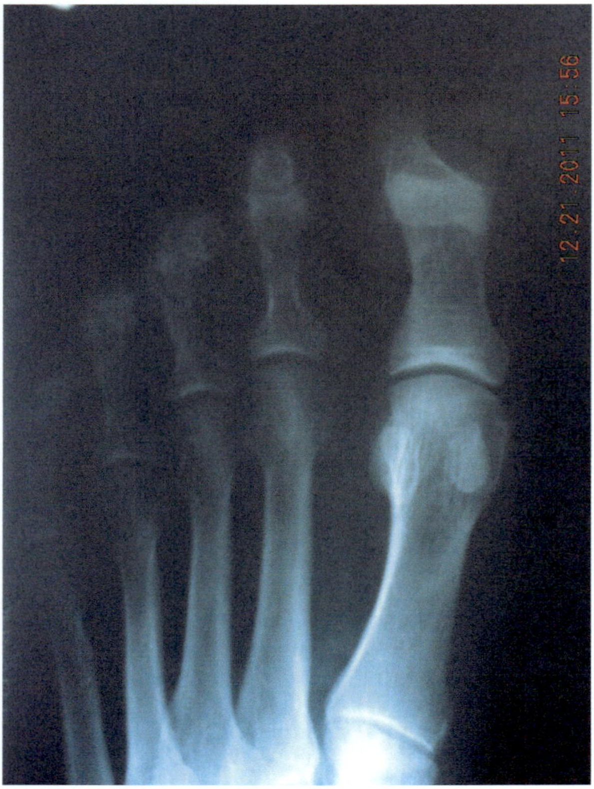

Photo 16.1 A preoperative AP radiograph demonstrating well-maintained metatarsalphalangeal joints 1–5 and flexion contractures of the proximal interphalangeal joints 1–5. Note the flexion contracture of the distal interphalangeal joint too as well as varus rotation of the third, fourth, and fifth toes

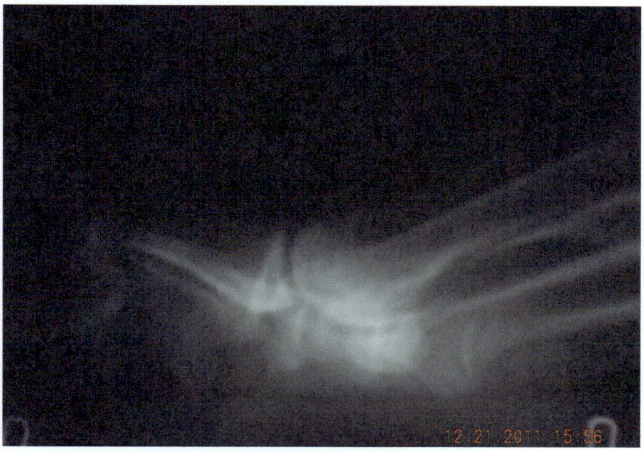

Photo 16.2 A lateral preoperative radiograph demonstrating flexion contracture at the interphalangeal joints

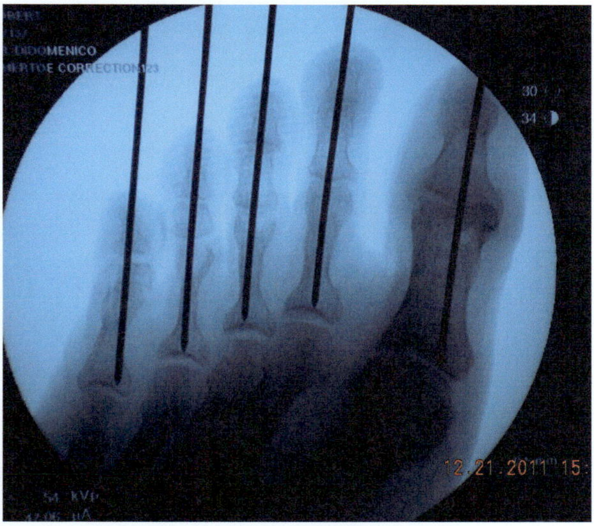

Photo 16.3 An intraoperative AP view following the performance of a flexor digitorum longus tendon transfer of second, third, fourth, and fifth toes as well as a flexor hallucis longus tendon transfer of the great toe. The toes are out to their natural length; each joint is preserved and well maintained

Case 2

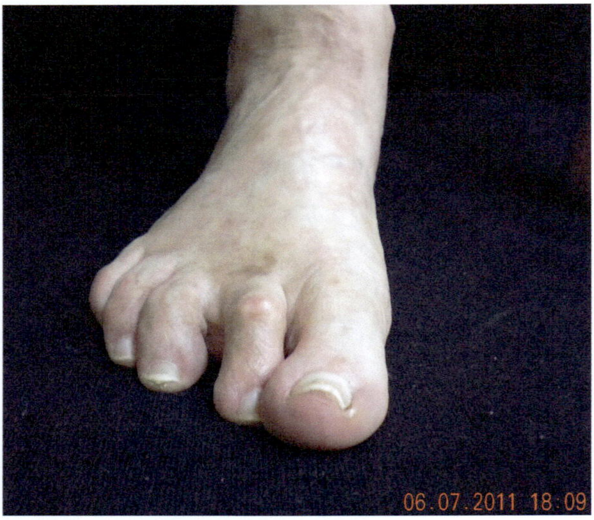

Photo 16.1 A clinical view of a patient who had previous surgery for hammertoe correction surgery done on the second and third toe. The patient now presents with a recurrent hammertoe of the second and third toe with the addition of hammertoe pain of the lesser toes

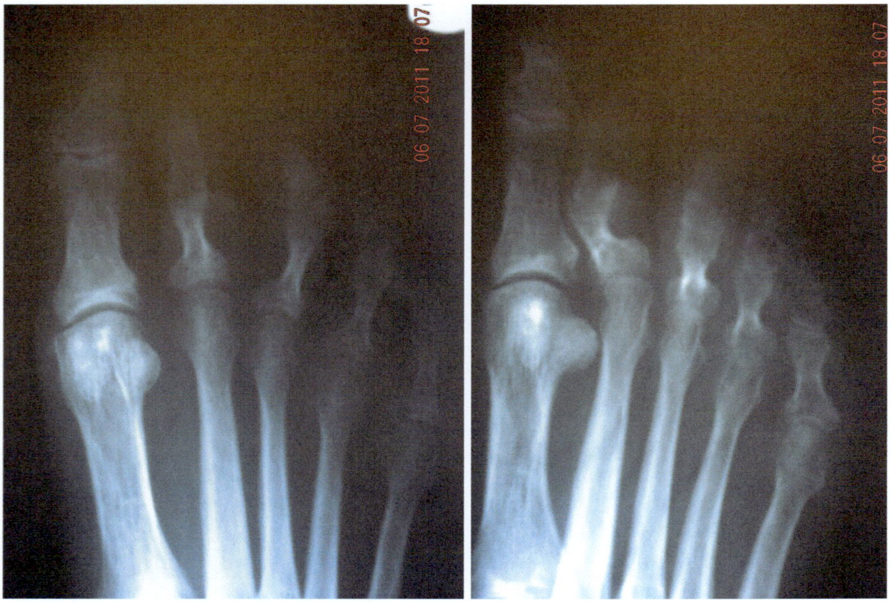

Photos 16.2 and 16.3 An AP and medial oblique preoperative radiograph demonstrating hammertoe deformities 2–5. Please note there is some medial pulling of the distal aspect of toes 3, 4, and 5

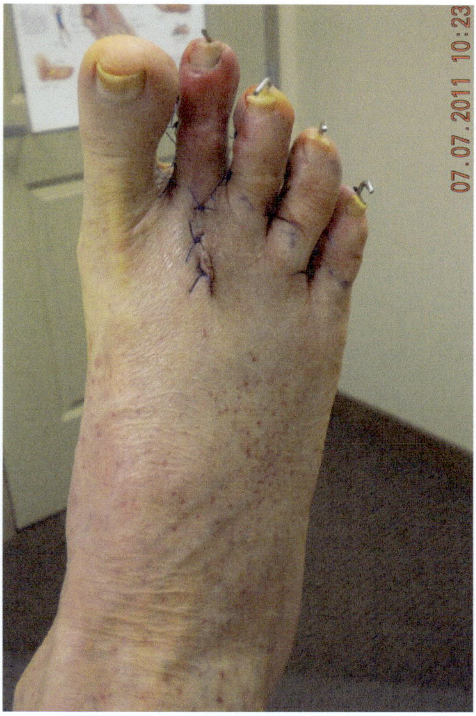

Photo 16.4 Postoperative view of this patient who underwent an extensor digitorum brevis to extensor digitorum longus tendon transfer coupled with a flexor digitorum longus tendon transfer of the second toe. This patient also had a flexor digitorum longus tendon transfer of the third, fourth, and fifth toes too

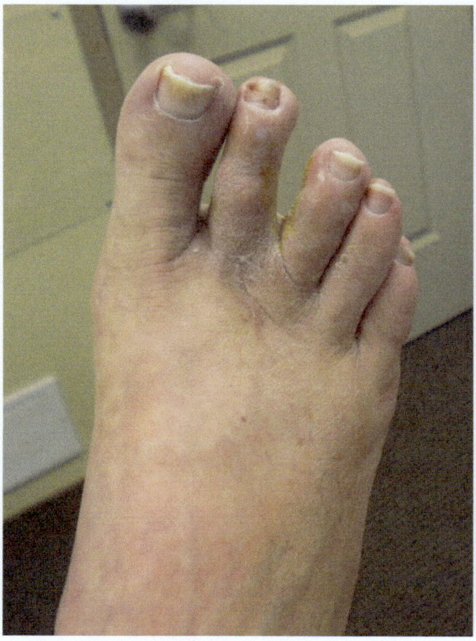

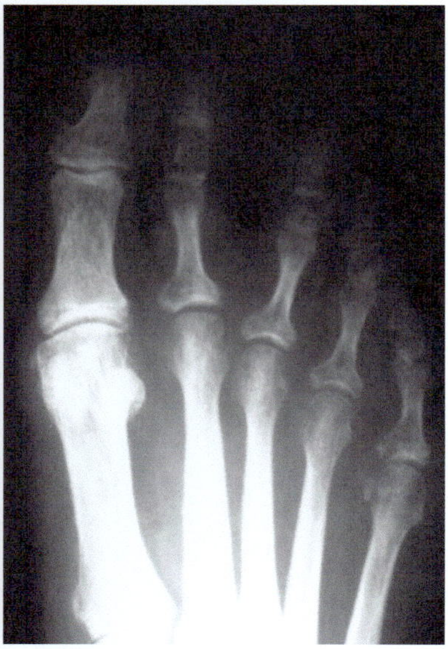

Photos 16.5 and 16.6 Clinical and radiographic postoperative following extensor digitorum brevis to extensor digitorum longus tendon transfer coupled with a flexor digitorum longus tendon transfer of the second toe. This patient also had a flexor digitorum longus tendon transfer of the third, fourth, and fifth toes too. Note on photo 6 how the toes lay more in a more neutral position and all the joint spaces are maintained

Case 3

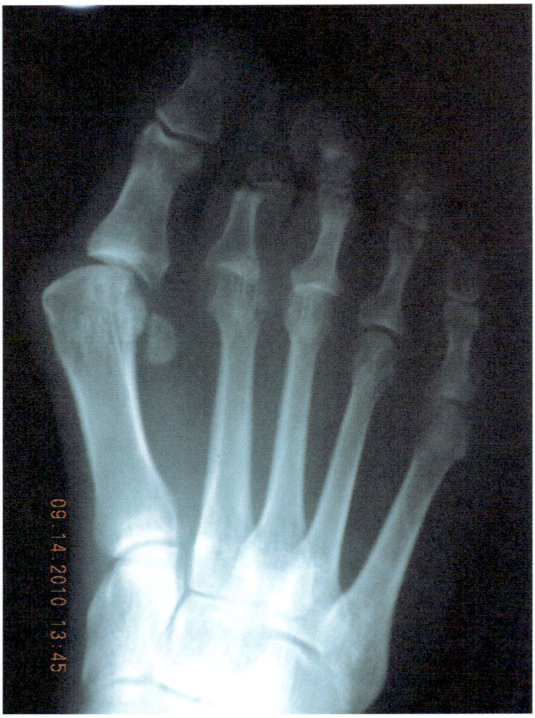

Photo 16.1 An AP radiograph of a patient who had previous bunionectomy and second hammertoe correction where an arthroplasty of the proximal interphalangeal joint of the second toe was done. Note the dorsal dislocation of the base of the proximal phalanx on the second and third toes on the second and third metatarsals. The patient presents with a recurrent bunion and second hammertoe

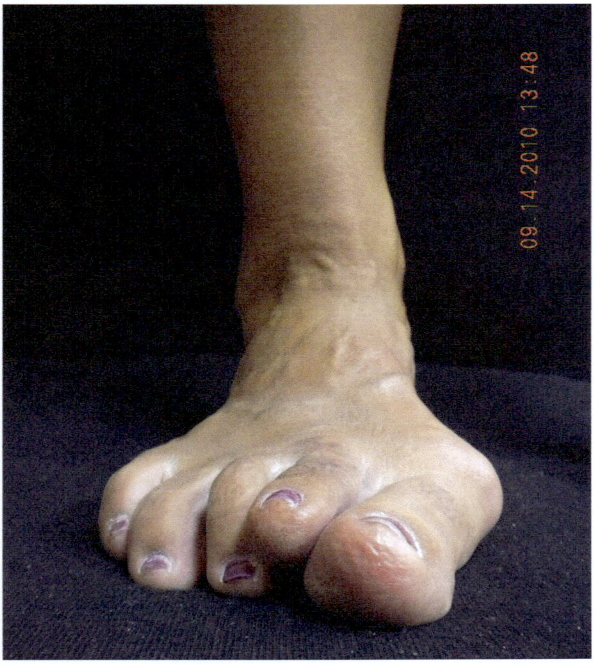

Photo 16.2 This suffers from a recurrent bunion and second hammertoe and a plantar plate tear of the second and third metatarsalphalangeal joint

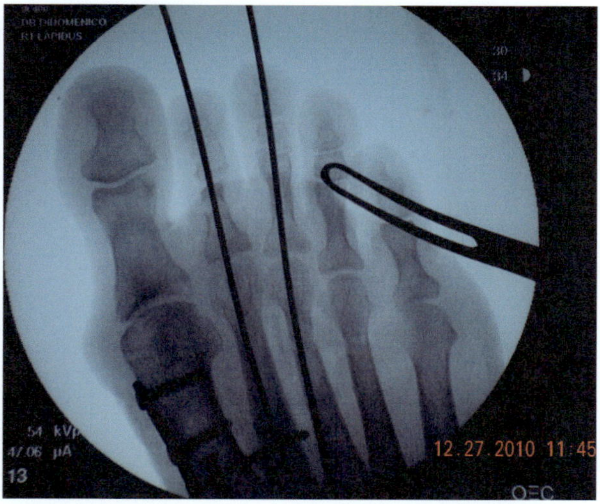

Photo 16.3 An intraoperative AP view demonstrating post bunion reduction, K-wire fixation of second and third toes. This patient underwent and extensor digitorum brevis to extensor digitorum longus tendon transfer coupled with a flexor digitorum longus tendon transfer of the second toe and third toe. In this view, an Allis clamp is visualized from a lateral approach which would be holding the flexor digitorum longus tendon prior to transferring the flexor digitorum longus to the extensor hood

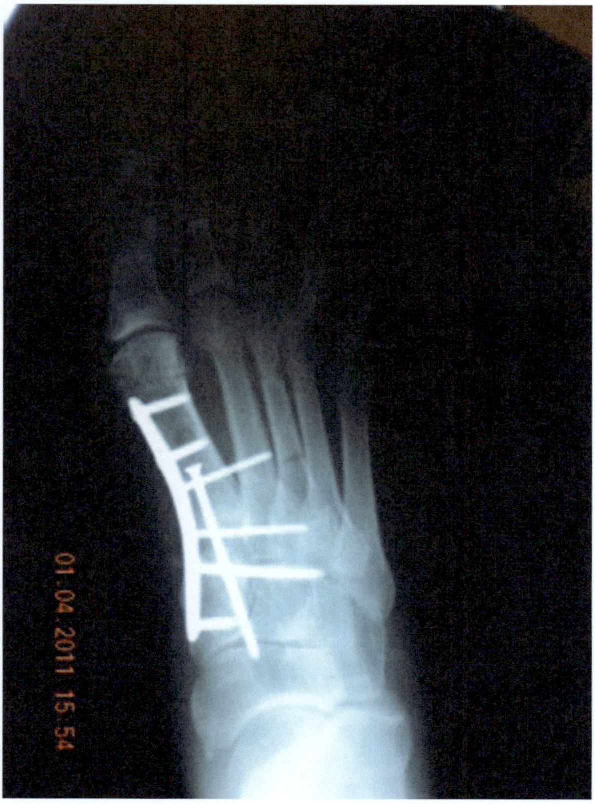

Photo 16.4 A postoperative AP view demonstrating post Lapidus bunionectomy and hammertoe correction of the second and third toes. This patient underwent a Lapidus bunionectomy and extensor digitorum brevis to extensor digitorum longus tendon transfer coupled with a flexor digitorum longus tendon transfer of the second toe and third toe for the plantar plate tears and hammertoe deformities

Case 4

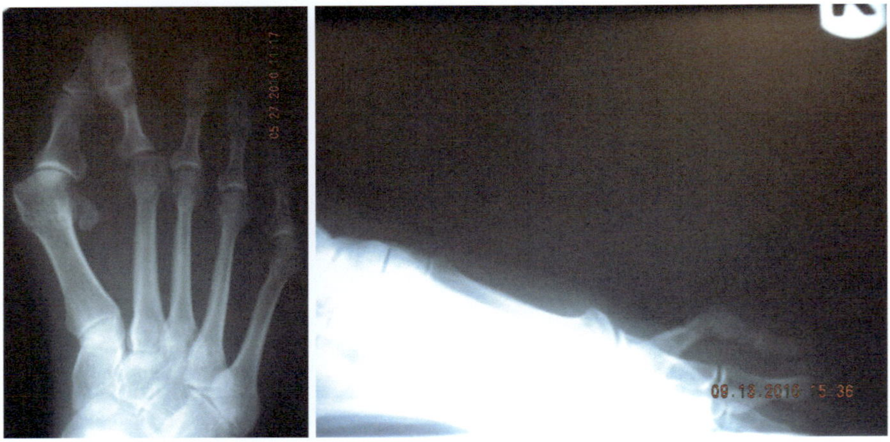

Photos 16.1 and 16.2 An AP preoperative and lateral X-ray demonstrating a large hallux abducto valgus deformity along with a crossover hammertoe. An MRI demonstrates a plantar plate tear of the second metatarsalphalangeal joint

Photo 16.3 A postoperative AP view demonstrating post Lapidus bunionectomy and hammertoe correction of the second toe. This patient underwent an HAV reduction via a Lapidus bunionectomy and extensor digitorum brevis to extensor digitorum longus tendon transfer coupled with a flexor digitorum longus tendon transfer of the second toe for the plantar plate tear and hammertoe deformity

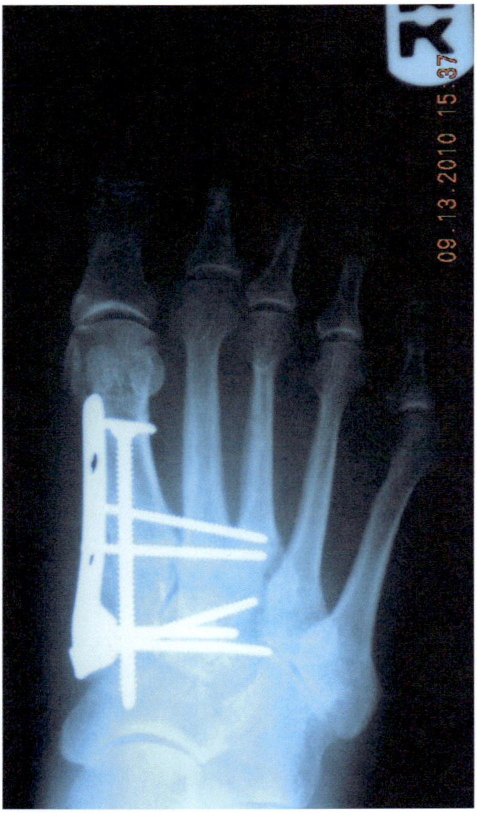

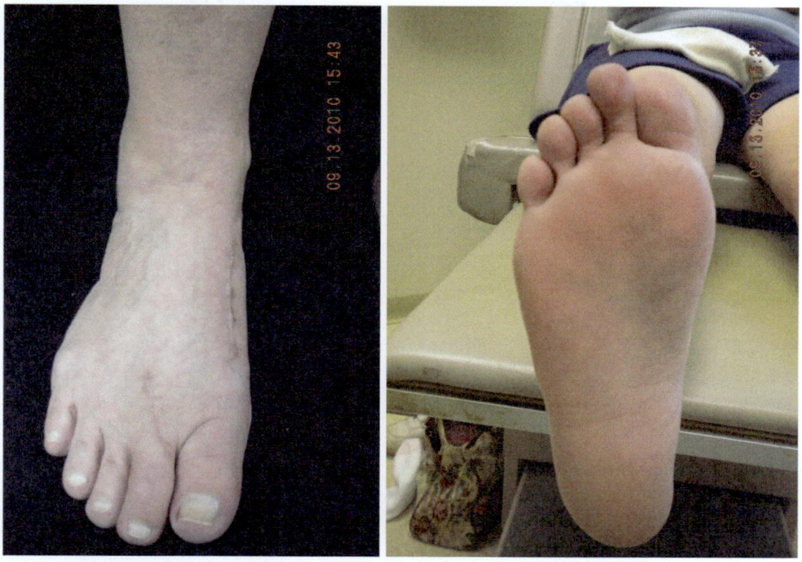

Photos 16.4 and 16.5 Postoperative clinic views demonstrating post Lapidus bunionectomy and hammertoe correction of the second toe. This patient underwent an HAV reduction via a Lapidus bunionectomy and extensor digitorum brevis to extensor digitorum longus tendon transfer coupled with a flexor digitorum longus tendon transfer of the second toe for the plantar plate tear and hammertoe deformity

Case 5

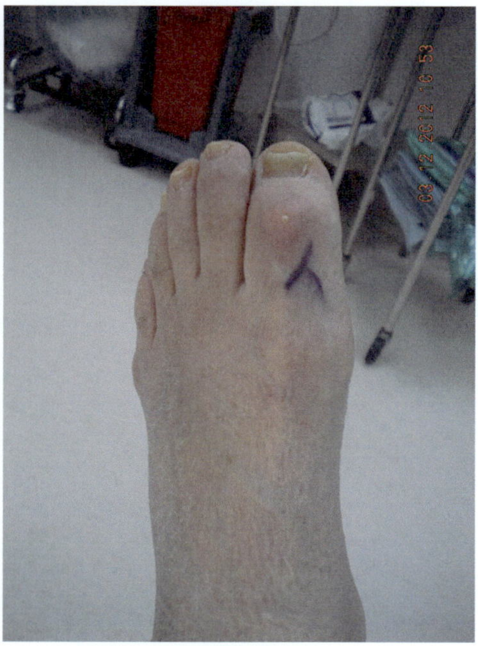

Photo 16.1 A preoperative clinic view of a diabetic patient who gets a recurrent ulcer at the dorsal aspect of the interphalangeal joint of the hallux secondary to a dynamic flexor contraction during gait

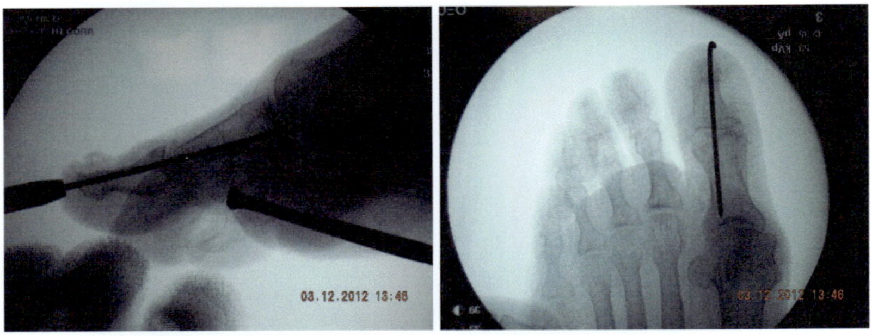

Photos 16.2 and 16.3 Intraoperative AP and lateral views demonstrating K-wire fixation following a flexor hallucis longus tendon transfer of the great toe. The tendon transfer removes the underlying cause of a flexion contracture. Note the interphalangeal joint is reduced and well maintained

Case 6

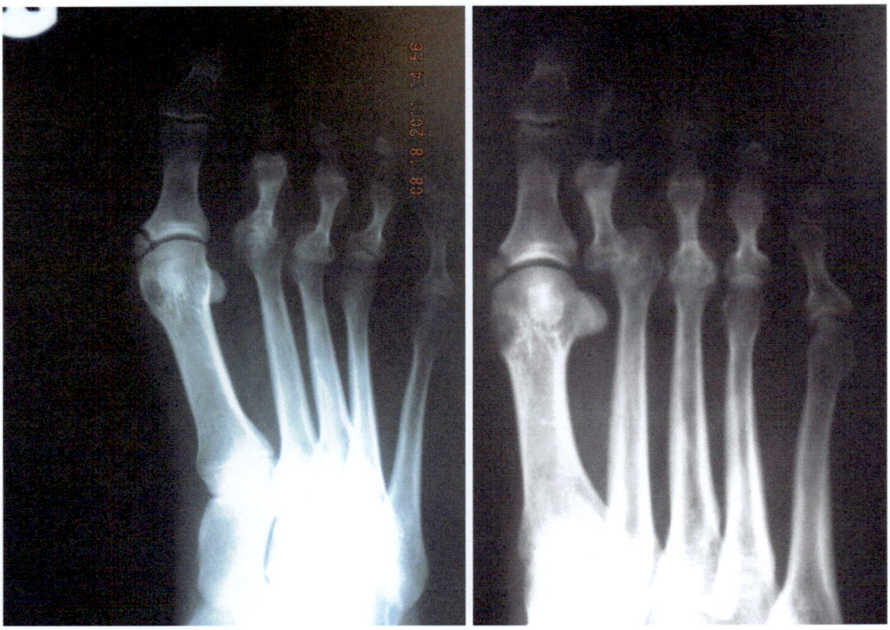

Photos 16.1 and 16.2 AP and medial oblique radiographs demonstrating hammertoe deformities of digits 2, 3, 4, and 5. This patient also has a plantar plate tear of the second and third metatarsal-phalangeal joint

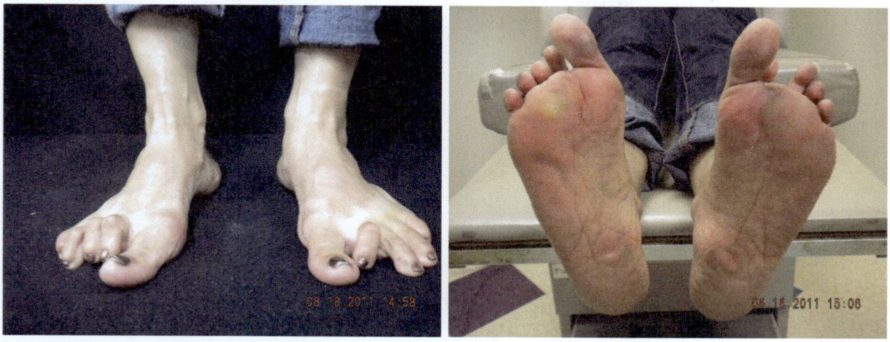

Photos 16.3 and 16.4 Clinical views of this patient who suffers from bilateral hammertoe deformities, plantar plate tears, and painful plantar lesions of the foot secondary to severe hammertoe deformities and plantar plate tears

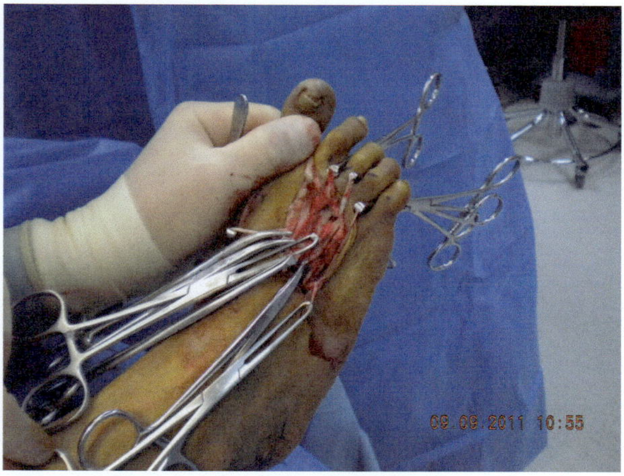

Photo 16.5 An intraoperative view of a modified Hibbs being performed to correct the severe hammertoes 2–5 and plantar plate tears/ deformities of the second and third metatarsal-phalangeal joint

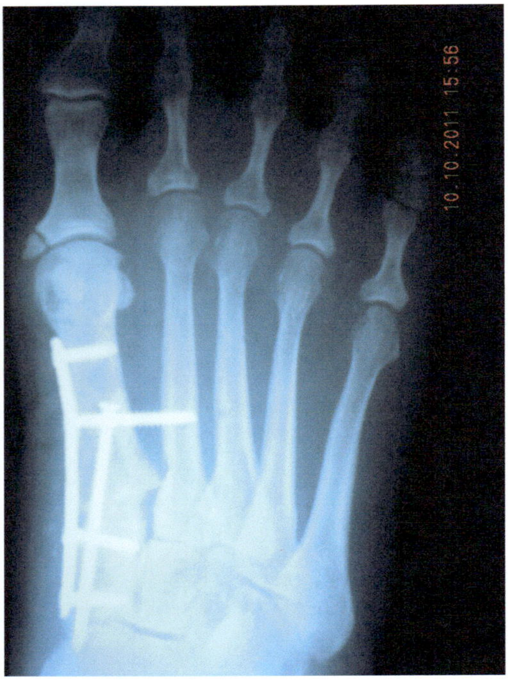

Photo 16.6 An AP postoperative X-ray demonstrating good anatomic alignment following a Lapidus arthrodesis (to stabilize the first tarsal-metatarsal joint) and a modified Hibbs and flexor tendon transfer of toes 2–5. Note that the metatarsalphalangeal joints as well as the interphalangeal joints are well aligned and reduced appropriately

Case 7

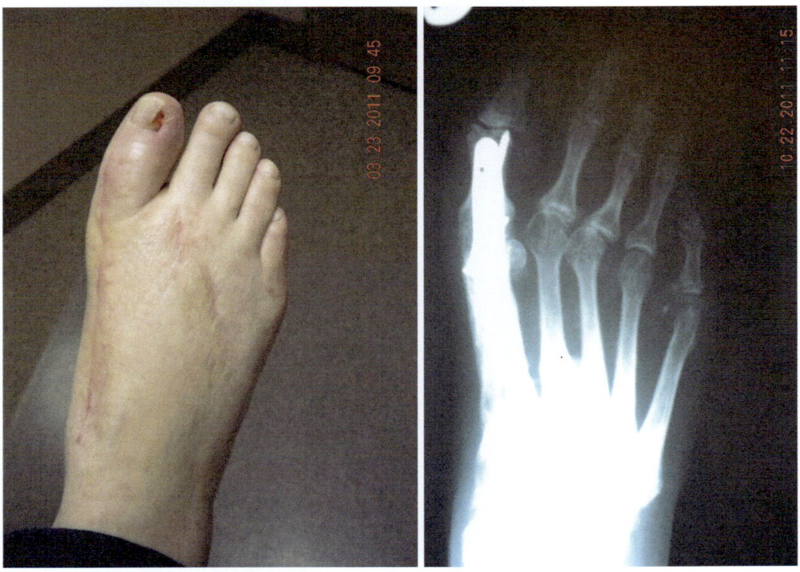

Photos 16.1 and 16.2 An AP X-ray and clinical view of a rheumatoid patient who underwent an arthrodesis of the first metatarsalphalangeal joint along with a modified Hibbs and flexor tendon transfer of toes 2–5

Case 8

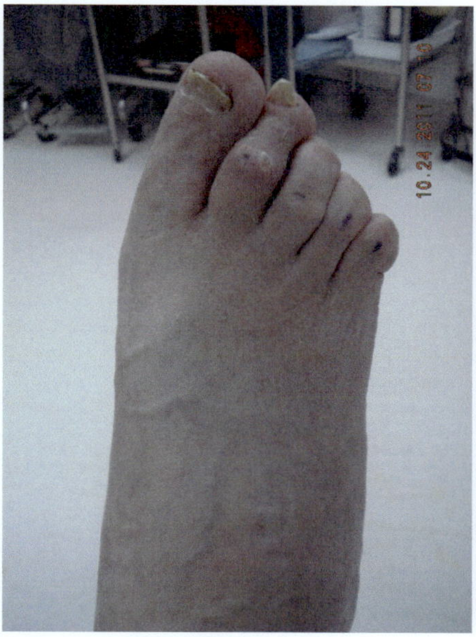

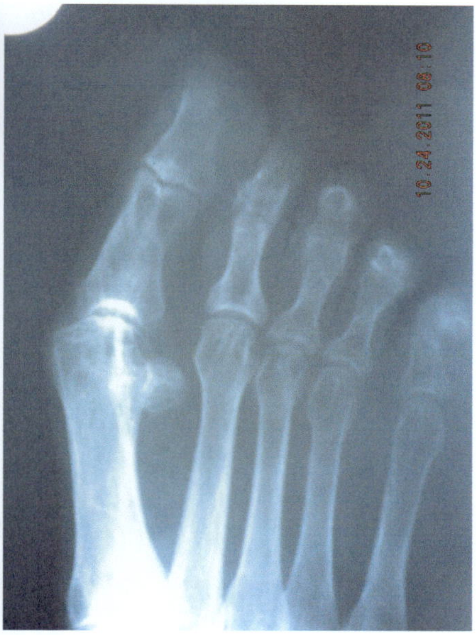

Photos 16.1 and 16.2 A clinical photo demonstrating marked flexion contracture at the proximal interphalangeal joints of toes 2–5. A pre-op AP X-ray demonstrating flexion contractures at the proximal interphalangeal joints 2–5. Please note the well-maintained joint space at the metatarsal-phalangeal joint demonstrating a lack of pathological changes at metatarsalphalangeal joints 2–5

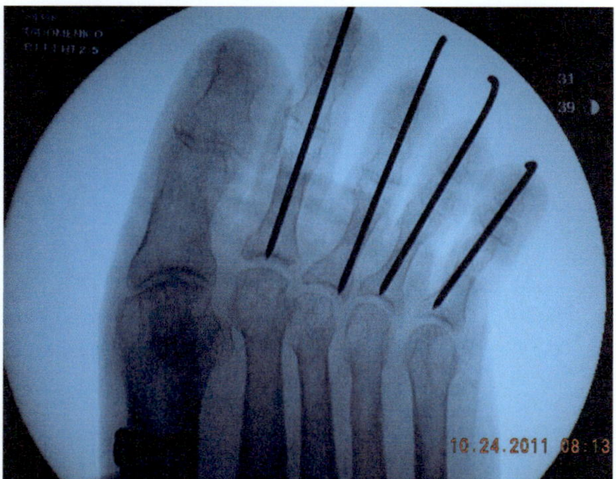

Photo 16.3 An intraoperative AP X-ray demonstrating correction of the flexion contractures at the proximal interphalangeal joints 2–5 via flexor tendon transfers. Note there is no loss of cubic volume of bone, the interphalangeal joints are stabile as the medial and collateral ligaments were left intact, and the joint spaces of the metatarsalphalangeal joints, PIPJ and DIPJ, are all maintained

Case 9

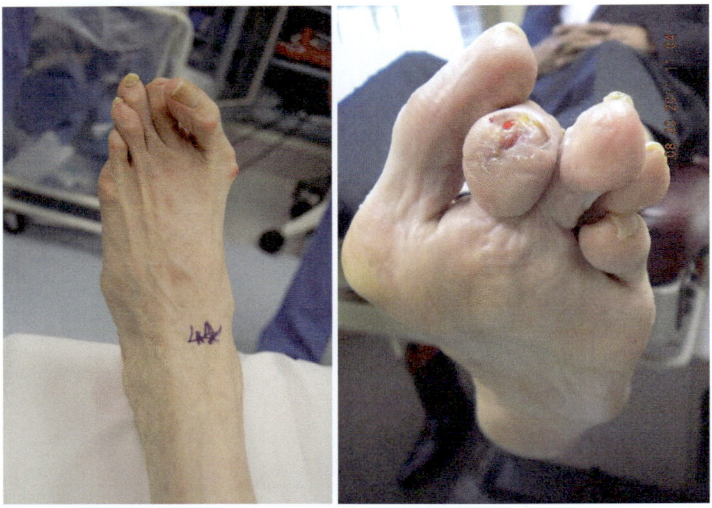

Photos 16.1 and 16.2 Preoperative clinical views of a neuropathic patient who experiences recurrent ulcers secondary to multiple plane digital deformities and a hallux valgus deformity

Photo 16.3 An intraoperative view while performing the modified Hibbs procedure. This view demonstrates the distal stump of extensor digitorum longus tendons 2, 3, and 4 being held by Allis clamps placed in the first, second, and third web spaces, respectively. The proximal portion extensor digitorum brevis tendons 2, 3, and 4 are reflected proximal and held by Allis clamps. Mosquito hemostats are holding the proximal portion of the extensor digitorum longus tendons 2 and 3. In this photo a Mosquito hemostat is not holding the fourth extensor digitorum longus tendon. The fifth extensor digitorum longus tendon is being held within the pickups

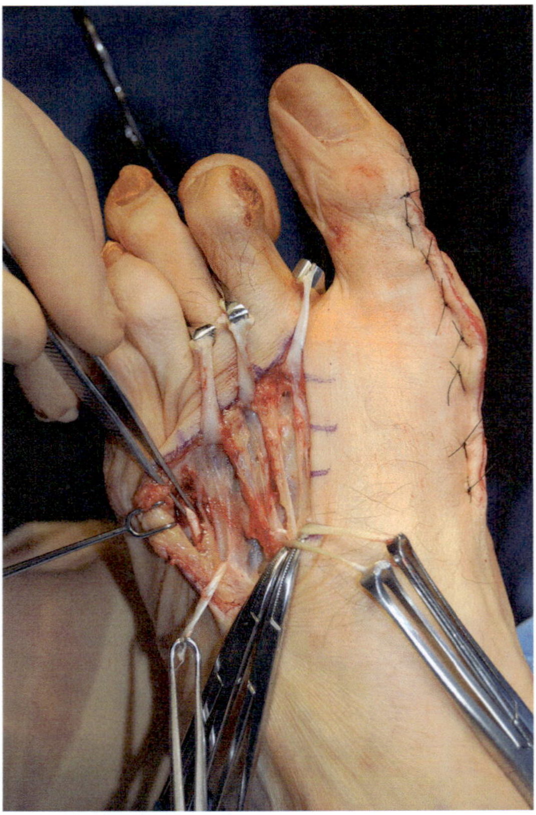

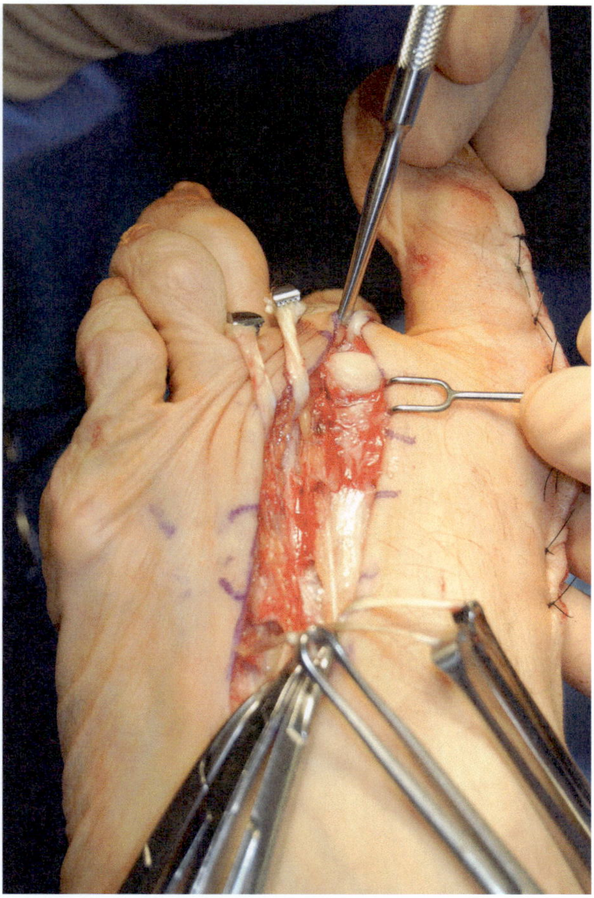

Photo 16.4 An intraoperative view while performing the modified Hibbs procedure demonstrating the access the surgeon has to the metatarsalphalangeal joints. In this photo, the second metatarsal head is exposed

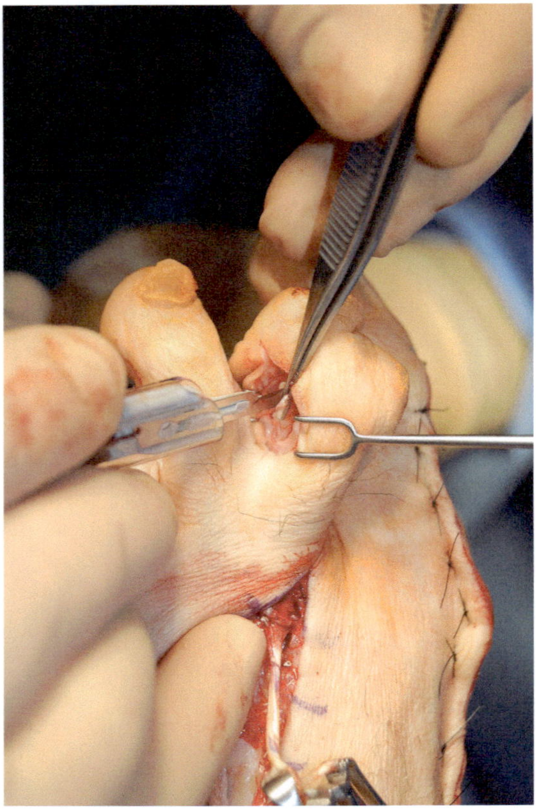

Photo 16.5 An intraoperative view of performing a flexor digitorum longus transfer on the lateral aspect of the second toe. The flexor digitorum longus tendon is identified and the soft tissues are freed from the tendon

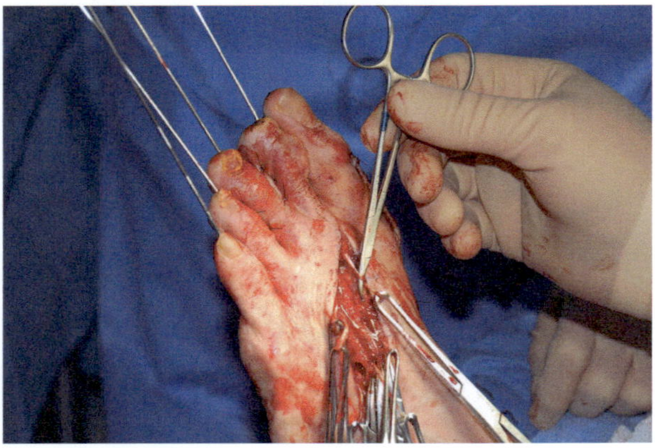

Photo 16.6 An intraoperative view while performing the modified Hibbs dissection and completion of flexor tendon transfer of digits 2, 3, 4, and 5. Note the toes are placed in the desired anatomic position and the extensor tendons are now being transferred. In this photo a vasectomy clamp is within the distal stump of the second extensor digitorum longus tendon and to receive the proximal stump of the second extensor digitorum brevis tendon being held by the an Allis clamp

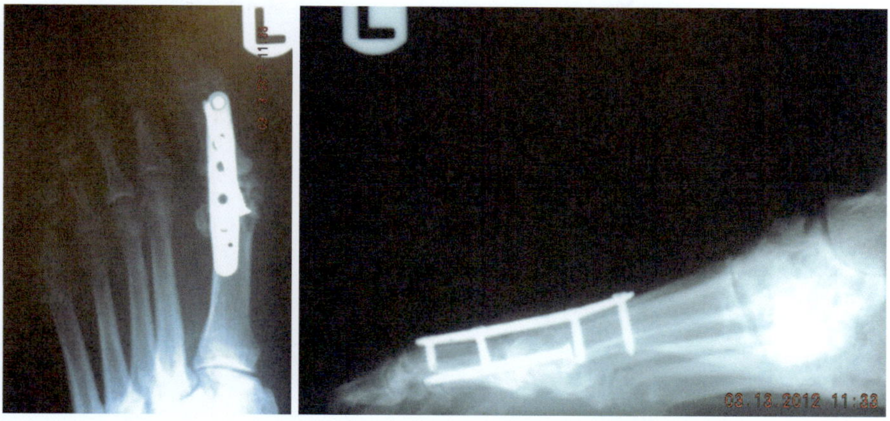

Photos 16.7 and 16.8 A postoperative AP and lateral X-ray demonstrating good anatomic alignment following an arthrodesis of the first MTP, a modified Hibbs procedure of digits 2–5, flexor tendon transfers 2–5

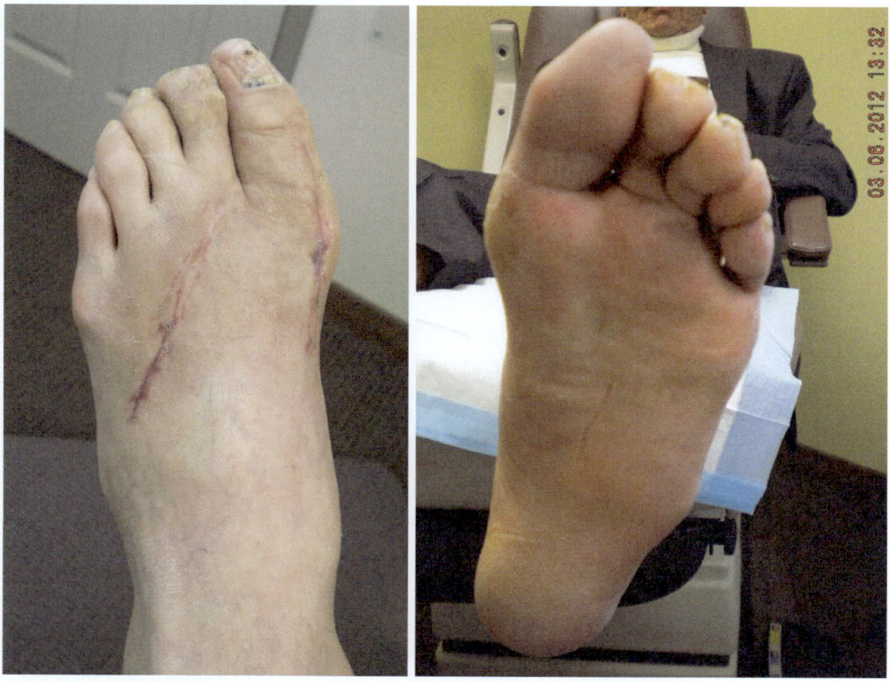

Photos 16.9 and 16.10 Postoperative clinical views following an arthrodesis of the first MTP, a modified Hibbs procedure of digits 2–5, flexor tendon transfers 2–5

References

1. Shirzad K, Kiesau CD, DeOrio JK, et al. Lesser toe deformities. J Am Acad Orthop Surg. 2011;19:505–14.
2. Coughlin MJ. Lesser toe abnormalities. Instr Course Lect. 2003;52:421–44.
3. Dipreta JA. Metatarsalgia, lesser toe deformities, and associated disorders of the forefoot. Med Clin North Am. 2014;98:233–51.
4. Boberg J, Eilts C. Lesser digital deformities: etiology, procedure selection, and arthroplasty. In: McGlamry's comprehensive textbook of foot and ankle surgery. Philadelphia: Lippincott; 2013. p. 117–23.
5. Mizel M. Correction of hammertoe and mallet toe deformities. Oper Tech Orthop. 1992;2(3):188–94.
6. Coughlin M, Dorris J, Polk E. Operative repair of the fixed hammertoe deformity. Foot Ankle Int. 2000;21(2):94–104.
7. Biyani A, Jones DA, Murray J. Flexor to extensor tendon transfer for curly toes-43 children reviewed after 8 (1–25) years. Acta Orthop Scand. 1992;63(4):451–4.
8. Niklas B. Surgical Management of Digital Deformities. In: Hallux Valgus and forefoot surgery. New York: Churchill; 1994. p. 359–77.
9. Nery C, Coughlin M, Baumfeld D, Mann T. Lesser metatarsophalangeal joint instability: prospective evaluation and repair of plantar plate and capsular insufficiency. Foot Ankle Int. 2012;33(4):301–11.
10. Coughlin M. Review article- common causes of pain in the forefoot in adults. J Bone Joint Surg. 2000;82-B(6):781–90.
11. Busa S, Maasb M, de Langc A, Michelsa R, Levia M. Elevated plantar pressures in neuropathic diabetic patients with claw/hammer toe deformity. J Biomech. 2005;38(9):1918–25.
12. DiDomenico L, Rollandini J. A closer look at tendon transfers for crossover hammertoe. Podiatry Today. 2014;27(6):44–51.
13. Boberg JS. Surgical decision making in hammertoe surgery. In: Vickers NS, et al., editors. Reconstructive surgery of the foot and leg: update '97. Tucker, GA: Podiatry Institute; 1997. p. 3–6.
14. Bouchard JL, Castellano BD. Clawtoe deformities and contractures of the forefoot. In: Camasta CA, Vickers NS, Ruch JA, editors. Reconstructive surgery of the foot and leg, update 88. Tucker, GA: Podiatry Institute Publishing; 1998. p. 14–21.
15. Hibbs RA. An operation for "clawfoot". JAMA. 1919;73:1583–5.
16. Hansen S Jr. Transfer of the extensor digitorum communis to the midfoot. In: Functional reconstruction of the foot and ankle. Philadelphia: Lippincott; 2000. p. 451.
17. Rosenbaum AJ, Lisella J, Patel N, et al. The cavus foot. Med Clin N Am. 2014;98:301–12.
18. Ford L, Collins K, Christensen J. Stabilization of the subluxed second metatarsophalangeal Joint: flexor tendon transfer versus primary repair of the plantar plate. J Foot Ankle Surg. 1998;37(3):217–22.
19. Yao L, Do H, Cracchiolo A, Farahani K. Plantar plate of the foot: findings on conventional arthrography and MR imaging. AJR Am J Roentgenol. 1994;163:641–4.
20. Schwend RM, Drennan JC. Cavus foot deformity in children. J Am Acad Orthop Surg. 2003;11:201–11.
21. Piazza S, Ricci G, Ineco EC, et al. Pes cavus and hereditary neuropathies: when a relationship should be suspected. J Orthop Traumatol. 2010;11:195–201.
22. Baravarian B, Thompson J, Nazarian N. Plantar plate tears: a review of the modified flexor tendon transfer repair for stabilization. Clin Podiatr Med Surg. 2011;28:57–68.
23. Bhatia D, Myerson M, Curtis M, Cunningham B, Jinnah R. Anatomical restraints to dislocation of the second metatarsophalangeal joint and assessment of a repair technique. J Bone Joint Surg Am. 1994;76-A(9):1371.
24. Gonzalez A, Bayod J, Prados-Frutos JC, Losa-Inglesias M, Jules K, Bengoa-Vallejo RB, Doblare M. Finite-element simulation of flexor digitorum longus or flexor digitorum brevis tendon transfer for the treatment of clawtoe deformity. J Biomech. 2009;42:1697–704.

25. Boyer M, DeOrio J. Transfer of the flexor Digitorum longus for the correction of lesser-toe deformities. Foot Ankle Int. 2007;28(4):422–30.
26. Gazdag A, Cracchiolo A. Surgical treatment of patients with painful instability of the second metatarsophalangeal joint. Foot Ankle Int. 1998;19(3):137–43.
27. Ruch JA. Surgical classification of the cavus foot deformity. In: Camasta CA, Vickers NS, Ruch JA, editors. Reconstructive surgery of the foot and leg. Update 43. Podiatry Institute Publishing: Tucker, GA; 1994. p. 205–9.
28. Vlachou M, Beris A, Dimitriadis D. Modified Chuinard-Baskin procedure for managing mild-to-moderate cavus and claw toe deformity in children and adolescents. J Foot Ankle Surg. 2008;47(4):313–20.
29. Brody PJ, Grumbine N. Peroneus tertius reconstruction for flexible clawtoes associated with cavus deformity: a preliminary report. J Foot Surg. 1984;23(5):357–61.
30. Boffeli TJ, Tabatt JA. Minimally invasive early operative treatment of progressive foot and ankle deformity associated with Charcot-Marie-tooth disease. J Foot Ankle Surg. 2015;54:701–8.

Chapter 17
Plantar Plate Repair via a Plantar Approach

Eric G. Powell, Melinda A. Bowlby, and Jeffrey C. Christensen

Clinical Presentation

Subjective Complaints

Typically, patients with plantar plate pathology will describe insidious onset of submetatarsal pain and toe dysfunction that occurs over months to years; however, specific traumatic events can induce acute plantar plate dysfunction. Focal submetatarsal pain consistent with metatarsalgia is typically an early sign of plantar plate inflammation. The patient typically complains of pain with digital range of motion, especially dorsiflexion, swelling, digital deformity, footwear limitations, difficulty walking on hard surfaces, and activity limitations [1]. The pain to the joint can be severe, and the edema can apply increased pressure to the adjacent nerve yielding a clinical presentation similar to that of a neuroma [2, 3]. As the plantar plate degenerates or tears, the toe will lose stability, the patient may simply complain of an isolated hammer or clawtoe, or that the toe no longer purchases the ground. Isolated transverse plane toe deviation is seen with partial tears of the plantar plate. The presence of a hammertoe can exist concomitantly at various stages of plantar plate pathology.

Etiological Mechanisms

The plantar plate is the most important sagittal plane static stabilizer of the metatarsophalangeal joint; however, the deep transverse intermetatarsal and collateral ligaments are also important joint stabilizers as well [4, 5]. The etiological mechanisms that

E. G. Powell · M. A. Bowlby · J. C. Christensen (✉)
Podiatric Section: Department of Orthopedics, Swedish Medical Center, Seattle, WA, USA

E. A. Cook, J. J. Cook (eds.), *Hammertoes*,
https://doi.org/10.1007/978-3-319-16552-3_17

Table 17.1 Etiological mechanisms

Long lesser metatarsal
Short first metatarsal
First ray hypermobility
Elevated first metatarsal
Hallux valgus deformity
Mid-/hindfoot hypermobility with medial column overload
Direct trauma or repetitive stress
Localized or systemic arthropathy
Malunion metatarsal fracture
Corticosteroid-induced failure
High-fashion footwear

result in failure are multifactorial (Table 17.1), with the majority of mechanisms caused by an underlying structural abnormality that creates uneven load patterns to the forefoot. Structurally, the deformity is commonly seen with a concomitant hallux abductovalgus deformity (Fig. 17.1). Biomechanically, the instability across the first ray due to the unlocking mechanism imparts overloading on the lesser metatarsals [6]. Progressive abutment pressure of the hallux against the second digit, will eventually cause elevation of the lesser toe which in turn places increased pressure on the plantar plate via retrograde force to the metatarsal head that can over time accelerate the pathology. Although not exclusively seen, accompanying the first ray instability is a long metatarsal to the affected digit with the plantar plate tear [7]. The long metatarsal imparts a greater dorsiflexory force to the digit and over time causes attenuation and tear to the plantar plate along with mechanical trauma to the plate itself from the pressure of the long metatarsal onto the plantar plate tissues (Fig. 17.2). Pronation that leads to overloading of the lesser metatarsophalangeal joints has also been described as a mechanism leading to plantar plate injury. Repetitive stress to the forefoot from shoe gear and activity can also impart damage to the plantar plate leading to injury of the ligament. Crossover toe deformity can involve a partial plate deficiency as well as focal injury to the tie-bar system (deep transverse intermetatarsal ligament and collateral ligaments of the metatarsophalangeal joint) [8, 9]. There is attenuation of the lateral collateral ligaments of the metatarsophalangeal joint along with capsular thinning on the lateral side. The medial structures of the metatarsophalangeal joint are often adapted to shortening of the structures. As the toe is in a dorsomedial position, this puts the pull of the extensor digitorum longus, the flexor digitorum longus, and the interossei medially deviated to the central axis of the metatarsophalangeal joint which further contributes to accentuation of the deformity (Fig. 17.3).

Other non-biomechanical causes of plantar plate tear include inflammatory arthropathies, avascular necrosis of the metatarsal head, neuromuscular disease, and generalized hypermobility syndromes [3]. Injection of steroid into the joint or the intermetatarsal spaces can cause softening of the tissues resulting in iatrogenic attenuation and tearing of the plantar plate or the associated pericapsular structures. Essentially any insult to the joint that causes any form of joint imbalance or overload can potentiate a plantar plate injury.

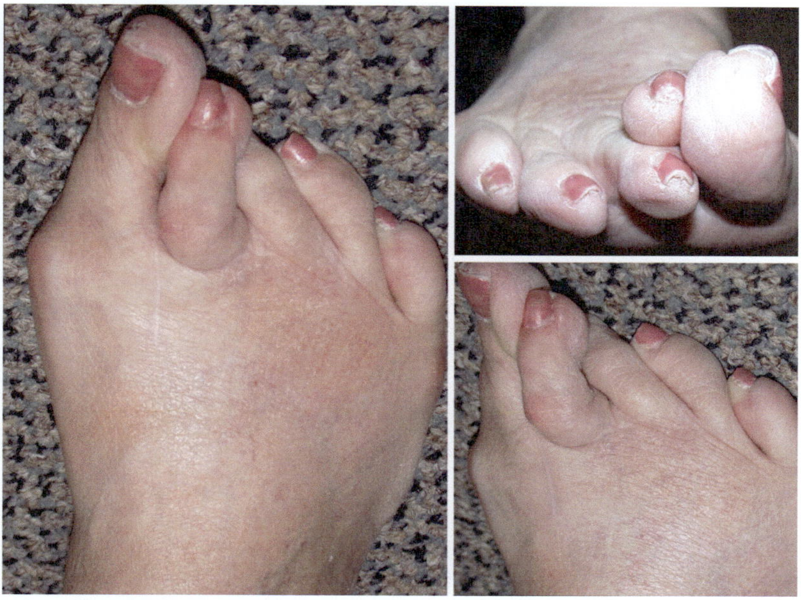

Fig. 17.1 Patient with hallux valgus (failed previous McBride bunionectomy) and rupture of plantar plate of the second toe. Note the stacked toe deformity of the second and third toes. With the valgus rotation of the hallux, the second toe was unable to cross over the hallux. In this case the third toe crosses under, supporting the second toe deformity

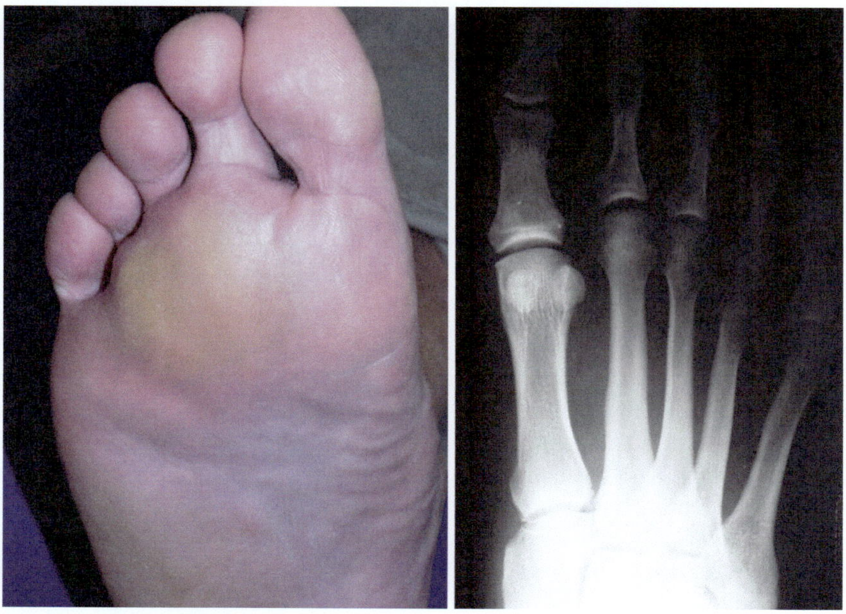

Fig. 17.2 Morton's foot with a relative long second metatarsal. Lesser metatarsal overload predisposes this patient to elevated lesser metatarsal loads during ambulation and is a risk factor for eventual plantar plate dysfunction

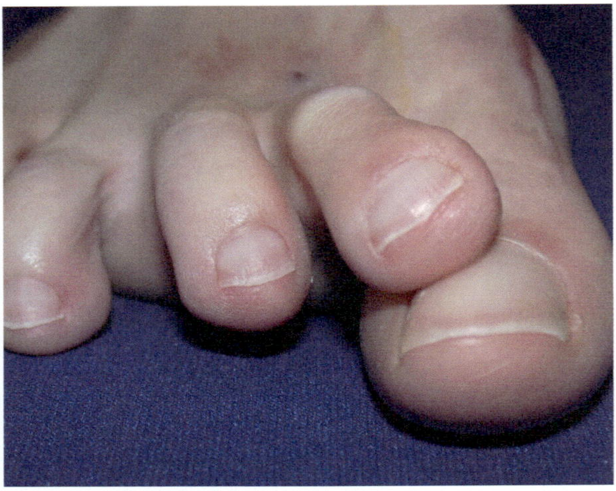

Fig. 17.3 Crossover toe deformity that occurred within 6 months after successful bunionectomy. The bunionectomy created shortening of the metatarsal segment exposing the second metatarsal to excess loads

Diagnosis

Objective Findings

When trying to find solutions for digital problems, understanding the functional anatomy and evaluating plantar plate integrity are of critical importance and require manual examination. In the early stages of plantar plate dysfunction, a patient will present with marked inflammation to the area with palpable calor and edema. It is valuable to simulate weightbearing by manually loading the foot and observing relative digital movement of the lesser digits. Persistent dorsiflexion of the proximal phalanx is at minimum, an indicator of central thinning of plantar plate. However, a dorsal drawer test of the lesser metatarsophalangeal joint (lesser digital Lachman's maneuver) should be performed with toe-held rectus (Fig. 17.4). A positive Lachman's is classically described as subluxation of the joint dorsally greater than 50% of the joint space or greater than 2 millimeters [10]. Lachman's maneuver is a confirmatory test for evaluating plantar plate integrity and not if a tear is present or not, as there are situations where the plantar plate is attenuated and not torn.

The static and dynamic digital stabilizers should be examined weightbearing. The plantar plate and the plantar fascia slip are the primary static stabilizers of the toe. When the static stabilization is intact, the digit will firmly contact the ground via the reverse windlass mechanism and will resist any passive dorsiflexion by the examiner. In contrast, an attenuated or torn plantar plate will not tension which affects toe purchase and the reverse windlass, allowing the affected toe to be passively dorsiflexed with ease (Fig. 17.5). Dynamic purchase may be assessed using the "paper pull-out test," where a narrow sheet of paper is inserted under the involved toe and the patient is directed to grasp the sheet with their toe as the examiner attempts to pull the paper away [1].

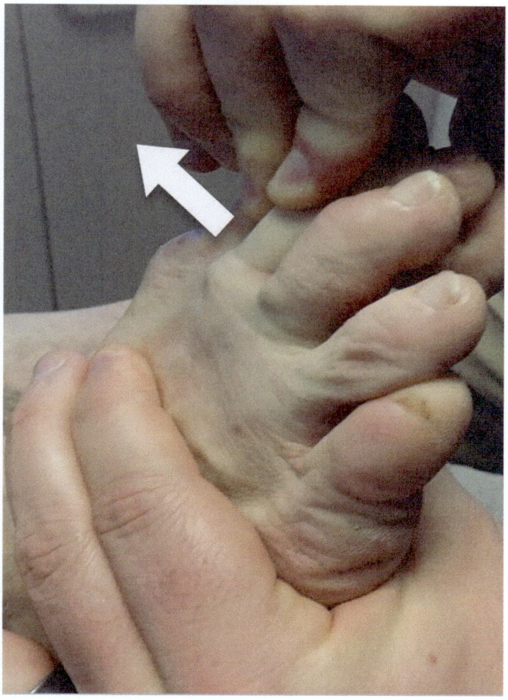

Fig. 17.4 Demonstration of the lesser digital drawer maneuver (Lachman). Examiner resists digital dorsiflexion with the maneuver. Note the dorsal bulge of the phalanx subluxing on the metatarsal head

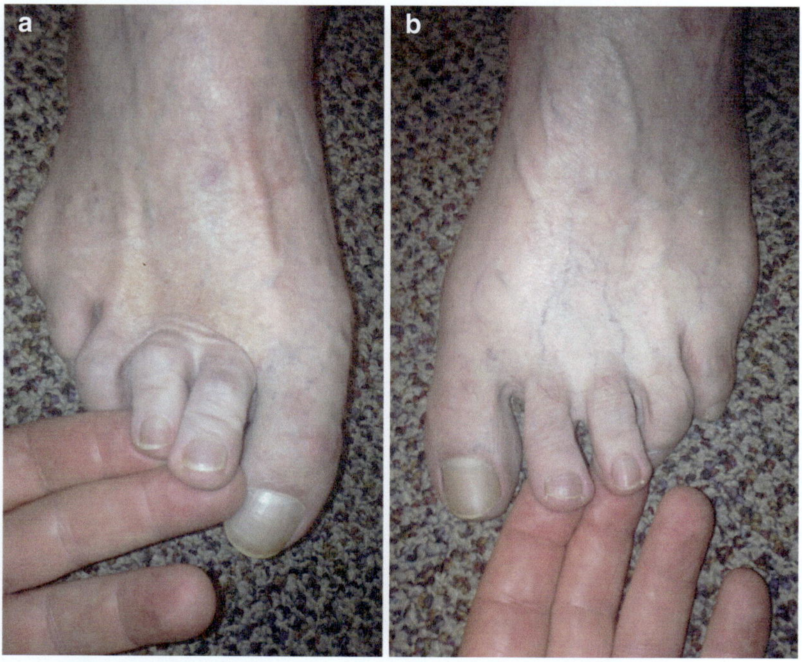

Fig. 17.5 (**a**, **b**) Testing of static stabilizers on a patient with clawtoes 2 and 3 on the right foot (**a**); normal-appearing toes on left foot (**b**). The clawtoes pose no resistance to dorsiflexion (suggestive of plantar plate dysfunction), while the normal toes resist dorsiflexion

In the typical crossover toe, there is deviation of the digit which is dorsal and medial and medial drift of the adjacent toe as well. The vast majority of crossover toe deformities have a positive drawer test [11].

Radiographs

The full examination should include proper weight-bearing foot radiographs. Assessment of the structure of the foot includes careful evaluation of the metatarsal parabola, digital position, metatarsophalangeal joint alignment and joint space symmetry, and first ray and hallux position. Structural abnormalities are correlated with associated symptoms.

Arthrogram

Lesser metatarsophalangeal joint arthrogram wherein a radiopaque dye is injected into the joint under fluoroscopic guidance has diagnostic utility when there are tears in the plate [12] (Fig. 17.6). Due to the proximity of the flexor tendon and its sheath to the plantar plate, any tear to the plate will allow dye to leak from the joint space

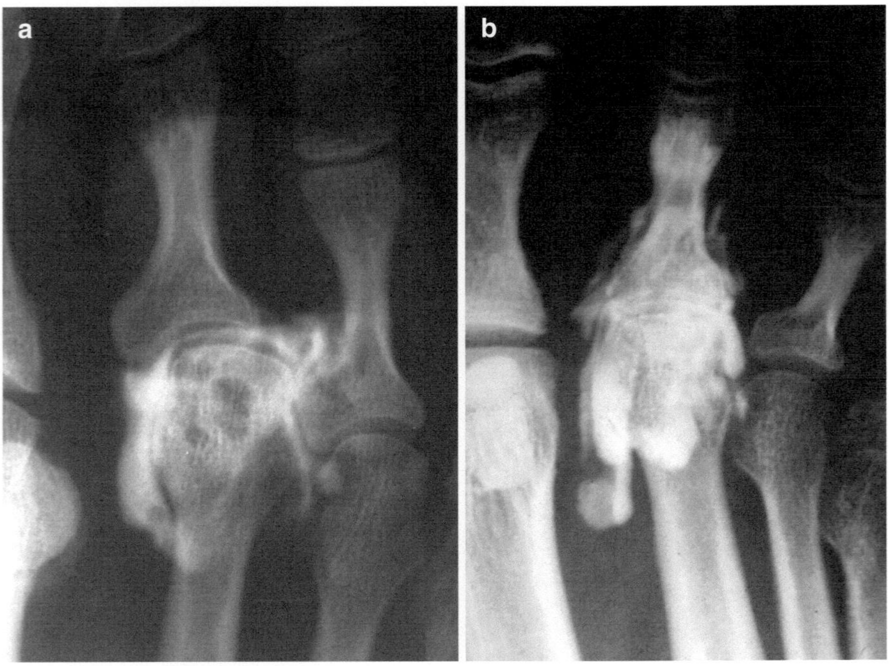

Fig. 17.6 (**a**) Normal second metatarsophalangeal arthrogram. (**b**) Abnormal second metatarsophalangeal arthrogram. Note the presence and absence of flexor tendon filling from dye leakage

into the flexor tendon sheath. On the fluoroscopic image, one would expect to see radiopaque dye proximal to the expected joint capsule tracking up the flexor tendon sheath or extravasating out of the joint capsule. The main disadvantage of this technique are the false negatives seen in joints with attenuated plantar plates that do not have discrete tears as there is no dye leakage into the flexor sheath.

Ultrasound

Diagnostic ultrasound has utility when screening patients with resistant forms of metatarsalgia and suspected plantar plate tears [2, 13–15]. Longitudinal ultrasound has been shown to be 90% accurate in the diagnosis of a tear to the plantar plate, but there is inaccuracy in being able to locate the tear. Performing dynamic ultrasound seems to increase the accuracy of diagnosis of subtle plantar plate tears [16]. Ultrasound is more cost-effective than advanced imaging techniques. With the popularity of in-office handheld ultrasound machines that provide a consistent and quick assessment, ultrasound has a place in the workup and diagnosis of plantar plate tears. If there is doubt and the patient is a surgical candidate, MRI can always be undertaken for definitive diagnosis.

MRI

MRI is an effective tool to accurately diagnose and locate plantar plate tears as well as evaluate plate attenuation [2, 13–15]. The accuracy was at 96% with MRI, and MRI was concluded to be superior to confirming tears along with localization of the tear.

The addition of contrast dye into the joint can further augment and add to the accuracy of visualization of plantar plate tears with MRI as well (Fig. 17.7 *MRI*) [17].

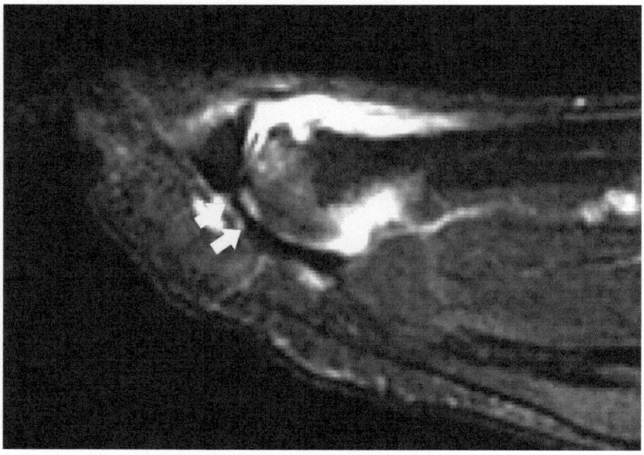

Fig. 17.7 Sagittal MRI slice of the second metatarsophalangeal joint. Note plantar plate attenuation (arrow)

The major drawback to this method is cost and the amount of variation of the joint. Bursa formation, extravasation through the capsule puncture site, and normal variant capsular recesses can attribute to an increased volume of injectable without the presence of a plantar plate tear, and results need to be interpreted carefully.

Surgical Treatment

Treatment Rationale

The plantar plate is a broad disk-shaped structure that extends the cup shape to the osseous portion of the proximal phalanx base where it is firmly attached. It is a unique structure as it is designed to withstand tensile forces via the windlass mechanism alternating with compressive forces via the load path of the metatarsal segment. Plantar plate repair is usually only a part of the surgical plan that also addresses the predisposing mechanical factors that led to the plantar plate failure. These predisposing factors such as long metatarsal, hypermobile first ray, hallux valgus, and gastrocnemius equinus need to be simultaneously addressed at the time of plantar plate repair to ensure a durable repair with less risk for subsequent failure. Direct repair techniques can also address postoperative complications associated with floating toe (Fig. 17.8).

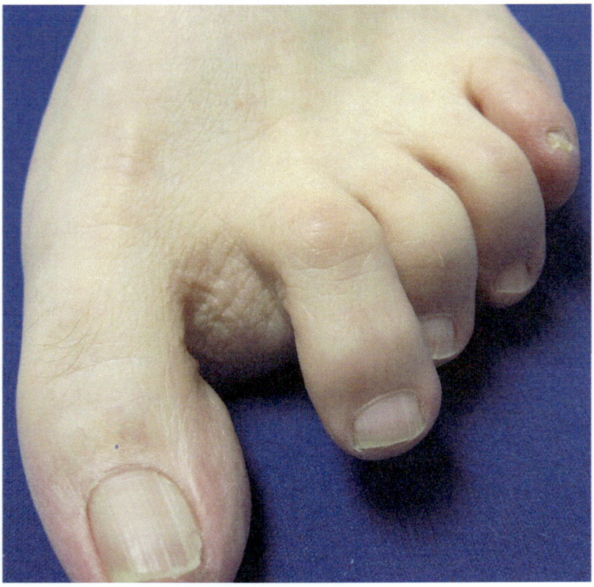

Fig. 17.8 Example of floating digit of the second toe

Surgical Procedure

A direct plantar approach affords the most straightforward method of repair of the plantar plate (Fig. 17.9 a-d). For optimal healing and visualization, it is recommended that the incision is predominantly longitudinal in orientation. It can be

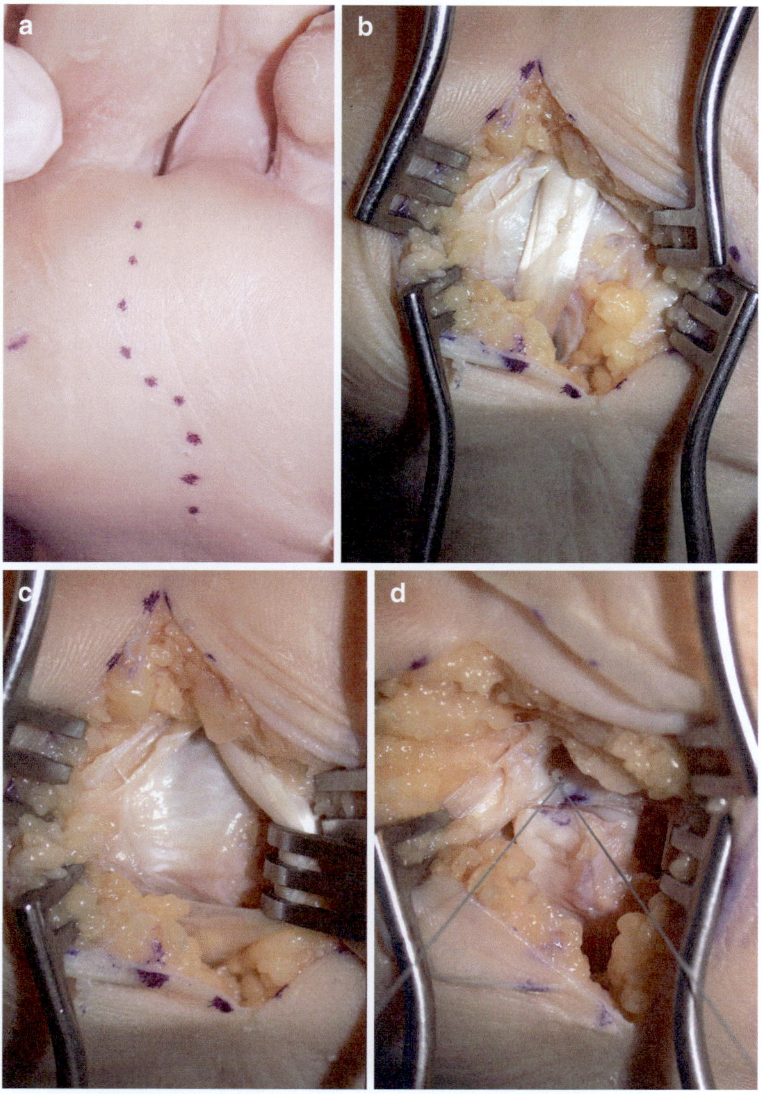

Fig. 17.9 (**a**) Planned incision for direct plantar plate repair. (**b**) Dissection exposing flexor tendon sheath. (**c**) Retraction of flexor tendons exposing attenuated plantar plate. (**d**) Plate was detached and advanced removing thinned attritional zone

longitudinal, s-shaped, or step-down in appearance; however, as the incision crosses the position of the metatarsophalangeal joints, it should cross between the metatarsal heads [1, 18]. Sharp dissection is performed through the fat pad to maintain the fibrous organization as much as possible. The incision is carried obliquely toward the plantar aspect of the head to reach the underlying flexor sheath. The sheath is longitudinally released to allow for tendon retraction, allowing full visualization of the plantar plate. The pathological appearance follows a spectrum of attenuation, partial tear, or complete tear; the tear typically transverses at either mid-substance or at the proximal phalanx insertion [1]. The type of repair is dictated by the pattern of tissue injury and degree of digital deformity. A mid-substance tear is often repaired with a 2–0 or 3–0 absorbable or nonabsorbable orthopedic suture in a figure-eight technique. In this approach, simple and complex tears of the plantar plate can be repaired. A small wedge of plate tissue can be removed during the repair to address mild transverse plane digital deformity. Tears of the base of the proximal phalanx require use of a mini bone anchors or trans-osseous suturing (Fig. 17.10). The same technique is used if the surgeon chooses to reflect the tissues off the base of the proximal phalanx to advance an attenuated plantar plate. It should be noted that with advancement, the collateral ligaments need to be released to achieve enough movement of the plate and then sutured back to the plate pad. It is recommended after placing the first suture that simulated loading of the foot is performed to determine if the toe deformity is reduced [1]. If not, it is recommended that a section of tissue be excised from the plate. Often pinning the toe in a plantarflexed position is necessary to protect the plate repair, particularly in revision situations or when the quality of the tissue is compromised. Protected

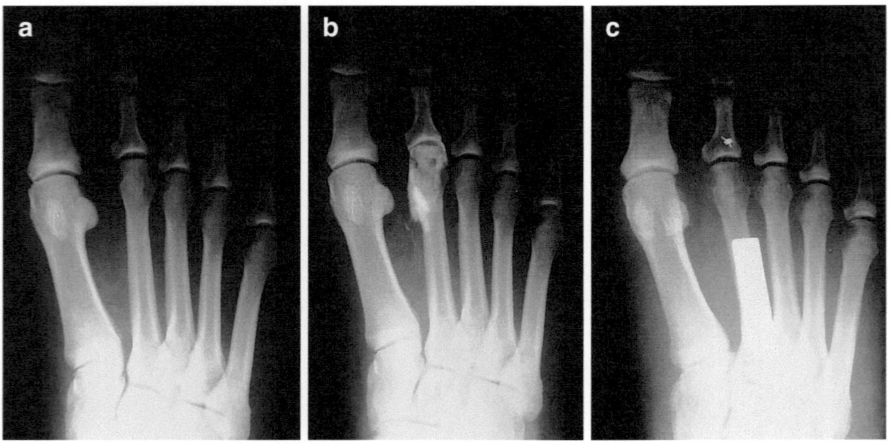

Fig. 17.10 (**a**) Case example patient with relatively long second metatarsal and intractable metatarsalgia. (**b**) Positive arthrogram for plantar plate tear. (**c**) Cylindrical shortening of the second metatarsal combined with mini anchor into the second proximal phalanx base to reattach the plantar plate

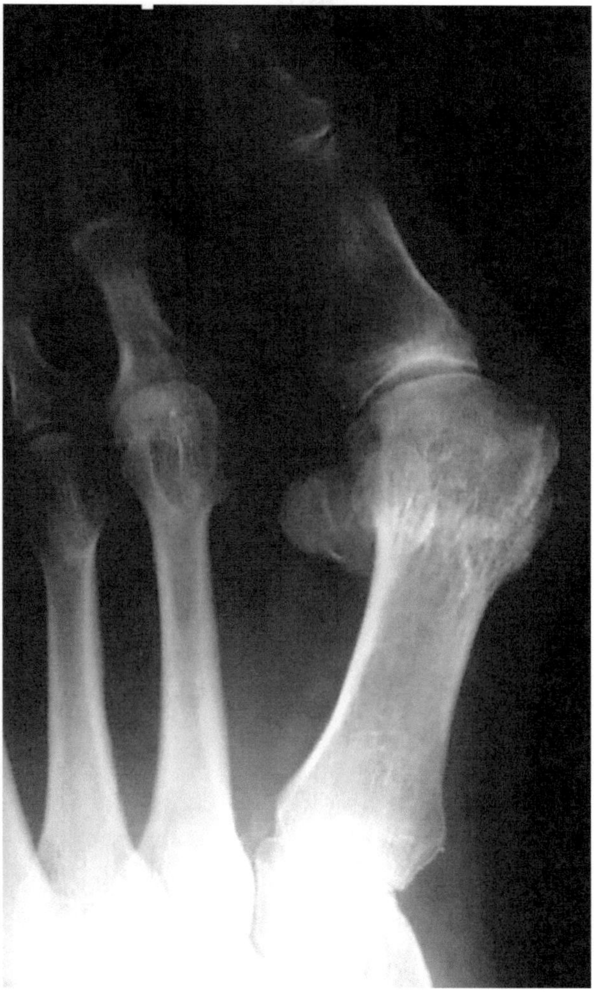

Fig. 17.11 Radiograph of the foot with severe hallux valgus and dislocated second toe

non-weightbearing for 4–6 weeks is recommended postoperatively to ensure adequate strength of the repair. Long term, the patient should be supported with orthotics for off-loading to maintain long-term durability.

Digital dislocation is the end stage of hammertoe deformity with complete rupture of the plantar plate (Fig. 17.11). While a direct approach can be made in attempt to repair the plantar plate. It is generally not possible to relocate the toe with a plantar approach. In these situations, the quality of the plantar plate remnants is generally poor. If it is known or discovered that the plantar plate is not repairable, then flexor digitorum longus transfer to the proximal phalanx base is recommended as a substitute for the plantar plate [19].

Clinical Pearls

- Direct repair of the plantar plate is a useful technique in revision hammertoe surgery or floating toe after shortening metatarsal osteotomy where the length-tension relationship of the plantar plate has been altered.
- Flexor digitorum longus tendon transfer to the proximal phalanx can be used to augment a plantar plate repair especially when the quality of the repair is in question.
- In transverse plane digital deformity with plantar plate insufficiency, an oblique transpositional osteotomy is helpful in combination with plantar plate repair to rebalance the soft tissues.
- Some surgeons prefer to use a cylindrical shortening osteotomy when performing direct plantar plate repair to reduce dorsal scaring that could impede sagittal plane digital correction.

Clinical Pitfalls

- Arthrofibrosis and risk for vascular compromise of the digit are complications that may be encountered with the use of dual incisions that cross the metatarsophalangeal joint.
- Fat pad atrophy is a risk of direct plantar plate repair; thus, blunt dissection of the fat pad is discouraged.
- Isolated direct repair of the plantar plate is generally not performed, as this technique is typically combined with other procedures. Neutralizing dynamic deforming forces and normalizing structural and functional defects of the foot can reduce destructive forces crossing the plantar plate.

References

1. Bouché RT, Heit EJ. Combined plantar plate and hammertoe repair with flexor digitorum longus tendon transfer for chronic, severe sagittal plane instability of the lesser metatarsophalangeal joints: preliminary observations. J Foot Ankle Surg. 2008;47:125–37.
2. Klein EE, Weil L Jr, Weil LS Sr, et al. Clinical examination of plantar plate abnormality: a diagnostic perspective. Foot Ankle Int. 2013;34:800–4.
3. Yu GV, Judge MS, Hudson JR, Seidelmann FE. Predislocation syndrome: progressive subluxation/dislocation of the lesser metatarsophalangeal joint. J Am Podiatr Med Assoc. 2002;92:182–99.
4. Suero EM, Meyers KN, Bohne WHO. Stability of the metatarsophalangeal joint of the lesser toes. A cadaveric study. J Orthop Res. 2012;30:1995–8.
5. Wang B, Guss AD, Ghalayon O, et al. Deep transverse metatarsal ligament and static stability of lesser metatarsophalangeal joints. Foot Ankle Int. 2015;36:573–8.
6. Christensen JC, Jennings MM. Normal and abnormal function of the first ray. Clin Podiatr Med Surg. 2009;26:355–71.
7. Klein EE, Weil L Jr, Weil LS Sr, Knight J. The underlying osseous deformity in plantar plate tears: a radiographic analysis. Foot Ankle Spec. 2013;6:108–18.

8. Coughlin MJ, Schutt SA, Hirose CB, et al. Metatarsophalangeal joint pathology in crossover second toe deformity. A cadaveric study. Foot Ankle. 2012;33:133–40.
9. Deland JT, Lee KT, Sobel M, DiCarlo EF. Anatomy of the plantar plate and its attachments in the lesser metatarsophalangeal joint. Foot Ankle Int. 1995;16:480–6.
10. Thompson FM, Hamilton WG. Problems of the second metatarsophalangeal joint. Orthopedics. 1987;10:83–9.
11. Kaz AJ, Coughlin M. Crossover second toe: demographics, etiology, and radiographic assessment. Foot Ankle Int. 2007;28:1223–37.
12. Blitz NM, Ford LA, Christensen JC. Second metatarsophalangeal joint arthrography: a cadaveric correlation study. J Foot Ankle Surg. 2004;43:231–40.
13. Gregg J, Silberstein M, Schneider T, Marks P. Sonographic and MRI evaluation of the plantar plate: a prospective study. Eur Radiol. 2006;16:2661–9.
14. Klein EE, Weil L Jr, Weil LS Sr, Knight J. Magnetic resonance imaging versus musculoskeletal ultrasound for identification and localization of plantar plate tears. Foot Ankle Spec. 2012;5:359–65.
15. Klein EE, Weil L Jr, Weil LS Sr, Knight J. Musculoskeletal ultrasound for preoperative imaging of the plantar plate: a prospective analysis. Foot Ankle Spec. 2013;6:196–200.
16. Feuerstein CA, Weil L Jr, Weil LS Sr, et al. Static versus dynamic musculoskeletal ultrasound for detection of plantar plate pathology. Foot Ankle Spec. 2014;7:259–65.
17. Mazzuca JW, Yonke B, Downes JM, Miner M. Fluoroscopic arthrography versus MR arthrography of the lesser metatarsophalangeal joints for the detection of tears of the plantar plate and joint capsule: a prospective comparative study. Foot Ankle Int. 2013;34:200–9.
18. Blitz NM, Ford LA, Christensen JC. Plantar plate repair of the second metatarsophalangeal joint: technique and tips. J Foot Ankle Surg. 2004;43:266–70.
19. Ford LA, Collins KB, Christensen JC. Stabilization of the subluxed second metatarsophalangeal joint: flexor tendon transfer versus primary repair of the plantar plate. J Foot Ankle Surg. 1998;37:217–22.

Chapter 18
Weil Osteotomy and Its Modifications

Jeremy J. Cook and Emily A. Cook

Presentation/History

Case 1: A 57-year-old female was surgically treated with multiple distal oblique metatarsal osteotomies 2 years prior to presentation to our clinic. The original treatment was for metatarsalgia. Several months after resuming normal weight-bearing activity, she developed forefoot pain diagnosed as a neuroma, this time treated with cortisone injections and off-loading orthotics. After an extended period of time, she presented to our clinic with continued diffuse forefoot pain and subjective numbness. Upon examination there is distal fat pad atrophy and prominence of both the second and third metatarsal heads. Pain upon palpation is evident at these locations. Sensation is preserved in the second interspace despite the subjective complaint of numbness (Fig. 18.1).

Diagnosis/Assessment

Tanaka and Maestro are largely credited with describing the importance of disruption of the metatarsal parabola [1, 2]. Their cumulative work contributed to our understanding that optimal functional mechanics of the forefoot require somewhat constant spatial metatarsal relationships relative to each other. Deviations lead to imbalance, which in turn contribute to digital deformities, MTP instability, soft tissue attenuation, and other forefoot pathology.

J. J. Cook (✉) · E. A. Cook
Harvard Medical School, Division of Podiatry,
Department of Surgery, Mount Auburn Hospital, Cambridge, MA, USA
e-mail: jeremycook@post.harvard.edu

E. A. Cook, J. J. Cook (eds.), *Hammertoes*,
https://doi.org/10.1007/978-3-319-16552-3_18

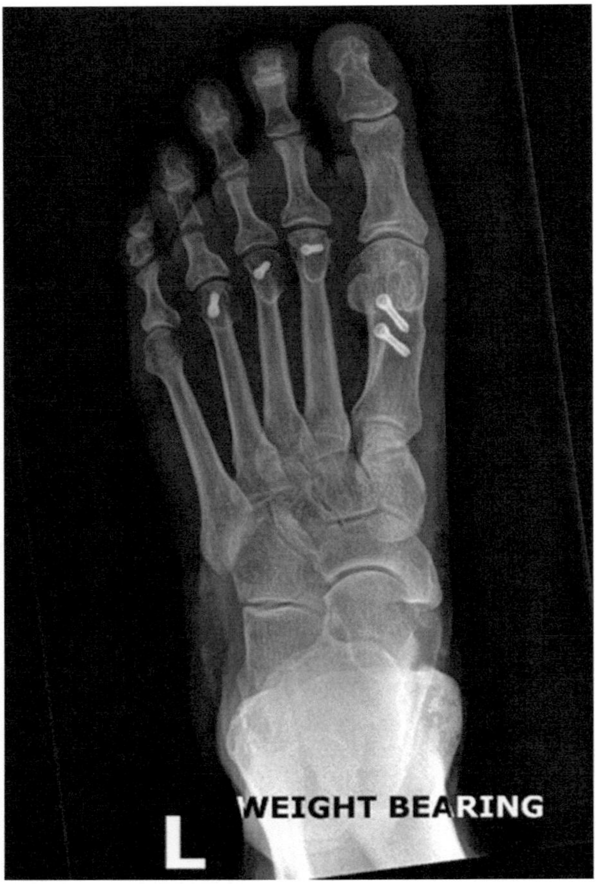

Fig. 18.1 Anterior-posterior weight-bearing radiograph status post 2-year multiple DOMOs by previous surgeon

Clinically correlated symptoms in conjunction with plain radiographs, including the anterior-posterior (AP) and sesamoid-axial, can provide a baseline screening for more overt metatarsal parabola dysfunction. Radiographs are sufficient imaging modalities for the vast majority of cases. Sometimes, advanced imaging is considered in more subtle cases and can help rule out other etiologies such as a stress fracture. Although a CT image is more precise in evaluating the metatarsal parabola, if advanced imaging is ordered, our tendency is to obtain an MRI which also permits inspection of the soft tissue structures including the collateral ligaments, plantar plate, and possible presence of a space-occupying mass such as a neuroma or bursa. In this current revision case, coronal MRI (Fig. 18.2) shows the prominent second and third metatarsals. This dysfunctional parabola was the result of significant proximal translocation of the capital fragments following original distal oblique metatarsal osteotomies. As a result, the vertical height of the metatarsals was increased and contributed to increased plantar pressures. The clinical symptoms and imaging guided treatment to a surgical correction which used distal parallel metatarsal osteotomies (DPMO) to treat the deformities. The specific technique is discussed in the subsequent text (Fig. 18.8).

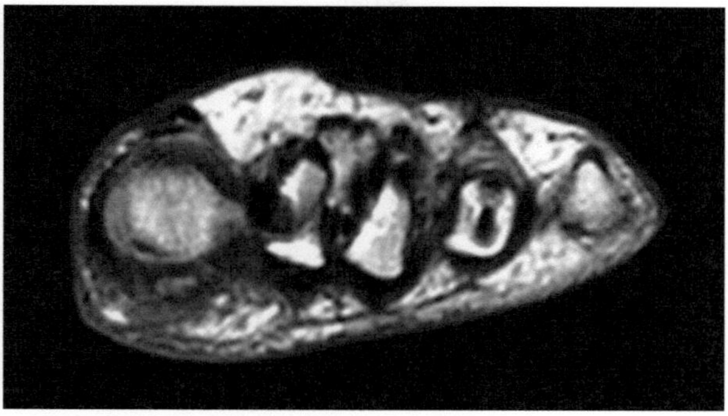

Fig. 18.2 Coronal MRI of the case patient. The image clearly demonstrates the significant abnormal prominence of the second and third metatarsals relative to the weight-bearing surface

Surgical Technique

The surgical treatment varies based on the type of distal oblique metatarsal osteotomy (DOMO) that is necessary as detailed in the next section. Surgical incision is surgeon preference and pathology specific and may be linear, curvilinear, or a skin plasty to address skin contractures. When multiple lesser metatarsal osteotomies are necessary, center the incision in the adjacent interspace (Fig. 18.3). Start the incision just proximal to the dorsal edge of the webspace and extend it proximally. If possible avoid entering the webspace with the incision as skin healing is usually more difficult here. This incision tends to be much longer than with the single osteotomy incisions in order to reduce the pressure applied to the skin edges to provide adequate exposure. Following the preferred surgical incision, the neurovascular structures are retracted as encountered down to the extensor hood. After the hood is incised, retract the tendons away to visualize the joint capsule.

The capsulotomy is dependent upon concomitant procedures and may be an inverted U if a concomitant MTPJ reconstruction is planned or anticipated. If an inverted U capsulotomy is performed, the surgeon should apply coaxial distraction to the toe to pucker the joint and to avoid joint damage while making the capsulotomy. If the surgeon performs a linear capsulotomy, the surgeon should dorsiflex the MTPJ to prevent damage to the articular cartilage. Next assess the articular cartilage and note any pathology. Raise a limited subperiosteal flap for the osteotomy extending from the dorsal articular margin proximally no more than 1 cm. Preservation of the collateral ligament attachments is not only important to digital stability but if left intact will provide a mechanism to control the capital fragment's position post-osteotomy.

MTPJs with severe dorsal contracture or frank dislocation may require more extensive periarticular release. In long-standing deformities, adhesions of the plantar structures may occur. In these limited cases, a small McGlamry elevator may be inserted partially in order to prevent excessive dissection that can destabilize the joint and lead to poor digital purchase. Complete insertion can strip the proximal insertion point of the plantar plate from the metatarsal head and is not recommended.

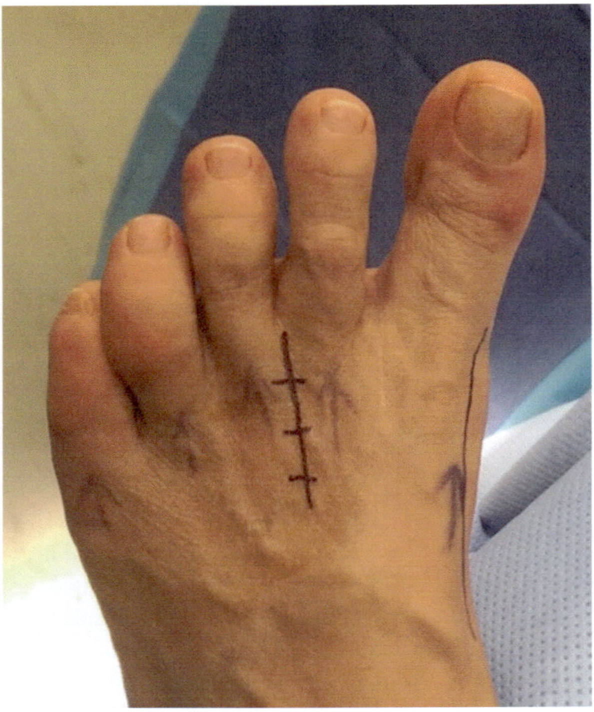

Fig. 18.3 Incision placement for multiple metatarsal osteotomies is centered in the adjacent interspace

For a traditional Weil osteotomy, the osteotomy is started within the articular surface, ~2–3 mm below the dorsalmost margin of the metatarsal head (Fig. 18.4). Please note that the authors no longer perform a traditional Weil osteotomy and now perform a modified version described within the next section. The osteotomy should be neutral in both frontal and transverse planes and oriented as close to parallel to weight-bearing surface as possible relative to the sagittal plane (Fig. 18.5). The more vertically oriented the osteotomy, the greater the translation within the sagittal plane. If not performed in this manner, less shortening occurs, and instead the capital fragment becomes more plantarly prominent.

Once the osteotomy is complete, the capital fragment will often seek its own level, migrating proximally and plantarly. If it moves to a level that makes sense based on preoperative assessment, then it is acceptable to fixate at that level. However, "seeking its own level" does not guarantee the best position. Studies have shown that translocation of >3 mm will result in clinically significant plantarflexion and increased vertical height of the metatarsal head, leading to a plantarly prominent metatarsal head clinically and plantar shift of the MTPJ center of rotation [3]. If manually translocating the capital fragment, be cognizant that the greater the translocation, the greater the degree of shortening and plantarflexion.

Once the capital fragment is in the necessary position, a temporary k-wire (depending on the size of the metatarsal) can be used to prevent movement. Fixation is surgeon dependent, but we prefer cannulated screws for this procedure. The guide

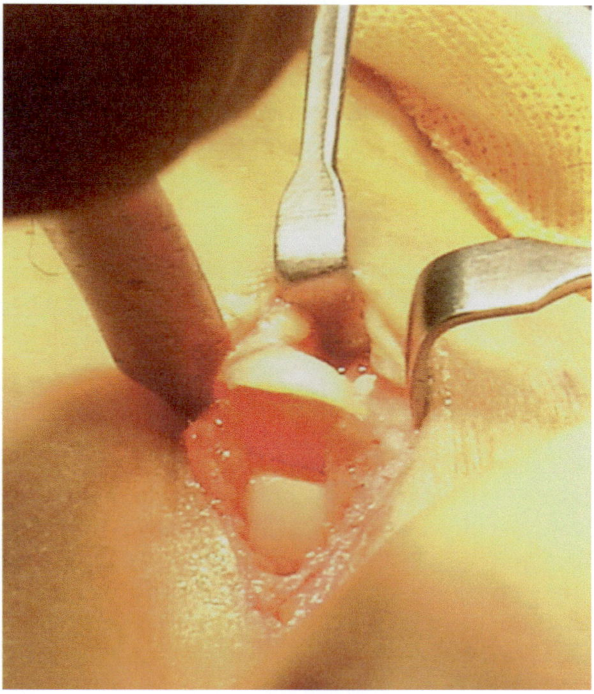

Fig. 18.4 Intra-operative image showing the thickness of the dorsal shelf created by the distal oblique osteotomies. The techniques which use multiple cuts will result in a thinner dorsal shelf

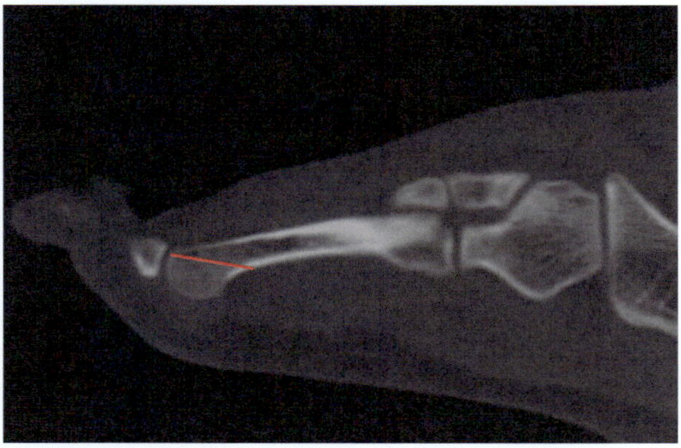

Fig. 18.5 CT image demonstrating the standard position of the DOMO (Weil osteotomy). This is a single-cut intra-articular osteotomy and should be neutral in both frontal and transverse planes and oriented as close to parallel to weight-bearing surface as possible relative to the sagittal plane. The more vertically oriented the osteotomy, the greater the translation within the sagittal plane

wire is oriented perpendicular to the osteotomy and it's usually ~ 1 cm from the articular surface. Drill, countersink, and measure are per manufacturer protocol. A 12 mm or 14 mm screw is usually used, but be sure that the measurement doesn't permit intra-articular penetration. Remove the temporary k-wire. Finally, use a rongeur and resect the distal overhang to contour the edge. Typically a single 2.5 mm screw is adequate for fixation but is more vulnerable to rotation than two screws. Supplement with either a 2.5 mm or 2.0 mm screw to avoid rotation. There should be at least one screw head width distance between each screw head to prevent stress riser. In cases where translocation of more than 3 mm is needed, it is more typical to use a two-screw construct along with a MTPJ reconstruction for soft tissue rebalancing.

With fixation complete, irrigation and closure are performed as dictated by the concomitant procedures with absorbable suture deep and skin closure [4].

Iterations of the Osteotomy

Although the classic "Weil" osteotomy is not technically difficult, overtime it became evident that the Weil osteotomy had intrinsic limitations, which not only were less effective, but actually contributory to suboptimal results and complications such as, a floating toe and transfer metatarsalgia [5].

As noted above, excessive translocation can lead to plantar prominence, but another important impact is the influence this has on the center of rotation (COR) of the MTPJ. As presented by Trnka et al., translocation of the capital fragment simultaneously moves the MTPJ center of rotation (COR). In a normally aligned toe, the COR is coplanar with the adjacent interosseous tendon. In contrast, a digit dorsally contracted at the MTPJ will have the interosseous tendon axis dorsally deviated such that it functions above the COR and is unable to aid with MTPJ plantarflexion [4]. Following a standard distal oblique metatarsal osteotomy, the axis of the interosseous tendon improves, but the COR remains well below the tendon which contributes to the "floating toe" frequently associated with these osteotomies. This is further exacerbated by aggressive translocation. Dr. Barouk is credited with recognizing some of these issues and introduced a modification deemed the "second layer Weil osteotomy." [3] Essentially, this modification added a second osteotomy cut to the original Weil osteotomy. The second osteotomy was made plantar and slightly off-axis from the first osteotomy resulting in a plantar-posterior-based wedge (Fig. 18.6). With the wedge of bone removed, the COR assumed better position relative to the intrinsic muscles. The second layer technique is somewhat difficult to perform resulting in variability in wedge thickness. If the wedge was made too thin, then it failed to adequately address the previously noted problems.

If the wedge was made too thick, it created two distinct issues. The first was that the available articular surface area and functional cartilage available for ROM was significantly reduced. The second issue was that it resulted in overly aggressive elevation of the metatarsal head causing a dysfunctional loading surface. This latter problem was further compounded when multiple osteotomies were performed resulting in disruption of the functional metatarsal parabola.

Although a significant improvement over the original Weil osteotomy, the second layer technique was still vulnerable to the above mentioned shortcomings. Another

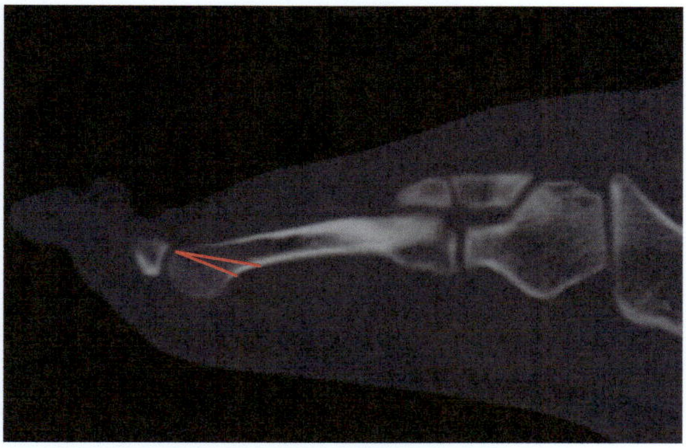

Fig. 18.6 CT image demonstrating the standard position of the "second layer Weil osteotomy." This is a multiple-cut intra-articular osteotomy which results in a plantar-posterior-based wedge. As with the DOMO, both cuts should be neutral in both frontal and transverse planes

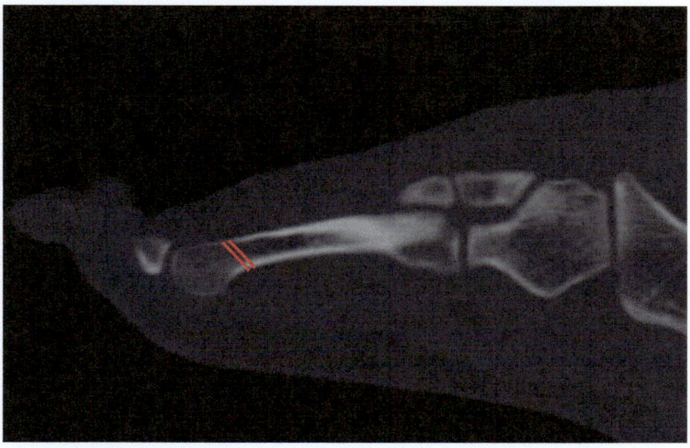

Fig. 18.7 CT image demonstrating the standard position of the Maceira osteotomy. Unlike the other techniques described, this multiple-cut osteotomy is purely extra-articular. The cuts are parallel to each other and nearly perpendicular to the longitudinal axis of the metatarsal. The resultant shortening minimizes the plantar prominence of the head even in significant length changes

solution was the technique as described by Maceira which used parallel cuts within the metatarsal neck. It differs from the prior techniques since it is an extra-articular osteotomy within the longitudinal axis of the metatarsal (Fig. 18.7). The primary benefit of the technique was that it is a purely shortening procedure that doesn't convert the intrinsic muscles into dorsiflexors of the MTPJ. Since the osteotomy does not alter the COR, the procedure remains vulnerable to a post-operative floating toe. The main limitation of the technique is achieving stable fixation. Due to the location and more vertical orientation of the cuts, there is a smaller osteotomy surface area available for fixation [3, 6, 7].

The final modification has been used in our practice for several years and is simply a merger of the Maceira and the second layer Weil osteotomy, simply called a "Weil with a Wafer." Instead of taking a wedge, parallel osteotomies are made intra-articularly at the typical location and orientation. The second cut is made parallel

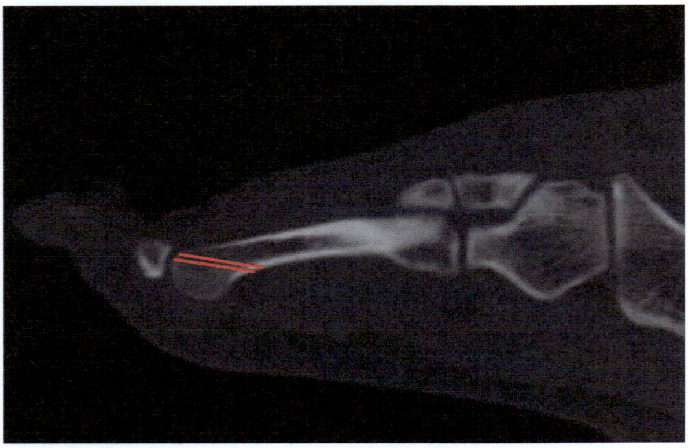

Fig. 18.8 CT image demonstrating the orientation of the distal parallel metatarsal osteotomy (DPMO). This is the authors' preferred technique, which is also called a "Weil with a Wafer." As with prior iterations, this is a multiple-cut intra-articular osteotomy that is neutral in both frontal and transverse planes. It preserves MTPJ center of rotation and minimizes the increase in plantar prominence

but 1–2 mm plantar to the normal osteotomy (Fig. 18.8). The resulting wedge is 1–2 mm in thickness and allows for greater shortening while restoring the COR into a more anatomically correct position. The capital fragment translates as with the traditional Weil osteotomy, but with the wafer removed, the metatarsal head translates dorsally as well. Unlike the traditional Weil osteotomy, the vertical height of the metatarsal is not significantly increased by a mere 3 mm displacement. And unlike the "second layer Weil," this distal parallel metatarsal osteotomy (DPMO) doesn't trade functional cartilage for correction. The DPMO can be fixated with 1–2 screws. The primary limitation is the technical difficulty in creating precise parallel osteotomies in such a small space. Commercially produced guides such as the Metatarsal Osteotomy Guide (MOG) are available to help with this technique and to produce a greater degree of precision.

Outcomes

The role of a dysfunctional metatarsal parabola in digital deformity genesis is indisputable [1, 2]. Hofstaetter et al. reported that after 7 years of follow-up, 88% of patients rated their outcome as good to excellent despite moderate to severe joint stiffness in 68% in patients with a mean shortening of 4.3 mm [8]. Although the traditional Weil osteotomy has been successful in treatment of metatarsalgia, it has a duplicitous impact on the treatment of hammertoe deformities. The traditional Weil osteotomy has been a standard of care for years but is frequently associated with floating toes. Frequency of this complication is variable and has been reported with a frequency of 20–68% [4, 8–10]. Those numbers must be considered within context. None of the studies statistically controlled for the amount of shortening that occurred in surgery. As noted before capital fragment translocation of more than 3 mm has significant biomechanical consequences. O'Kane and Kilmartin performed Weil osteotomies with an average shortening of 5.2 mm, and this resulted in floating toe in 42% of patients [11]. Flint et al. performed 138 Weil osteotomies with an average shortening of 2.4 mm resulting in a postoperative floating toe rate of 18% [12].

Pérez Muñoz and colleagues performed 314 Weil osteotomies with the secondary resection technique in a patient population needing >4 mm of shortening and found a satisfaction rate of 80% and floating toe occurrence of 4%. The most common complaint was stiffness in 60.2% of patients [13].

References

Clinical Pearls/Pitfalls

- Each metatarsal declination angle changes moving laterally, and the declination angle becomes more parallel with the weight-bearing surface. This has several significant consequences. The risk of the saw blade running up the shaft increases. Another consequence is that the osteotomy becomes longer. Finally, as you move laterally, the physical barrier of the foot itself will cause the angle of the osteotomy to become more vertically oriented. This is generally well tolerated because less translation is usually necessary in the third and fourth metatarsals in order to achieve correction of the metatarsal parabola.
- If the dorsal osteotomy isn't at least 2 mm below the dorsal distal articular surface, then the thickness of the dorsal shelf can be too thin and more prone to stress risers (Fig. 18.4).
- When performing multiple osteotomies, start medial and move lateral in order to preserve the metatarsal parabola relationship.
- Don't forget to consider the roles of the plantar plate and collateral ligaments in MTPJ stability and prevention of floating toe.

1. Tanaka Y, Takakura Y, Kumai T, Samoto N, Tamai S. Radiographic analysis of hallux valgus. A two-dimensional coordinate system. J Bone Joint Surg Am. 1995;77:205–13.
2. Maestro M, Besse J, Ragusa M, Berthonnaud E. Forefoot morphotype study and planning method for forefoot osteotomy. Foot Ankle Clin. 2003;8:695–710.
3. Barouk LS. Forefoot reconstruction. 2nd ed. Paris: Springer; 2005.
4. Trnka J, Nyska M, Parks BG, Myerson MS. Dorsiflexion contracture after the Weil osteotomy: results of cadaver study and three-dimensional analysis. Foot Ankle Int. 2001;22:47–50.
5. Maceira E, Farinas F, Tena J, Escobar R, Baltes JL. Analisis de la Rididez Metatarso-falangica en las Osteotomias de Weil. Rev Med Cir Pie. 1988;XII(2):35–40.
6. Espinosa N, Myerson MS, Fernandez de Retana P, Maceira E. A new approach for the treatment of metatarsalgia: the triple Weil osteotomy. Tech Foot Ankle Surg. 2009;6:254–63.

7. Hofstaetter SG, Hofstaetter JG, Petroutasas JA. The Weil osteotomy: a seven-year follow-up. J Bone Joint Surg Br. 2005;87:1507–11.
8. Migues A, Slullitel G, Bilbao F, Carrasco M, Solari G. Floating-toe deformity as a complication of the Weil osteotomy. Foot Ankle Int. 2004;25(9):609–13.
9. Perez HR, Reber LK, Christensen JC. The role of passive plantarflexion in floating toes following Weil osteotomy. J Foot Ankle Surg. 2008;47(6):520–6.
10. O'Kane C, Kilmartin TE. The surgical management of central metatarsalgia. Foot Ankle Int. 2002;23(5):415–9.
11. Flint WW, Macias DM, Jastifer JR, Doty JF, Hirose CB, Coughlin MJ. Plantar plate repair for lesser metatarsophalangeal joint instability. Foot Ankle Int. 2017;38(3):234–42.
12. Pérez Muñoz I, Escobar-Antón D, Sanz-Gómez TA. The role of Weil and triple Weil osteotomies in the treatment of propulsive metatarsalgia. Foot Ankle Int. 2012;33:501–6.
13. Roukis TS. Central metatarsal head-neck osteotomies: indications and operative techniques. Clin Podiatr Med Surg. 2005;22(2):197–222.

Chapter 19
Lesser MTPJ Reconstruction

Emily A. Cook, Jeremy J. Cook, and Robin Cook

Presentation/History

Rupture, attenuation, and/or imbalances of the collateral ligaments and plantar plate lead to sagittal, frontal, and/or transverse subluxation of the proximal phalanx resulting in various deformities including hammertoes, crossover toes, and transverse plane digital deviations (Fig. 19.1a–d). Many of the traditional techniques which address MTPJ stability, including extensor tendon lengthenings, MTPJ releases, flexor digitorum longus tendon transfers, and Weil osteotomies, have been known to potentially lead to less predictable outcomes including floating toes, malalignment, continued pain, and dissatisfaction (Fig. 19.2). The poor predictability of lesser MTPJ rebalancing is likely due to the fact that underlying etiologies are often multifactorial, complex, and vary widely between patients. Rebalancing of the soft tissue structures surrounding the MTPJ and reestablishing the center of rotation of the MTPJ are technically difficult. The physical size of the structures and confined space as well as limitations in specialized surgical instrumentation has made MTPJ rebalancing particularly challenging. As a result, nonanatomic repairs and releases, often combined with temporary pinning of the MTPJ, are commonly performed procedures [1–6].

Advances in research have allowed foot and ankle surgeons to achieve a deeper understanding of MTPJ instability etiology. Surgical instrumentation developed from this research and biomechanic testing has improved the ability to restore anatomic alignment and function in a more predictable manner. We now know that the soft tissue construct comprised of both the plantar plate and the associated collateral ligaments play critical roles in the stability of the MTPJ. Therefore, a MTPJ repair should be at least considered whenever instability of the MTPJ is observed or created [7–9].

E. A. Cook (✉) · J. J. Cook · R. Cook
Harvard Medical School, Division of Podiatry, Department of Surgery, Mount Auburn Hospital, Cambridge, MA, USA
e-mail: ecook@mah.harvard.edu

E. A. Cook, J. J. Cook (eds.), *Hammertoes*,
https://doi.org/10.1007/978-3-319-16552-3_19

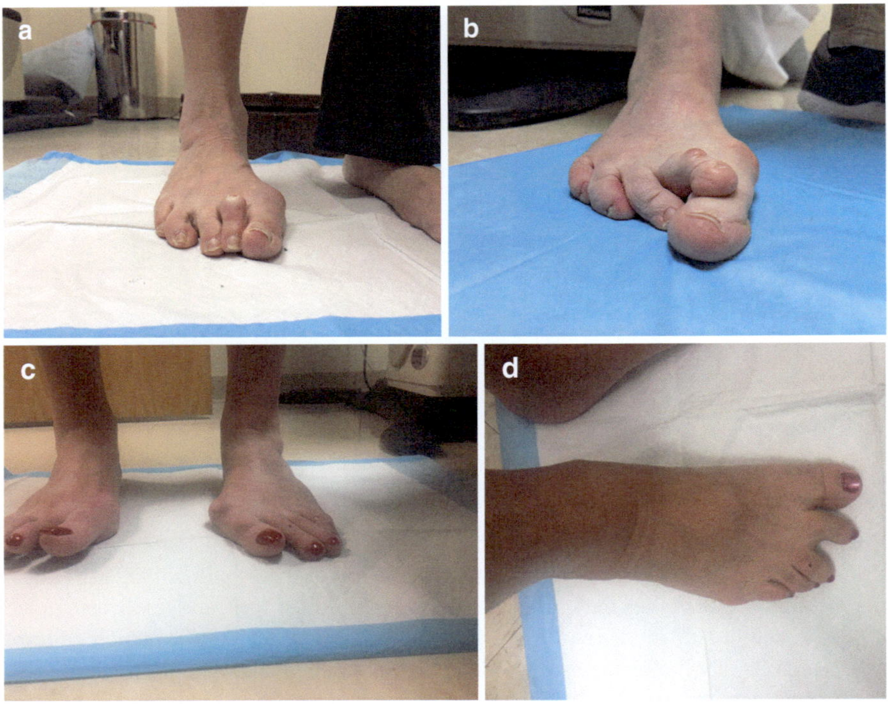

Fig. 19.1 The etiology of hammertoes is complex and can vary significantly between patients resulting in different pathologies including (**a**) a traditional hammertoe deformity; (**b**) crossover toe deformity; (**c**) lateral transverse plane deviation; and (**d**) deformities involving multiple MTPJs

Fig. 19.2 Floating toe after a bunionectomy, traditional Weil osteotomy, and PIPJ arthrodesis

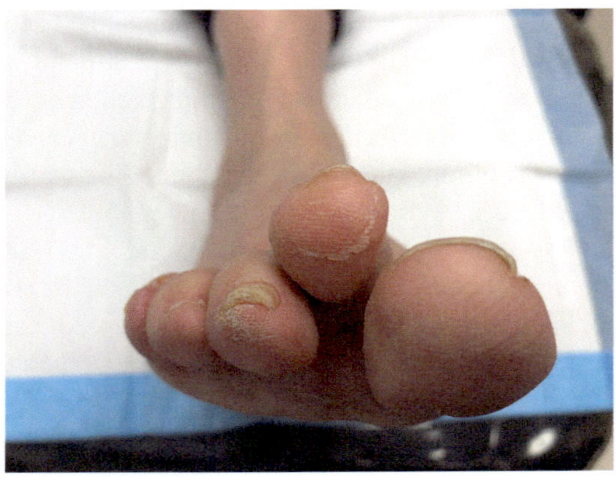

There is a significant and important distinction between a "plantar plate repair" and a MTPJ repair, and these two terms should not be used interchangeably. A plantar plate repair is based off of the traditional belief that there is a physical tear within the plantar plate, and this is directly or indirectly repaired. This chapter instead focuses on MTPJ repair which involves rebalancing the accessory and proper medial and lateral ligaments, in addition to an insufficient or torn plantar plate. Much like a Brostrom procedure, a stable tissue cuff is preserved on the metatarsal head proximally to plicate the distal soft tissue attenuation or compromise. In the current procedure, the attenuated or insufficient plantar plate and collateral ligaments are released from their insertions on the proximal phalanx as one unit and then anatomically reattached under physiologic tension to restore MTPJ alignment, balance, and function.

The history or clinical presentation of MTPJ pathology varies significantly depending on the underlying etiology, patient characteristics, and severity. Active or athletic patients may relate a traumatic event where there was a "pop" or pain beneath the toe during an activity or injury. More commonly, patients with longstanding hallux valgus or first ray pathology will present with 2nd MTPJ pathology. There may be pain association with the bunion or first ray, but this is frequently asymptomatic. Although medial column pathology is often asymptomatic it must be addressed in conjunction with the MTPJ pathology. Both hallux valgus and lesser toe deformities are more prevalent in females, and both deformities are believed to be highly heritable as assessed in 2446 adults in the Framingham Foot Study [10]. The examiner should also determine if there have been previous surgeries, infections, or wounds to this area. There should be no active wounds and infections if considering a lesser MTPJ repair.

Diagnosis/Assessment

Assessment and diagnosis of plantar forefoot pain or metatarsalgia can be challenging, and the biomechanic complexity of the MTPJ is often underestimated. While collateral ligament and plantar plate insufficiencies can be obvious when there is a crossover toe, they are often subtle and frequently missed in patients with intractable metatarsalgia. There should be a high index of suspicion of plantar plate and collateral ligament pathology in the setting of a corresponding hammertoe, first ray pathology, callus, or swelling beneath the metatarsal head or equinus.

One common condition in which MTPJ pathology is confused with is a neuroma. This is because pain can be present on palpation in the distal sulcus with both conditions. Splaying of the toes may also be interpreted as a positive Sullivan's sign when in reality there is insufficiency or rupture of the collateral ligaments and/or plantar plate. Distinguishing between a neuroma and MTPJ pathology is critical as administration of a corticosteroid injection can further weaken the MTPJ complex, and the patient may be exposed to a neuroma excision but still have pain postoperatively due to the primary pathologic process being within the MTPJ.

Additional differential diagnoses may include but are not limited to capsulitis without MTPJ or plantar plate insufficiency or rupture, distal metatarsal stress fracture, Freiberg's infraction, as well as any form of arthritis including rheumatoid, psoriatic arthritis, gout, osteoarthritis, infectious, or post-traumatic.

While additional laboratory testing and imaging may be helpful in certain cases, MTPJ instability and imbalances are clinical diagnoses. In our experience, a good history and clinical examination is often more reliable and sensitive than imaging or serologic tests. We frequently obtain weight-bearing radiographs of the foot to assess alignment but reserve additional testing only for when the diagnosis is not clear. When needing to confirm or rule out other differential diagnosis, additional tests may include but are not limited to advanced imaging such as a MRI or CT and serologic testing. One simple test that may help confirm MTPJ insufficiency, especially in subtle or acute cases, is to perform a digital strapping (Fig. 19.3). If stabilization of the toe with either a strap or tape reduces pain, this helps support the diagnosis of MTPJ insufficiency. Less frequently, we may supplement the exam by performing a local anesthetic diagnostic block either within the joint or interspace to further confirm the location of the pathology. But the history and clinical examination are the most crucial components of diagnosing MTPJ pathology.

This clinical examination should include assessment both in the non-weight-bearing and stance (or simulated stance) positions. While the patient is seated, visual examination may reveal a hammertoe or a lesser toe transverse plane deviation where the toe may abut another toe. However, there may be no obvious deformity in the case of a pre-dislocation syndrome [11]. There may or may not be edema, warmth, or pain with palpation directly beneath the metatarsal head or more commonly within the distal sulcus. MTPJ range of motion may be completely normal, smooth, and pain-free but depends on the severity of the deformity. If there is limited dorsiflexion, there is likely dorsal subluxation of the proximal phalanx on the metatarsal head. A dorsal drawer test can also be helpful in differentiating pain from other etiologies such as a neuroma. However, a dorsal drawer test is often performed and interpreted incorrectly. To correctly perform a dorsal drawer test, the examiner should use one hand to stabilize the metatarsal head. The other hand should grasp the proximal phalanx where the thumb applies an upward pressure in order to try to sublux the MTPJ. The amount of displacement should be compared to the adjacent joints and contralateral limb [12]. This displacement may not be visualized in cases where the joint is already maximally subluxed or in obese patients. Therefore, a positive test is when there is either greater displacement compared to non-painful intact lesser MTPJs, pain elicited during the test, or no additional subluxation due to a pre-existing proximal phalanx dorsal subluxation or dislocation. In more chronic cases, the dorsal drawer test is often not painful, yet the

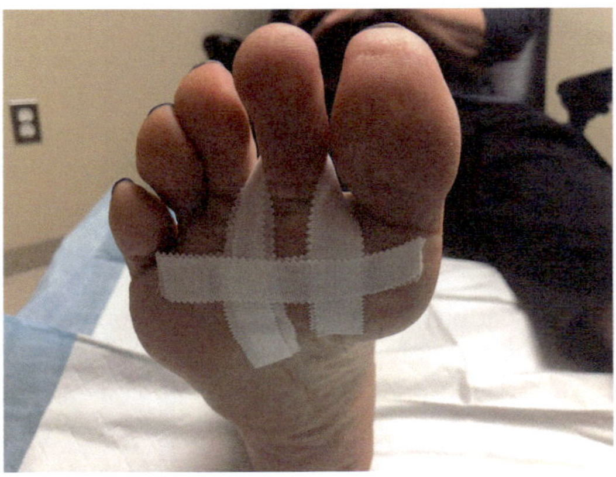

Fig. 19.3 A digital strapping is often performed to assess whether or not this provides temporary in recalcitrant metatarsalgia cases

examiner can easily dorsally displace the proximal phalanx. If the dorsal drawer test is truly negative, but the toe is transversely deviated, there should be a high suspicion for collateral ligament tear or imbalances.

Forefoot deformities often become more apparent during a stance evaluation or when the foot is loaded to simulate weight-bearing. A Kelikian push-up test can be performed by placing pressure beneath the metatarsal head and evaluating whether or not the lesser toe is in the correct alignment. On stance evaluation, the corresponding proximal phalanx may be dorsally and/or transversely subluxed. A second toe that is medially deviated and abutting the hallux and any crossover toe is pathognomonic for MTPJ instability.

Digital purchase should also be assessed, but there are no strict criteria in regard to this assessment. The lack of digital purchase may be visually apparent when the distal tuft of the lesser toe does not touch the ground during a stance examination. Another method for determining digital purchase is during a seated exam with the patient's hip, knee, and ankle at 90°. The patient is asked to push the toe down as much as possible for 3–4 s, while the examiner tries to slide a standard business card out from beneath the toe. There is good digital purchase if the patient can maintain purchase of the card. However, there is no degree of resistance specified for the examiner [13]. Even in the setting of good digital purchase, it is still quite possible to have MTPJ instability either within the collateral ligaments and/or plantar plate. Conversely, if there is no digital purchase, this helps confirm more severe MTPJ instability.

Weight-bearing radiographs can confirm clinical findings and provide quantitative angular measurements of MTPJ imbalances. While the physician may choose to perform an MRI to rule out other causes, an MRI is not necessary to diagnose MTPJ instability. MRIs often do not always show collateral ligament and plantar plate pathology even when it exists, especially in cases of attenuation and imbalances. To improve sensitivity and specificity of MRI, the digit may be strapped in a dorsiflexed position or one may order a 50% overlap or multiple overlapping thin slab/slice acquisition.

A vascular examination is performed on every surgical candidate and may include palpation of the pedal arteries, skin temperature, quality, and coloration assessment as well as capillary refill. It is important to consider that a chronic rigidly contracted toe can experience vasospasm once placed back into a rectus position acutely. Even with a normal vascular exam, although rare, it is possible to develop a vascular complication postoperatively. This is theoretically more common in a crossover toe or rigid deformity or if performing simultaneous adjacent MTPJ reconstructions given the degree of dissection necessary. In general, we rarely find that adjacent MTPJ reconstructions are necessary, even if multiple MTPJs are unstable, due to the vassal principle from the interconnectivity of the deep transverse metatarsal ligament, plantar fascia, as well as the extrinsic and intrinsic tendons. If there is a crossover toe, although not necessary the patient may be asked to perform tapings of the digit prior to surgery in order to improve flexibility of the digit and theoretically reduce the risk of vasospasm. However, if there is a very rigid and severe deformity, the patient is counseled on the possibility of vasospasm, and consideration is given toward a concurrent lesser metatarsal shortening osteotomy to help decompress tension placed on the proper digital arteries within the toes. If there are any vascular concerns identified on clinical exam, additional vascular consultation and/or testing is performed prior to consideration of any elective forefoot procedures.

Surgical Technique

A MTPJ repair is rarely performed in isolation and is frequently combined with correction of the major underlying etiology. Addressing the underlying etiology either surgically or conservatively is critical but beyond the scope of this chapter. Major culprits include first ray deformities such as a bunions, hammertoes, or metatarsal osteotomies when there is significant disruption to the metatarsal parabola. A gastrocnemius lengthening or other proximal procedures are sometimes necessary depending on the underlying etiology and severity. Many of these topics are covered in other chapters of this book.

A true MTPJ repair, as opposed to a "plantar plate repair" or "MTPJ release," consists of addressing the plantar plate and collateral ligaments by reefing these structures under appropriate physiologic tension in order to rebalance the MTPJ. The MTPJ reconstruction may also be combined with a PIPJ arthrodesis and/or lesser metatarsal osteotomy within the same ray as described in other chapters. When performed correctly, a MTPJ repair obviates the need for nonanatomic capsulotomies, capsulorrhaphies, MTPJ releases, flexor tendon, and extensor tendon transfers.

This surgical technique is system specific. We have outlined the technique for the system in which we have the most experience with utilizing. We favor this system for a multitude of reasons including that it is the only system to the authors' knowledge that has undergone rigorous mechanical testing both through computer simulation and cadaveric testing, addresses the collateral ligaments, and does not strip the plantar plate from its origin on the metatarsal head. Many of the other systems endorse stripping the origin of the plantar plate from the metatarsal head with a McGlamry elevator. We believe this is diametrically opposed to this surgery's intent of stabilization. Stripping of the metatarsal in this fashion allows for instability of the origin of the plantar plate.

Concomitant procedures are almost always performed first. An exception to this occurs when simultaneously performing a lesser metatarsal osteotomy or PIPJ arthrodesis with a MTPJ reconstruction. Under these circumstances, the dissection and suture tagging of the plantar plate and collateral ligaments is performed first, followed by the other concomitant procedures and ending with the remaining portions of the MTPJ reconstruction.

The MTPJ reconstruction begins with an incision over the affected MTPJ. The incision is based on surgeon preference which can be done in a longitudinal or curvilinear fashion or through a multitude of local flap options. The extensor hood is identified, and an extensor tenolysis is performed (Fig. 19.4a–b). The extensor tendons are either retracted or reflected with an open z-lengthening which is then later repaired during the soft tissue closure. The subcutaneous tissue is then bluntly separated from the capsule medially and laterally (Fig. 19.5a–c).

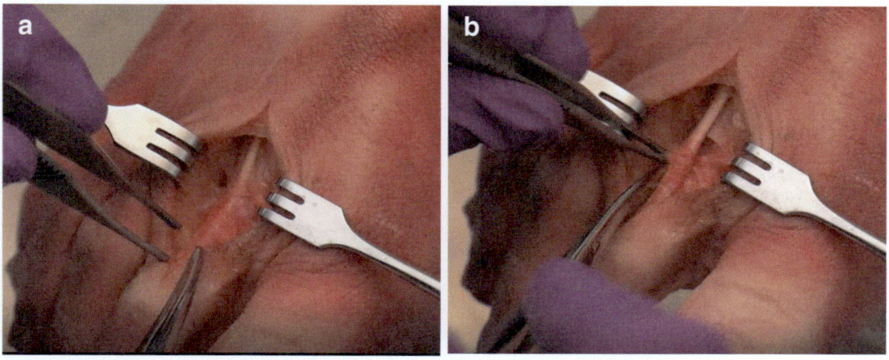

Fig. 19.4 (**a**) The extensor hood is identified and (**b**) a tenolysis is performed

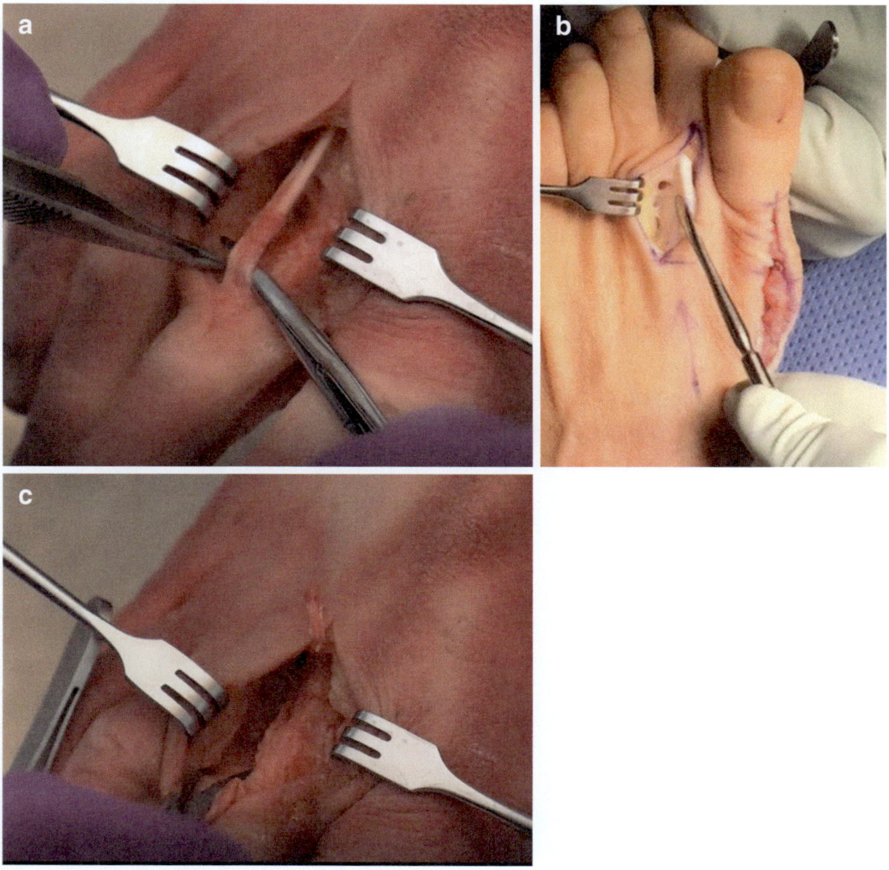

Fig. 19.5 Based on the extent of contracture or tension on the extensor tendons, they are either retracted to one side throughout the procedure or an open Z-lengthening is performed. (**a**) Testing of the degree of extensor tendon tension; (**b**) example of retracting extensors to one side; (**c**) example of performing an extensor tendon open Z-lengthening and subsequent blunt subcutaneous tissue separation of the MTPJ capsule

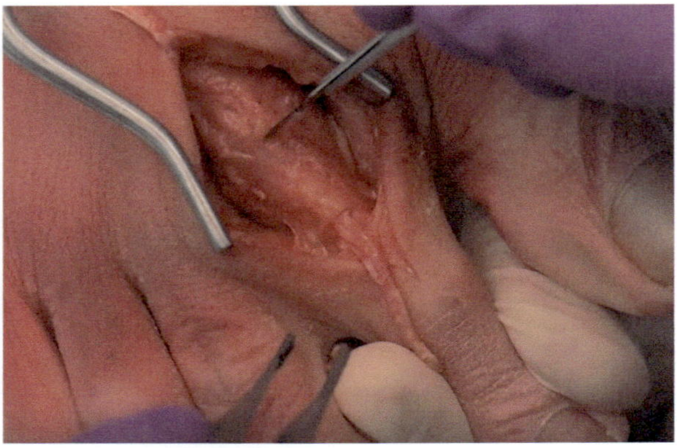

Fig. 19.6 An inverted U-capsulotomy is performed hugging the base of the proximal phalanx to ensure there is enough tissue accessible for suture tagging. This location becomes more apparent by distracting the toe and puckering the joint while performing the capsulotomy

The MTPJ is accessed through an inverted U-capsulotomy, which can lengthened longitudinally if a metatarsal osteotomy is also planned (Fig. 19.6). If performing a metatarsal osteotomy, we recommend only removing enough tissue to perform the osteotomy and to place osteotomy fixation through the tissue in order to preserve all medial and lateral collateral ligament attachments. The collateral ligaments and plantar plate are then detached from the proximal phalanx base in one intact sheet of tissue (Fig. 19.7a–d). The flexor tendon lies directly beneath the plantar plate, and therefore manual distraction of the toe with adequate visualization is necessary to avoid iatrogenic flexor tendon damage when releasing the plantar plate. There is a pin distractor that is also available for excessively contracted joints or if performing the procedure without an assistant (Fig. 19.8a–c). This is the most critical component of the dissection as it is easy to inadvertently shred the tissue resulting in a less ideal repair. A 60° beaver blade is sometimes helpful in releasing the soft tissue from the plantar aspect of the proximal phalanx. A blunt elevator also assists in freeing up the plantar plate from the flexor tendon enough so that the foot of the suture passer will be able to grasp the plantar plate. Finally, rasp the base of the proximal phalanx to create bleeding bone for the eventual repair to bond with during the postoperative period.

If performed correctly, even severely compromised tissue can be repaired. The final goal is to have a contiguous collar of tissue, consisting of the collateral ligaments and plantar plate that surrounds the metatarsal head. It is important to note that all proximal attachments are left intact, maintaining their respective anatomic metatarsal attachments (Fig. 19.9).

The tissue is then tagged with a specialized suture passer (Fig. 19.10a–d). Nonabsorbable 2–0 sutures are placed within the medial and lateral collateral ligaments as well as the medial and lateral portions of the plantar plate. To determine the best suture placement, visually bisect each collateral ligament and tag the collateral ligaments just plantar to their respective bisection (Fig. 19.11). We have found that if you tag the ligaments too high, then you risk subluxing the proximal

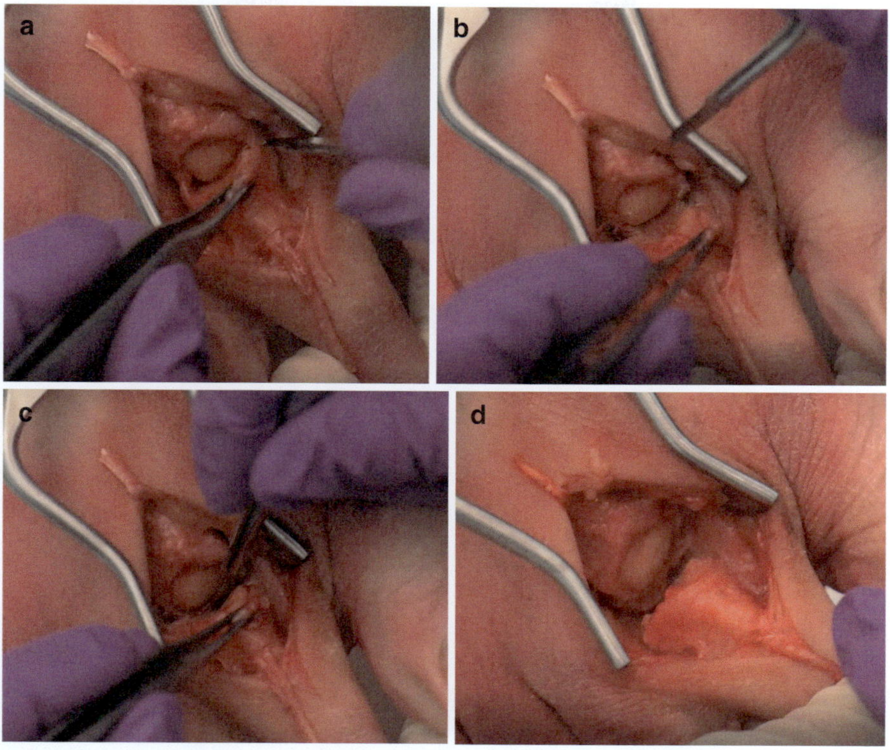

Fig. 19.7 Release of the MTPJ. (**a**) Both the accessory and proper collateral ligaments are released from the proximal phalanx base; (**b**) the plantar plate is now visualized which has a distinctive almond color; (**c**) the plantar plate is sharply released from the proximal phalanx base with care being taken to avoid shredding or creating layers within the plate and also to avoid iatrogenic injury to the flexor tendon; (**d**) final goal of creating a contiguous collar of tissue that surrounds the metatarsal head

phalanx dorsally during the tensioning phase. If you tag the collaterals too low, then you will achieve much less transverse plane correction. When tagging the plantar plate, be sure to avoid placing the suture in any pre-existing tears and ensure the tissue touches the back portion of the suture passer foot. Suture management is important, and we recommend placing the solid 2–0 sutures within the plantar plate and the striped 2–0 sutures within the collateral ligaments. A marking pen is then used to mark the sutures within the medial collateral ligament and medial portion of the plantar plate. Furthermore, the angle and trajectory of the needle for the suture passer run from superior to inferior. This allows grasping of difficult to reach tissue without damaging the articular cartilage.

A short and long drill guide is then utilized to create offset oblique tunnels through the proximal phalanx base (Fig. 19.12a, b). It is important to use the proper

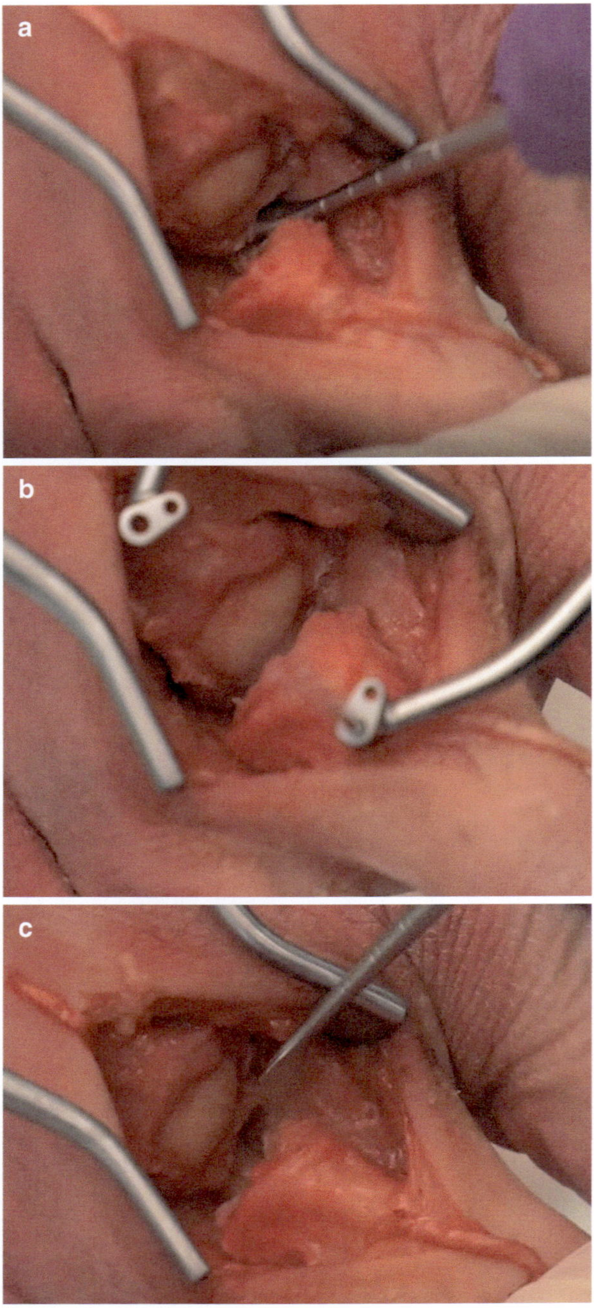

Fig. 19.8 (**a**) A blunt elevator helps separate the plantar plate from the flexor tendon for the suture passer. (**b**) Distraction is critical for visualization and a pin distractor is available if needed. (**c**) Care is taken to visually inspect the flexor tendon to ensure there was no iatrogenic injury while sharply releasing the plantar plate

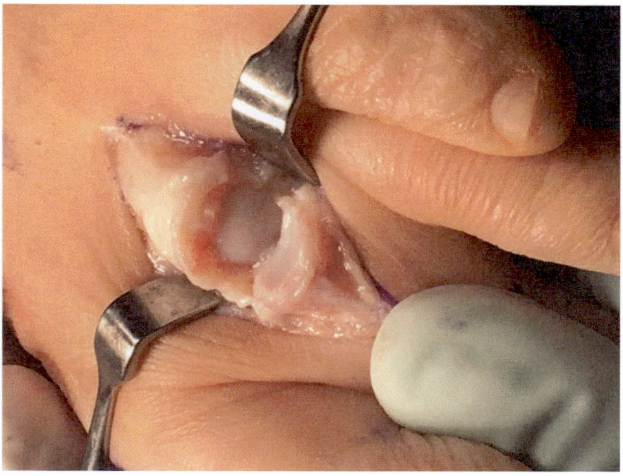

Fig. 19.9 A circumferential tissue cuff comprised of the plantar plate, collateral ligaments, and capsule surrounds the metatarsal head. All proximal attachments are left intact, and a McGlamry elevator is not used in this dissection

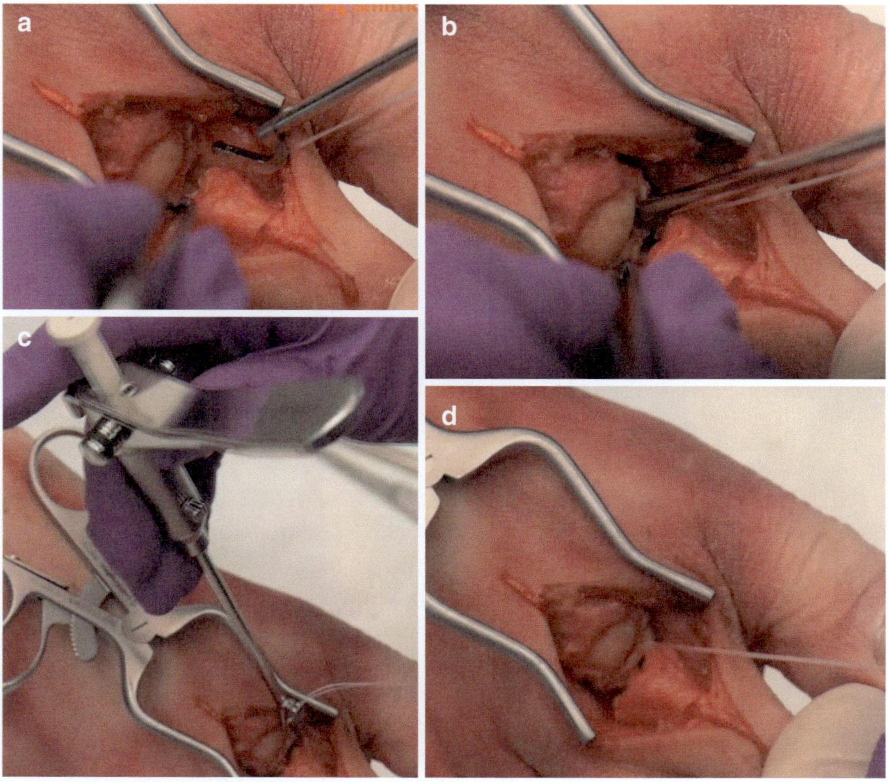

Fig. 19.10 2–0 Nonabsorbable suture is placed within the collateral ligaments and plantar plate (total of 4 sutures). The medial sutures are marked to aid in soft tissue rebalancing while tensioning later in the case. (**a**) A specialized suture passer is able to access the plantar plate through a dorsal approach without an osteotomy. (**b**) The suture passer places the suture within the desired position. (**c**) The hand rocks the suture passer away from the digits in order to prevent soft tissue entanglement with the suture. (**d**) The strength of the suture tag is tested

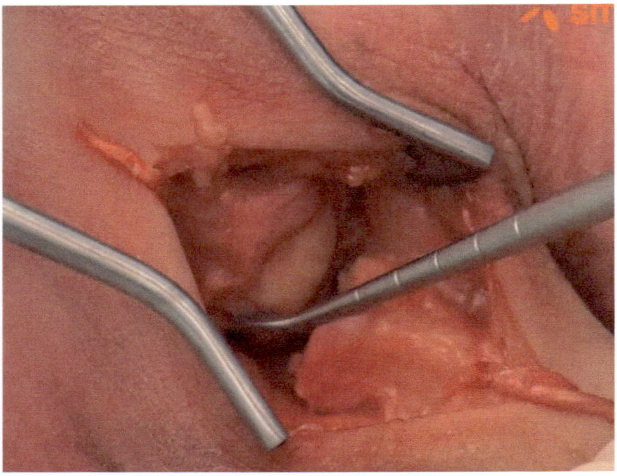

Fig. 19.11 Visually bisect each collateral ligament, and tag them just plantar to their respective bisection. An elevator is helpful in lightly assessing the integrity of the collateral ligaments

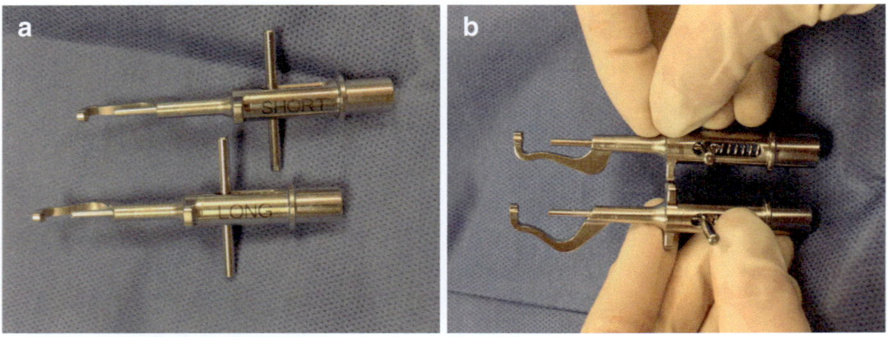

Fig. 19.12 (**a**) There is a short and a long drill guide. (**b**) Use the short drill guide first

sized drill pins as the tunnel diameter precisely fits both the 2–0 suture and interference rods at the end of the procedure. To properly seat each drill guide, ensure the plantar portion exits out each condyle. The convex portion of the guide should also sit flush against the concave portion of the proximal phalanx base (Fig. 19.13a, b). The short drill guide is used first. In the event, either drill guide is not properly seated, there is more room along the remaining portion of the phalanx for adjusting the long drill guide free hand. Drill each drill pin through the drill guide until the laser line is just buried and then remove the pin (Fig. 19.14a, b]. While avoiding any shifting of the drill guide, insert the suture shuttle through the guide until the collar of the suture shuttle touches the collar of the guide (Fig. 19.15a–c). This delivers a loop of suture to the plantar aspect of the proximal phalanx, and the suture shuttle is removed. The drill guide is removed leaving the loop of suture in place plantarly by cutting the suture between the distal suture knot and the guide (Fig. 19.16a, b). Alternatively, after placing the drill tunnels, a nitinol suture passer may be used in lieu of the shuttle. The medial plantar plate and collateral ligament are then pulled from plantar to dorsal through the tunnel using either the suture loop or nitinol suture passer. The lateral plantar plate and collateral ligaments are also pulled through their respective bone tunnel exiting out on the dorsal medial side of the proximal phalanx (Fig. 19.17a, b).

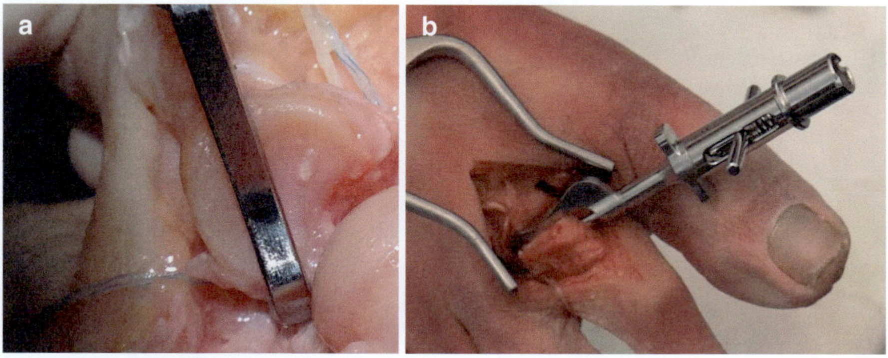

Fig. 19.13 (**a**) The drill guides are set at an oblique angle exiting out each plantar condyle. (**b**) The curvature of the drill guide must hug the concavity of the articular surface of the proximal phalanx base

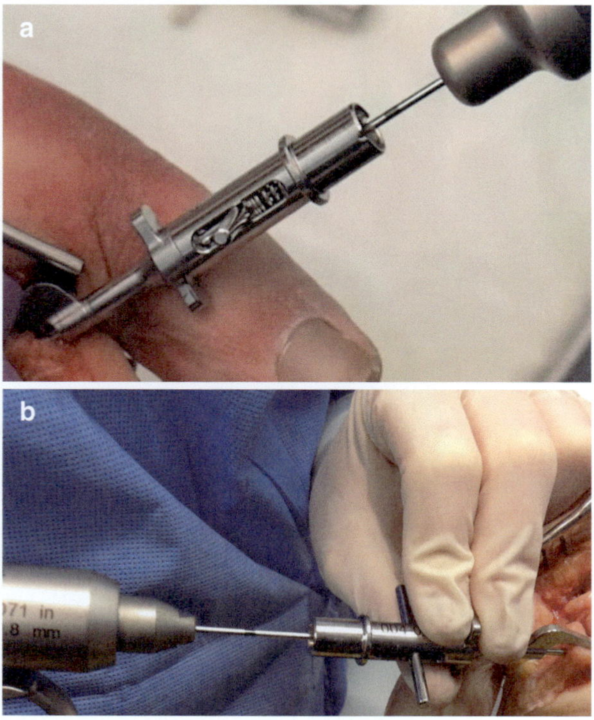

Fig. 19.14 (**a**) Use the properly sized wire to drill a bone tunnel to the laser line. (**b**) The surgeon must stabilize the drill guide while drilling. Avoid placing fingers on the longer drill guide arms as these will disengage the guide from the bone. Instead, please them on the smaller ledge below perpendicular to the longer retractable arm

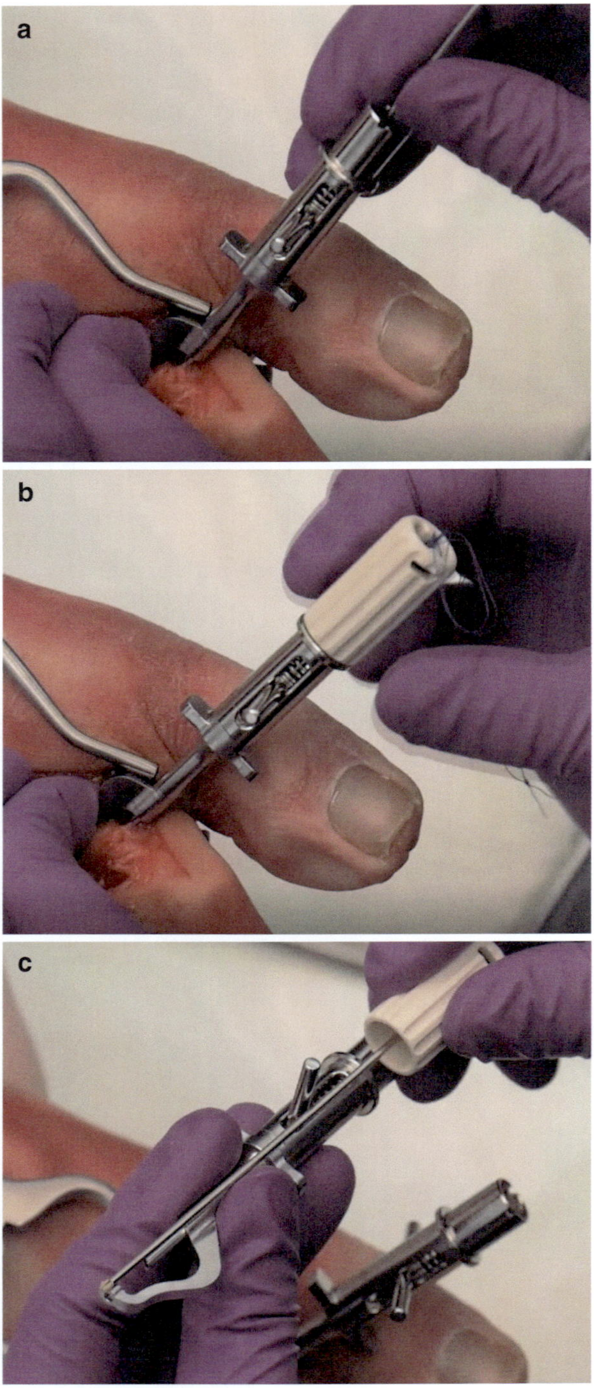

Fig. 19.15 (**a**) It is important to hold the suture shuttle similar to a dart as the shuttle must be placed centrally within the tunnel. (**b**) The shuttle is inserted until the collar abuts the drill guide metallic collar. (**c**) The shuttle is specifically designed to reach the end of the drill guide to deliver the suture plantarly

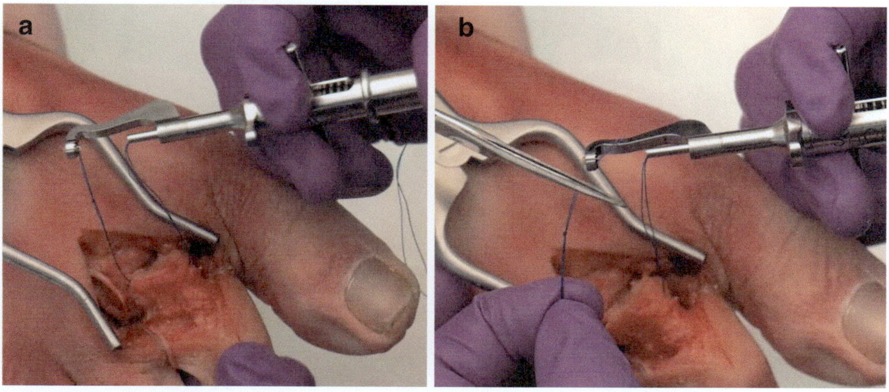

Fig. 19.16 (**a**) The drill guide can now be removed, leaving a loop of suture plantarly. (**b**) The drill guide is released by cutting the suture between the drill guide and knot

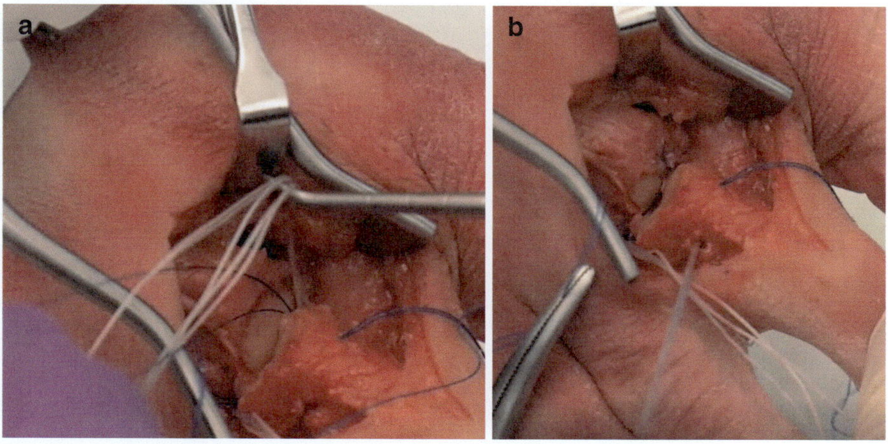

Fig. 19.17 (**a**) The two medial sutures (medial plantar plate and medial collateral ligaments) are placed through the suture shuttle loop. Slack is then applied in order to avoid suture bunching. (**b**) The suture shuttle then pulls these sutures from plantar to dorsal through the drill tunnel. This is repeated for the two lateral sutures

A tensioning device is used to achieve the necessary correction (Fig. 19.18a, b). Pass the sutures you wish to tension through the tensioning device (Fig. 19.19). Place the tensioner against the bone, remove all suture slack and clamp a needle driver on top of the tensioner (Fig. 19.20). Dial in the desired correction by stabilizing the tensioner base and by turning the tensioner head counterclockwise (Fig. 19.21). The desired correction is determined through a dorsal drawer test, medial and lateral stress testing, range of motion, and loading of the foot to ensure adequate deformity correction (Fig. 19.22). If physiologic tension and the desired

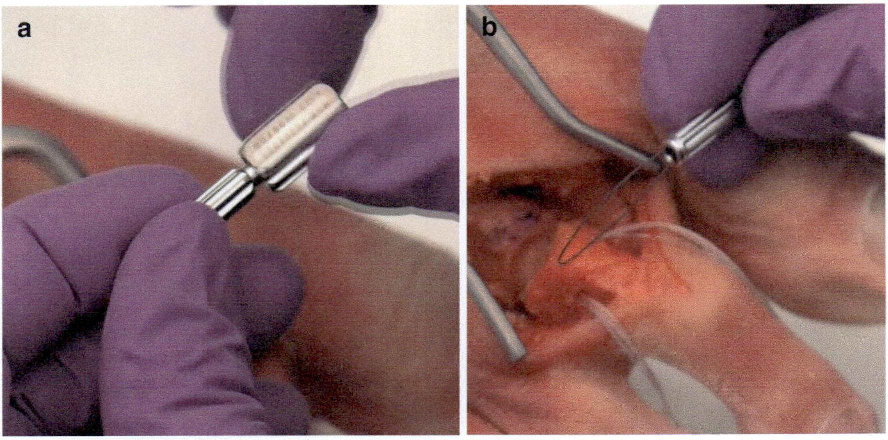

Fig. 19.18 (**a**) Ensure the tensioning device is closed down. (**b**) Place the nitinol suture passer through the tensioner

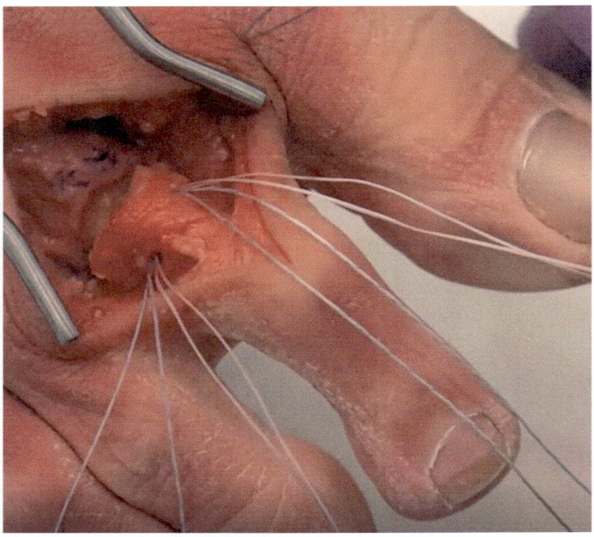

Fig. 19.19 Place the sutures with the greatest deformity through the tensioner. If there is severe dorsal contracture, we recommend placing both plantar plate sutures through the tensioner (medial and lateral). If there is medial transverse plane deformity, we recommend placing lateral collateral ligament and lateral plantar plate sutures through the tensioner (opposite for lateral transverse plane deformity)

deformity correction is not achieved, remove the tensioning device and repeat the tensioning process. Desired tension is achieved once there is correct alignment of the proximal phalanx in relation to the MTPJ without sagittal, transverse or frontal plane deviation. there is physiologic MTPJ range of motion and no instability detected with a dorsal drawer test or medial and lateral stress testing. It is critically important to avoid over-tighenting as this could lead to a painful stiff toe and joint degeneration. Once the desired tension and deformity correction is achieved, the correction is then held in place with threaded interference PEEK rods which are inserted into the bone tunnels with a drill until the threads are just buried. If the surgeon elected to leave either of the collateral ligament sutures outside of the previous tensioning step,

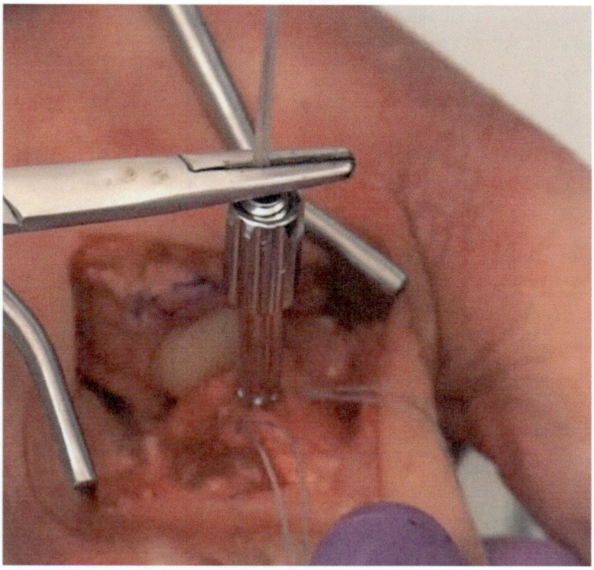

Fig. 19.20 The toe is held in the corrected position, all slack is removed from the suture, and a needle driver is clamped on the superior portion of the tensioner

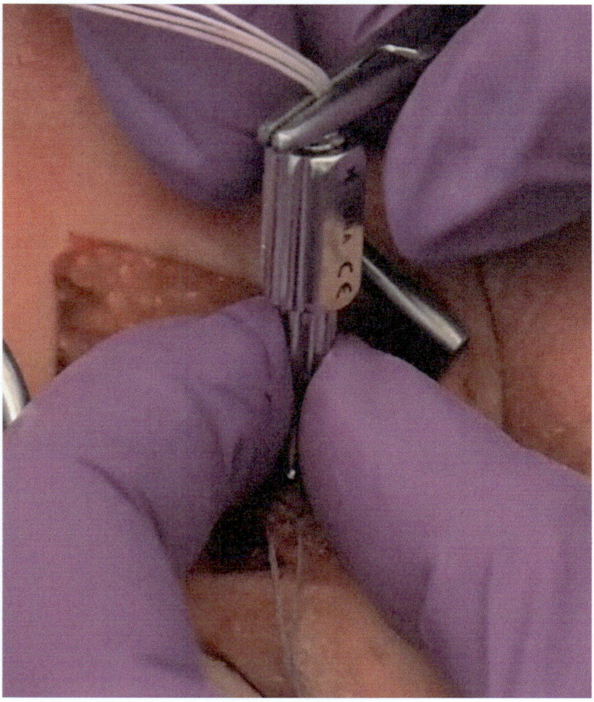

Fig. 19.21 The tensioner base is stabilized, while the head is turned counterclockwise until the desired amount of tension and deformity correction is achieved

for the expressed purpose of transverse plan correction, then these sutures are now tightened manually, while holding the digit in the correct position, by pulling on the sutures when inserting the threaded rods. The tensioner is then removed (Fig. 19.23).

Cut the threaded rods with a bone cutter, using the bone cutter tip to create a divot (Fig. 19.24). Tie the plantar plate and collateral ligament sutures, respectively

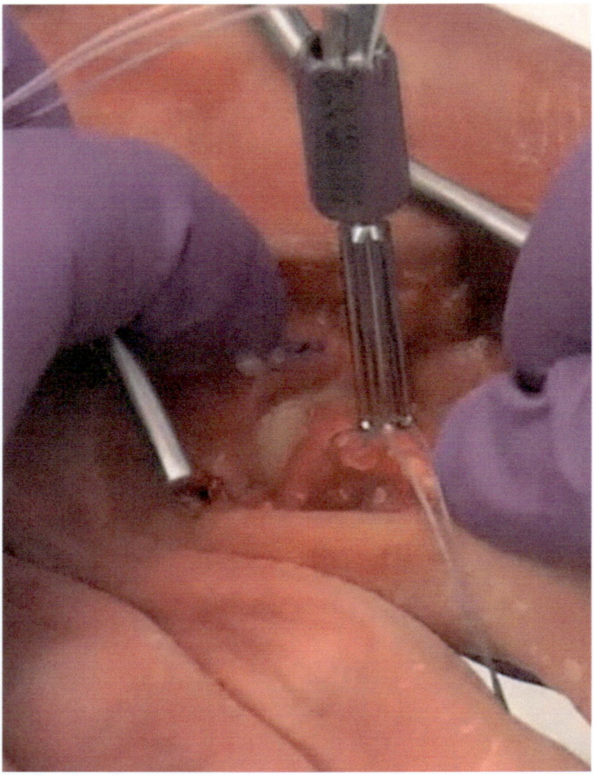

Fig. 19.22 A dorsal drawer test and medial and lateral stress testing is performed. The foot is loaded to ensure proper alignment, and the MTPJ joint range of motion is tested. If the desired correction is not achieved, the tensioner is removed and the tensioning step is repeated as necessary

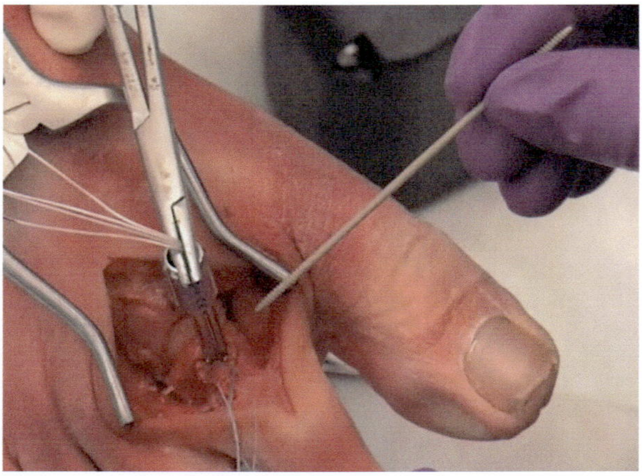

Fig. 19.23 A threaded interference anchor locks the correction into place

(two knots in total). To reduce knot prominence, slide each knot to the medial or lateral side into the divots made into the threaded rods.

The tensioner is used to tailor the correction to each individual deformity. Any number of sutures can be placed through the tensioner, but we have found that it is most helpful to place the sutures through the tensioner that address the most significant portion of the deformity. All remaining sutures are then manually tensioned by

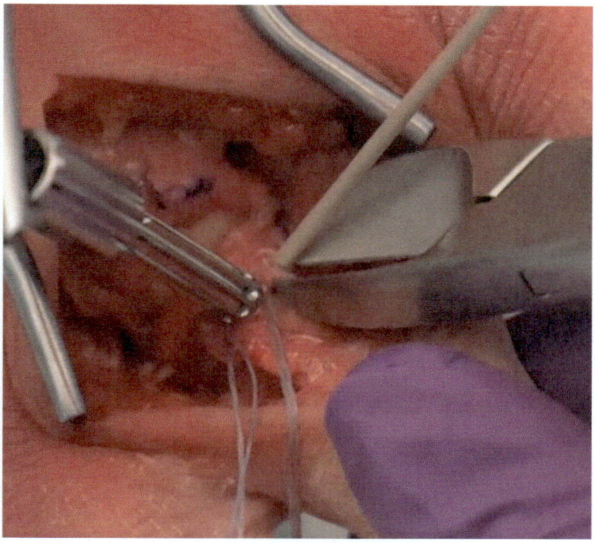

Fig. 19.24 Use the flat edge tip of a bone cutter to transect the interference rod. Suture over ties are then placed within each divot medially and laterally to avoid knot stack

pulling out all slack just before placing the threaded rods into the drill tunnels. For example, if there is a medially translocated second toe, the lateral collateral ligament and lateral plantar plate sutures would be placed through the tensioner. If done properly, the deformity will correct as the tension is "dialed in" with the tensioning device.

Outcomes

Multiple studies have found that both the plantar plate and collateral ligaments work in unison to provide multiplanar stability of a digit. Cadaveric mechanical studies have found that loss of the plantar plate led to an approximately 20% increase in dorsal displacement of a digit. And loss of just one additional collateral ligament resulted in ~60% increase in digital instability [7].

Clinical outcomes have also confirmed the importance of the collateral ligament and plantar plate complex in digital stability. A comparative study in 54 patients assessed digital stability following traditional rebalancing techniques versus the anatomic reconstruction outlined within this chapter (reconstruction of the collateral ligaments with plantar plate). Traditional rebalancing techniques were defined as the sequential MTPJ release and rebalancing until a negative push-up test was achieved. Specific traditional procedures included capsulotomies, capsulorrhaphies, plantar plate releases via a McGlamry metatarsal elevator, extensor hood releases, flexor tendon transfers, temporary MTPJ pinnings, and metatarsal osteotomies. Digital stability was defined as both a negative dorsal drawer and negative paper pull-out test. Patients treated with anatomic reconstruction had statistically significant greater digital stability (94% achieved good toe purchase, 100% achieved a negative dorsal drawer) compared to controls (traditional techniques) over the minimum 1-year follow-up duration, $p < 0.05$. All domains of the ACFAS Forefoot module scores were also higher in the anatomic group with the anatomic group maintaining better transverse plane radiographic alignment at final follow-up, $p < 0.05$ [14].

Outcome studies with variations of MTPJ reconstruction have also been reported. Combining a plantar plate repair with a Weil osteotomy through a dorsal incision has been associated with improved patient satisfaction and reduced pain in a small retrospective cohort of 13 patients [15]. In a larger prospective cohort of 91 patients, researchers found improved AOFAS scores, improved patient satisfaction, and a reduction in VAS over a mean 12-month follow-up period. Similar to Cook et al., all patients had a preoperative dorsal drawer exam with only 4.3% of this cohort still experiencing a positive dorsal drawer test postoperatively. But 18% of this cohort still had a floating toe, and 46% could not perform a paper pull-out test at final follow-up [16]. In another study, outcomes following a plantar plate repair with a FDL transfer through a plantar approach found to improve digital stability in all patients; however, 40% of this cohort had joint stiffness, and 30% had poor digital purchase [17].

Clinical Pearls/Pitfalls

- There is a high learning curve to properly perform this procedure and to maximize the deformity correction achieved. As with many complex procedures, it is recommended to become proficient with cadaveric dissections prior to performing a first case. But this developed skill is a worthwhile investment given the amount of correction and long-term stability that can be achieved with a difficult deformity.
- The soft tissue dissection technique is the most important yet challenging part of this procedure. This dissection is substantially different than traditional dissection techniques and is essential as any shredding of the tissues will result in a weak repair.
- The plantar plate can be over 5 mm thick, especially with long-standing pathology. While it is important to avoid iatrogenically damaging the underlying flexor tendon, it is also critical that you do not dissect into the plantar plate which would result in layering and shredding the structure. Furthermore, only grasp the plantar plate with an Adson-Brown forceps or place tension on it once a suture has been placed within it to avoid damaging it.
- The plantar plate is usually almond in coloration. Continue to transect this tissue being mindful in keeping it in one strong intact piece until you see a bright white structure just deep to it which is the flexor tendon. Be cautious to avoid iatrogenic laceration to the flexor tendon which can be adhered to the plantar plate. A 60 degree beaver blade or #66 blade can be useful when releasing the plantar plate [18].
- In some rare cases, especially when there was an aggressive concomitant metatarsal osteotomy, it is sometimes necessary to remove redundant plantar plate in order to ensure a strong reconstruction.

- In some rare, severe cases when there is absolutely no plantar plate, the plantar plate sutures are placed within the flexor tendon. However, usually the absence of a plantar plate is attributed to the dissection technique.
- To ensure an adequate bite of tissue with the specialized suture passer, the tissue must touch the back of the concave portion of the passer. The tissue has a tendency to be inadvertently pushed out of the passer during positioning of the suture passer. The use of an Adson-Brown forceps or pulling on previously sutured tissue can help keep the tissue from retracting proximally. Be careful when using any instrument that could cause shredding of the tissue.
- Suture organization is key to ensuring a smooth repair. By habit, we always place the solid colored suture in the plantar plate and the striped suture in the collateral ligaments. Furthermore, a marking pen is utilized to mark the medial sutures ("mark the medial sutures"). Therefore, it is clear which sutures to tension first after they are passed through the proximal phalanx.
- The long drill guide sits on the phalanx at a very oblique angle. To avoid guide interference with other toes, we will organize the drill guides so that the long drill guide will be angled toward the toes with the least amount of contracture. For example, if there are significantly hammered lesser toes laterally with a straight corrected bunionectomy, the long drill guide will be oriented so that the plantar portion exits out the lateral plantar condyle, and the drill guide will be angled medially toward the hallux.
- Ensure that the drill tunnels are oblique and exit out the proximal phalanx plantar condyles. If they are too vertical, the dorsal tunnel will be blocked by the tensioner eliminating the ability to place the interference rods.
- When pulling the sutures through the proximal phalanx bone tunnel, it is helpful to ensure they are not twisted and to leave some slack on the sutures before passing them to avoid bunching and tangling within the soft tissue and tunnel.
- Do not place the threaded rods into the bony drill tunnels until the desired correction has been achieved. Once the threaded rods are placed, the sutures are locked into place, and no additional correction can be obtained.
- Although conventional teaching advocates to overcorrect because some correction will be lost post-operatively, do not overcorrect a MTPJ reconstruction using this system. It is easy to make the toe too stiff with the tensioner. Given the composition of the plantar plate and its lack of elasticity, it does not "loosen up" postoperatively. The amount of correction achieved intraoperatively is usually the amount of correction maintained.

References

1. Barbari SC, Brevig K. Correction of clawtoes by the Girdlestone-Taylor flexor-extensor transfer. Foot Ankle. 1984;5:67–73.
2. Femino JE, Mueller K. Complications of lesser toe surgery. Clin Orthop Relat Res. 2001;391:72–88.
3. Dhukaram V, Hossain S, Sampath J, Barrie JL. Correction of hammertoe with an extended release of the metatarsophalangeal joint. J Bone Joint Surg Br. 2002;84:986–90.
4. Hofstaetter SG, Hoffstaetter JG. The Weil osteotomy: a 7 year follow up. J Bone Joint Surg Br. 2005;87:1507–11.
5. Migues A, Slullitel G, Bilbae F. Floating toe deformity as a complication of the Weil osteotomy. Foot Ankle Int. 2004;25:609–13.
6. Beech I, Rees S, Tagoe MJ. A retrospective review of the Weil osteotomy for lesser metatarsal deformities: an intermediate follow-up analysis. Foot Ankle Surg. 2005;44:358–64.
7. Suero EM, Meyers KN, Bohne WH. Stability of the metatarsophalangeal joint of the lesser toes; a cadaveric study. J Orthop Res. 2012;30:1995–8.
8. Deland JT, Lobel M, Arnockzky SP, Thompson FM. Collateral ligament reconstruction of the unstable metatarsophalangeal joint: an in vitro study. Foot Ankle Int. 1994;13:391–5.
9. Bhatia D, Myerson MS, Curtis MJ, Cunningham BW. Anatomical restraints to dislocation of the second metatarsophalangeal joint. J Bone Joint Surg Am. 1994;76A:1371–5.
10. Hannan MT, Menz HB Jordan JM, Cupples LA, Cheng C, Hsu Y. High heritability of hallux valgus and lesser toe deformities in adult men and women. Arthritis Care Res. 2013;65(9):1515–21.
11. Yu GV, Judge MS, Hudson JR, Seidelmann FE. Predislocation syndrome. progressive subluxation/dislocation of the lesser metatarsophalangeal joint. J Am Podiatry Med Assoc. 2002;92(4):182–99.
12. Coughlin MJ. Second metatarsophalangeal joint instability in the athlete. Foot Ankle. 1993;14:309–19.
13. Menz HB, Zammit GV, Munteanu SE, Scott G. Plantarflexion strength of the toes: age and gender differences and evaluation of a clinical screening test. Foot Ankle Int. 2006;27(12):1103–8.
14. Cook JJ, Johnson LJ, Cook EA. Anatomic reconstruction versus traditional rebalancing in lesser metatarsophalangeal joint reconstruction. J Foot Ankle Surg. 2018;57:509.
15. Weil L Jr, Sung W, Weil LS Sr, Malinoski K. Anatomic plantar plate repair using the Weil metatarsal osteotomy approach. Foot Ankle Spec. 2011;4(3):145–50.
16. Flint WW, Macias DM, Jastifer JR, Doty JF, Hirose CB, Coughlin MJ. Plantar plate repair for lesser MTP joint instability. Foot Ankle Int. 2017;38(3):234–42.
17. Bouche RT, Heit EJ. Combined plantar plate and hammertoe repair with flexor digitorum longus tendon transfer for chronic, severe sagittal plane instability of the lesser metatarsophalangeal joints: preliminary observations. J Foot Ankle Surg. 2008;47:125–37.
18. Roukis TS, Ringstrom JB. Lesser metatarsophalangeal release utilizing the #66 mini-blade. J Foot Ankle Surg. 1999;38(2):163–5.

Chapter 20
Lesion-Directed Fifth Toe Surgery

Mickey D. Stapp and Trevor S. Payne

Introduction

> You are not a good foot surgeon, until you are a good fifth toe surgeon.
> Thomas F. Smith, DPM

Deformities of the fifth toe and patient complaints associated with the fifth toe are very common occurrences. These deformities can be congenital or developmental. Most often, these deformities, in addition to associated complaints, are related to painful hyperkeratotic lesions. The underlying deformities causing these painful hyperkeratotic lesions are often bundled into a catchall category referred to as hammertoes. However, in reality, these deformities can have multifactoral and challenging components. The most common presentation of these hammertoes consists of contractures of the metatarsophalangeal joint (MTPJ) and the proximal interphalangeal joint (PIPJ), with or without varus rotation of the toe (Fig. 20.1) [1]. Other common presentations of these deformities may include hammertoe, mallet toe, claw toe, adductovarus rotation of the digit, overlapping toe, clinodactyly, and cock-up hammertoe. There are also incidences of lesions with no apparent causative structural deformity of the fifth toe (Figs. 20.2, 20.3, 20.4, 20.5, and 20.6). The majority of fifth toe surgery is directed at correcting the structural deformity and resolving the painful hyperkeratotic lesion [2] (Fig. 20.7). When conservative modalities have failed to rectify the patient's complaints, careful evaluation and appropriate procedure selection are paramount for a successful outcome.

M. D. Stapp (✉)
Private Practice, Augusta Foot & Ankle, PC, Evans, GA, USA

The Podiatry Institute, Decatur, GA, USA
e-mail: mickeystapp@comcast.net

T. S. Payne
Private Practice, Augusta Foot & Ankle, PC, Evans, GA, USA

E. A. Cook, J. J. Cook (eds.), *Hammertoes*,
https://doi.org/10.1007/978-3-319-16552-3_20

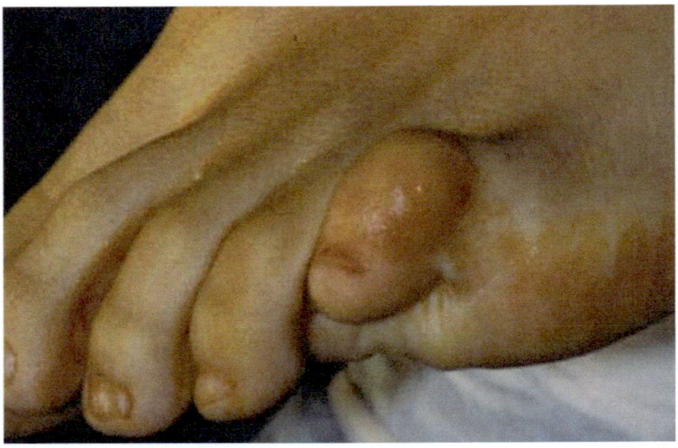

Fig. 20.1 Complex 5th hammertoe with dorsal contracture at the 5th MTPJ and plantar contracture at the 5th PIPJ

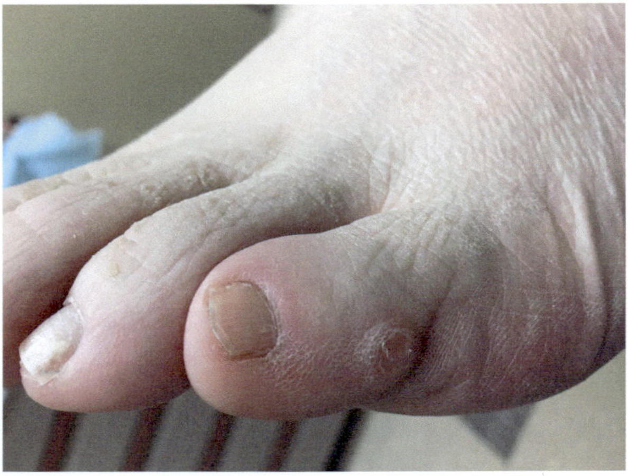

Fig. 20.2 Adductovarus deformity with lateral-based hyperkeratotic lesion

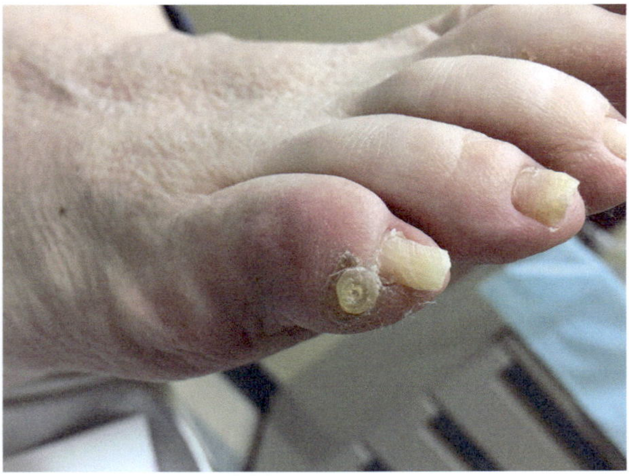

Fig. 20.3 Lister's corn

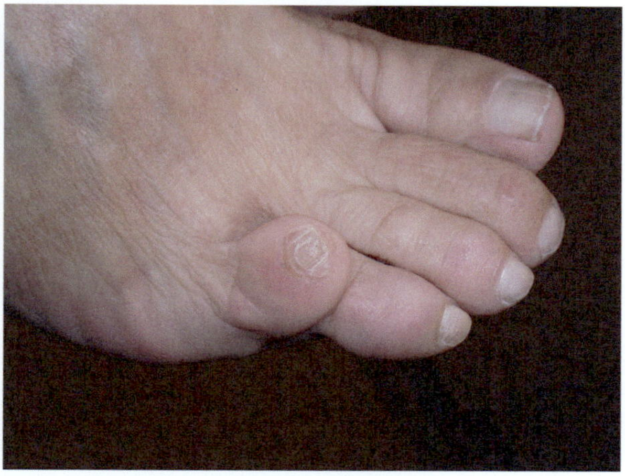

Fig. 20.4 Congenital overlapping 5th toe deformity

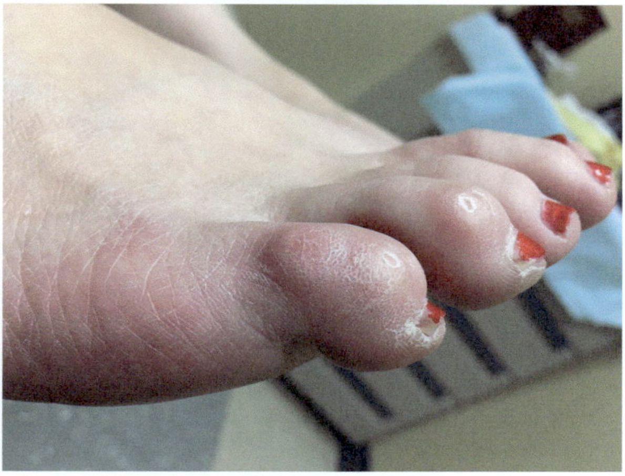

Fig. 20.5 Mallet toe deformity of 4th and 5th toes

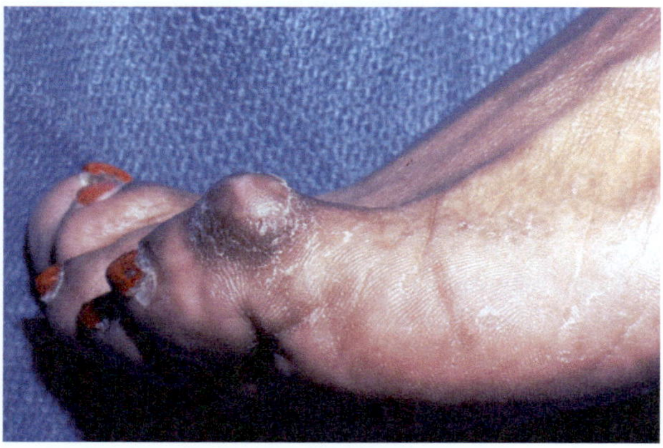

Fig. 20.6 Complex 5th hammertoe with hyperkeratotic lesion

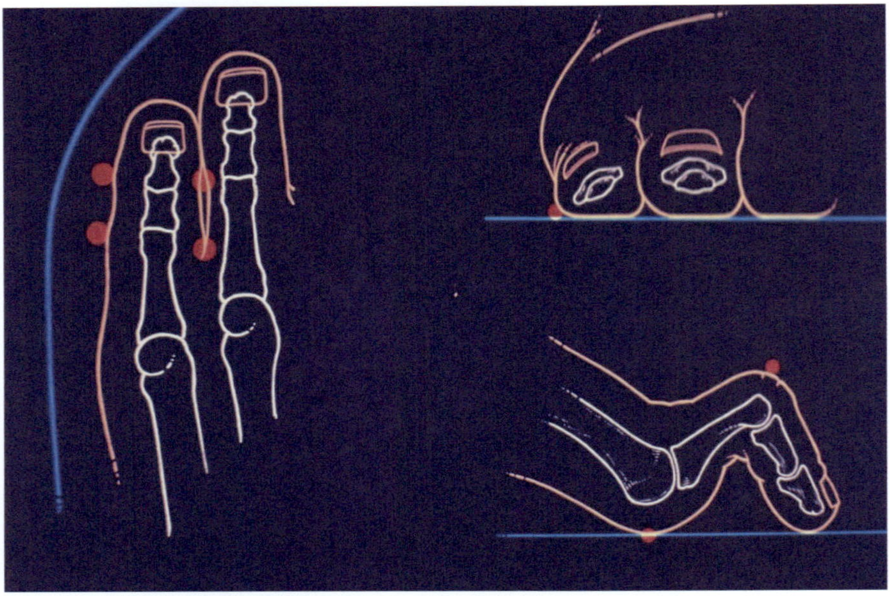

Fig. 20.7 Possible hyperkeratotic lesion locations of the 5th toe

The location of the lesion(s) and the structural deformity, evaluated in all three planes, will determine the appropriate procedure, or combination of procedures, to best address the patient's complaint and ensure long-term success. Simple excision of the painful lesion of a fifth toe alone is rarely successful. One exception is the deep interdigital corn between the fourth and fifth toes. This lesion may be addressed with skin surgery only without the need for osseous procedures and will be discussed later in this chapter. Most painful lesions will be addressed through a combination of osseous and soft tissue procedures, often times with an additional skin plasty. A simple arthroplasty through a linear midline incision will not be successful long term in many of these complex deformities. Early in our surgical training, we are taught that a simple arthroplasty will correct any type of fifth toe deformity and lesion pattern. This procedure may well be the first foot surgery performed in one's early training. The common statement, "it's only a little toe," brings on a new meaning much later in practice when this simple procedure has been performed and recurrence of the lesion and/or recurrent deformity of the fifth toe persists.

Anatomy

To better understand problems associated with a simple arthroplasty, it is critical to have a secure base of understanding related to the anatomy and biomechanics of the fifth toe complex. The extensor tendon dorsally has two points of insertion. The extensor digitorum longus (EDL) attaches at the wing-and-sling apparatus overlying the MTPJ and then attaches to the dorsal aspect of the base of the distal phalanx. There is no slip of the extensor digitorum brevis (EDB) to the fifth toe. The flexor tendons on the plantar aspect have two points of insertion. The flexor digitorum longus (FDL) attaches at the plantar aspect of the base of the distal phalanx and the flexor digitorum brevis (FDB) attaches at the plantar aspect of the middle phalanx. A simple arthroplasty is designed to relax the contractures of the flexor tendons at the PIPJ. If there is weakness of the flexor tendons, with dorsal contracture at the MTPJ, then a simple arthroplasty, without addressing the contracture at the MTPJ, will potentiate the weakness and result in a floating or cock-up toe.

Other anatomic structures about the fifth MTPJ produce more adductory forces than abductory forces. These forces, or imbalances thereof, usually result in the development of much of the deformity of the fifth toe. The fourth lumbrical and the third plantar interossei insert plantar-medial on the extensor sling and the plantar-medial base of the proximal phalanx, respectively, resulting in an adductory force. The directly opposing flexor digiti quinti and the abductor digiti minimi attach to the lateral and plantar-lateral aspect of the base of the proximal phalanx, respectively, causing abduction of the digit. With the absence of the EDB to the fifth toe, the flexors may have more power, and with the orientation and pull of the FDL tendon, the imbalance often results in adduction of the toe.

The fifth toe is made up of a proximal phalanx, middle phalanx, and distal phalanx. There are two joints of the toe, the PIPJ and distal interphalangeal joint (DIPJ). The base of the proximal phalanx articulates with the fifth metatarsal to form the fifth MTPJ. Collateral ligaments support each of these joints, medially and laterally. Repair of these collaterals, especially with an arthroplasty versus an arthrodesis, will aid in the transverse plane stability of the toe. Each of the three phalanges has condyles at their bases, but only the proximal and middle phalanges have epicon-

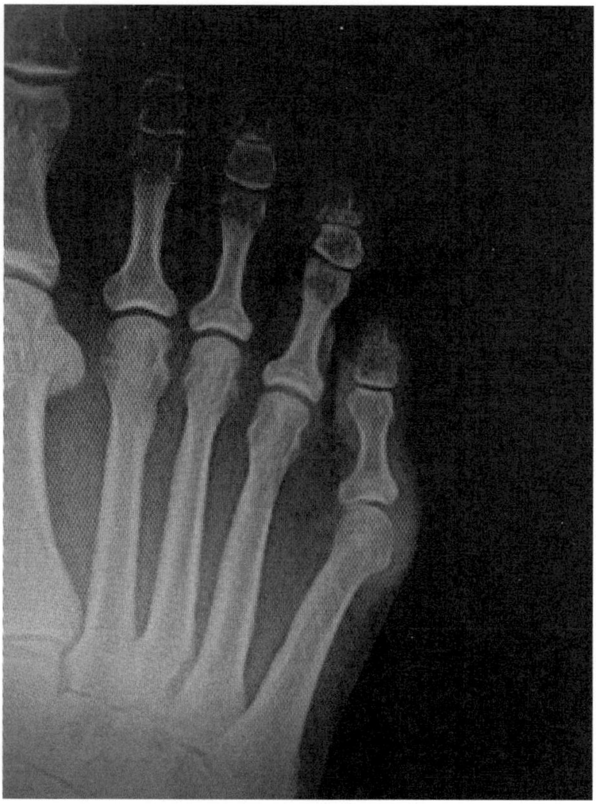

Fig. 20.8 Radiograph demonstrating synostosis of 5th distal interphalangeal joint

dyles at the heads of the bones. The distal phalanx has a specialized end of bone known as the tuft. There is a common anatomic variant demonstrated by a synostosis of the DIPJ being present in 37–76% of the population [4, 5] (Fig. 20.8). When this occurs, the fifth toe may be less flexible leading to an increased risk of hyperkeratotic lesions in shoes. The absence of this distal joint may also allow the toe to align unnaturally with adjacent fourth toe joints leading to higher incidence of interdigital hyperkeratotic lesions [4].

Discussion

It is important to understand that mastery of fifth toe surgery requires the foot and ankle surgeon to accept that an arthroplasty of the fifth toe PIPJ is not a "cure all" for every problem associated with the fifth toe. Even though an arthroplasty is usually performed when addressing the deformity of a fifth toe, it is often not sufficient alone to address all components of the deformity and lesion patterns. In contrast, an arthrodesis of the fifth PIPJ is rarely performed. An arthroplasty does relax the flexor contracture at the PIPJ but does not relax the extensor contracture at the MTPJ completely. In addition, unless a derotational skin plasty is incorporated with the arthroplasty, the arthroplasty has minimal frontal plane effect. An overaggressive resection of the head of the proximal phalanx may lead to a relative lengthening of the long flexor tendon and result in a floppy or non-purchasing toe (Fig. 20.9). The urge to resect more bone in an arthroplasty from the head of the proximal phalanx in an attempt to release continued intraoperative contracture, often times from

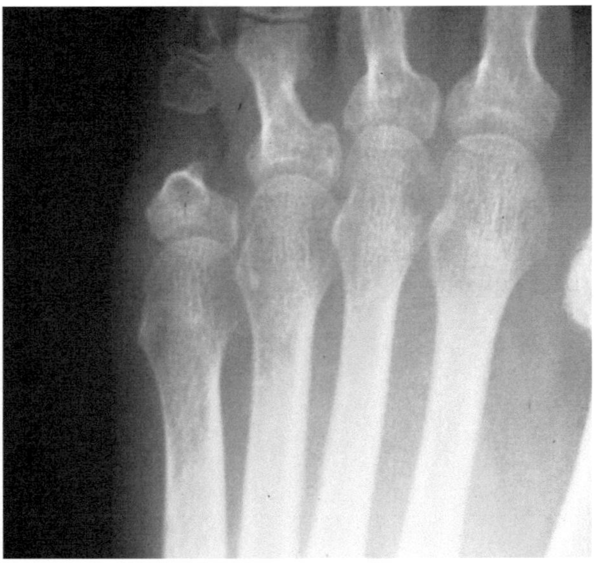

Fig. 20.9 Radiograph depicting overaggressive arthroplasty

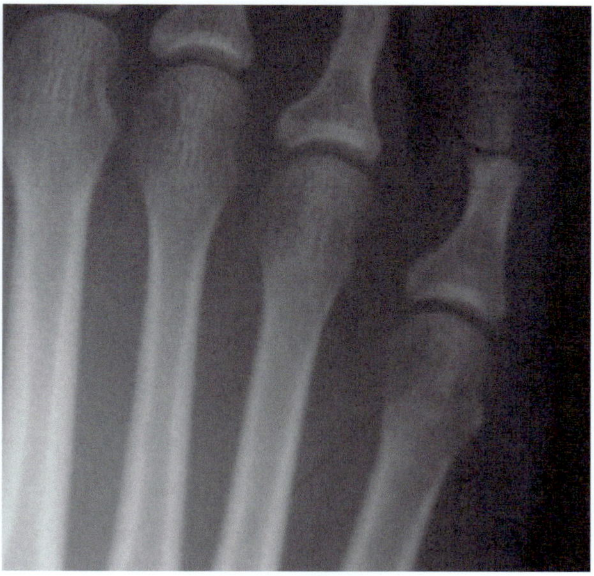

Fig. 20.10 Radiograph depicting retraction of middle and distal phalanges after resection of proximal phalangeal head

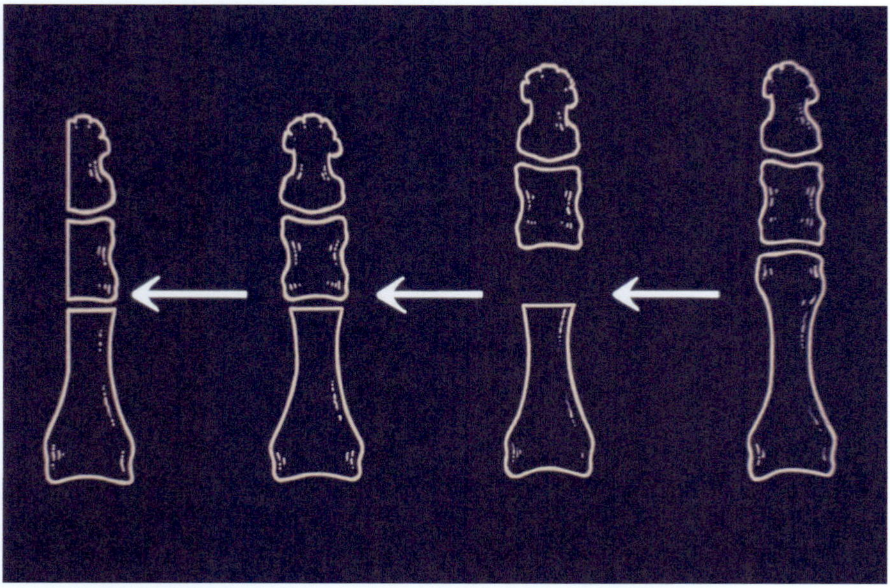

Fig. 20.11 Diagram representing simple arthroplasty with retraction of the more distal phalanges and narrowing of bony column after hemiphalangectomy has also been performed

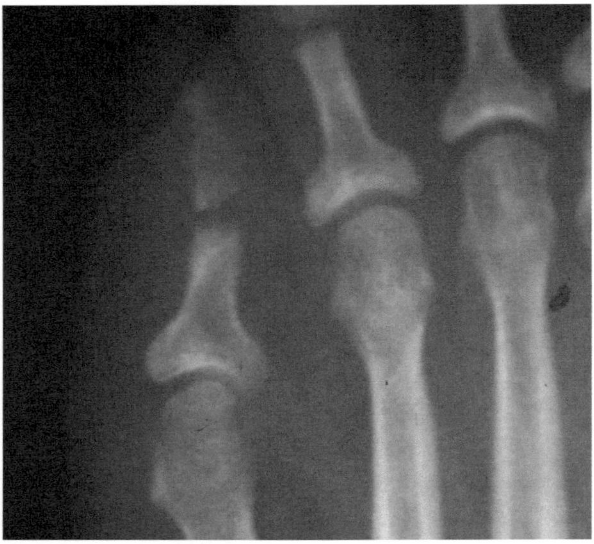

Fig. 20.12 Radiograph depicting hemiphalangectomy with PIPJ arthroplasty performed for lesions at the PIPJ and lateral aspect of the DIPJ

the MTPJ, should be avoided. The other consideration with a PIPJ arthroplasty is that the middle phalanx will drop back proximally, potentially replacing the head of the proximal phalanx. When this occurs, recurrent lesions are possible (Fig. 20.10). An arthroplasty also narrows the bony column at the PIPJ, but not at the middle phalanx or DIPJ (Fig. 20.11). This has to be taken into account when noting hyperkeratotic lesion patterns. A hemiphalangectomy may need to be combined when a hyperkeratotic lesion extends from the PIPJ and includes a lesion at either side of the DIPJ, or along the lateral aspect of the middle phalanx (Fig. 20.12). Lastly, the PIPJ arthroplasty does very little to balance the forces that created the deformity. These biomechanical forces must be evaluated and considered in the surgical plan of correction.

Evaluation of fifth toe complaints should include a thorough inspection, palpation of all joints involved, and passive range of motion of all the joints of the digit. The flexibility versus rigidity of each joint should be evaluated. The toe should be evaluated with the forefoot loaded to simulate weight bearing or inspection made of the deformity with the patient weight bearing. The deformity must be evaluated in all three planes. Failure to recognize contributing deforming force in one or more of the cardinal planes may lead to continued and/or recurrent deformity and lesions.

Digiti adductus occurs in the transverse plane. This is evaluated best from the top of the foot (Fig. 20.13). A pure transverse plane deformity may be associated with a Tailor's bunion deformity and usually shows interdigital lesion patterns. Correction of this transverse planal dominant deformity usually requires fifth metatarsal osseous procedures and rebalancing soft tissue procedures at the fifth MTPJ. Osseous procedures may need to be performed at the PIPJ level as well. Digiti extensus occurs in the sagittal plane. This is evaluated best from the side of the foot (Fig. 20.14). The sagittal plane deformity is often seen in a cavus foot type or with

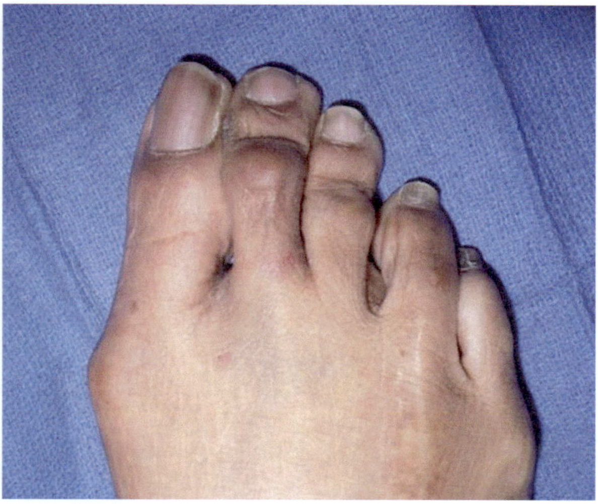

Fig. 20.13 Digiti adductus evaluated from the top of the foot. (Photo courtesy of Dr. Melissa Robitaille)

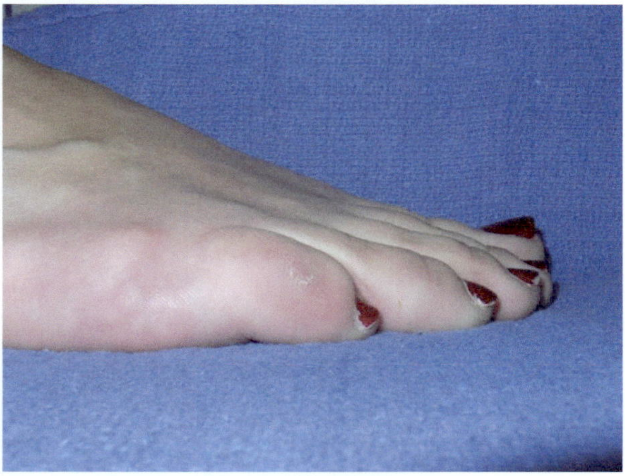

Fig. 20.14 Digiti extensus evaluated from the side of the foot. The dorsal contracture of the proximal phalanx may be difficult to appreciate clinically. (Photo courtesy of Dr. Melissa Robitaille)

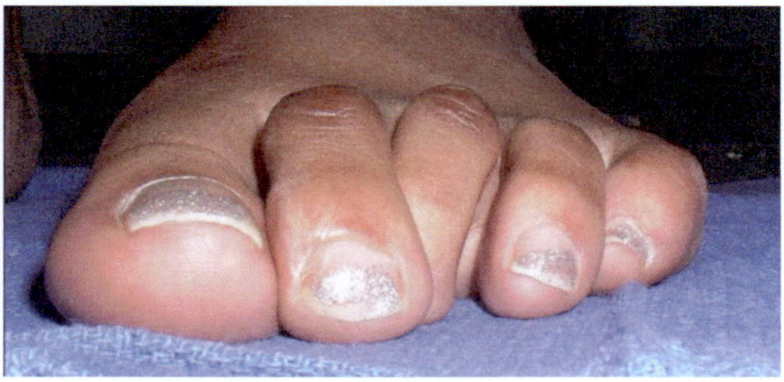

Fig. 20.15 Digiti varus evaluated from the front of the foot. (Photo courtesy of Dr. Melissa Robitaille)

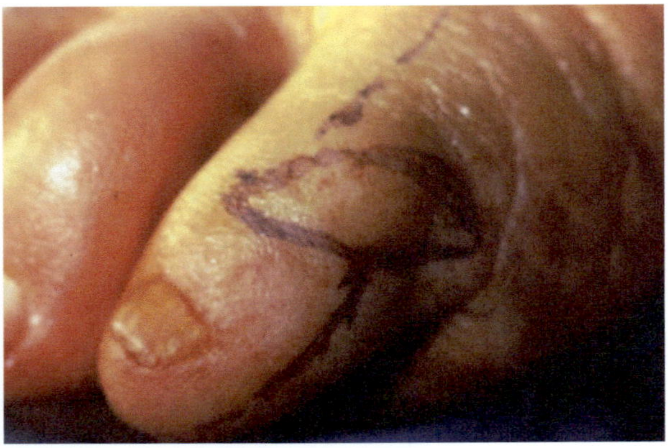

Fig. 20.16 Derotational skin plasty combined with other skin incisions

extensor substitution. This deformity usually shows a dorsal hyperkeratotic lesion at the PIPJ and sometimes beneath the fifth metatarsal head. Correction of this sagittal plane deformity requires full MTPJ release and osseous resection at the PIPJ. Digiti varus occurs in the frontal plane. This is best visualized from the front of the foot (Fig. 20.15). The frontal plane deformity is most common and is often seen in combination with one or both of the other planal deformities. The frontal plane fifth toe deformity is seen most often in pronated feet. Lesions may be present at the PIPJ and/or the DIPJ. If the rotation is severe, a periungual hyperkeratotic lesion, or Lister's corn, may be seen. The frontal plane component is corrected via some type of derotational skin plasty (Fig. 20.16).

Procedure Selection

Choices of surgical procedures for the fifth toe are multiple and must be adapted to each individual's pathology. Perhaps the simplest procedure, in that no osseous work is required, is the deep-seated hyperkeratotic lesion in the proximal aspect of the interdigital web space between the fourth and fifth toes. If this lesion, classically referred to as heloma molle, does not extend to the PIPJ of either the fourth or fifth digit, then a partial syndactyly can be performed without osseous surgery (Fig. 20.17a–e). If there is an interdigital hyperkeratotic lesion on any of the proximal or distal interphalangeal joints, then osseous surgery must be performed. Without other lesions or planal deformities, simple condylectomy of the condyle underlying the lesion may be sufficient. In extremely short fifth toes, the head of the proximal phalanx may have pressure and associated lesions with the lateral aspect of the base of the fourth proximal phalanx or the lateral aspect of the head of the fourth

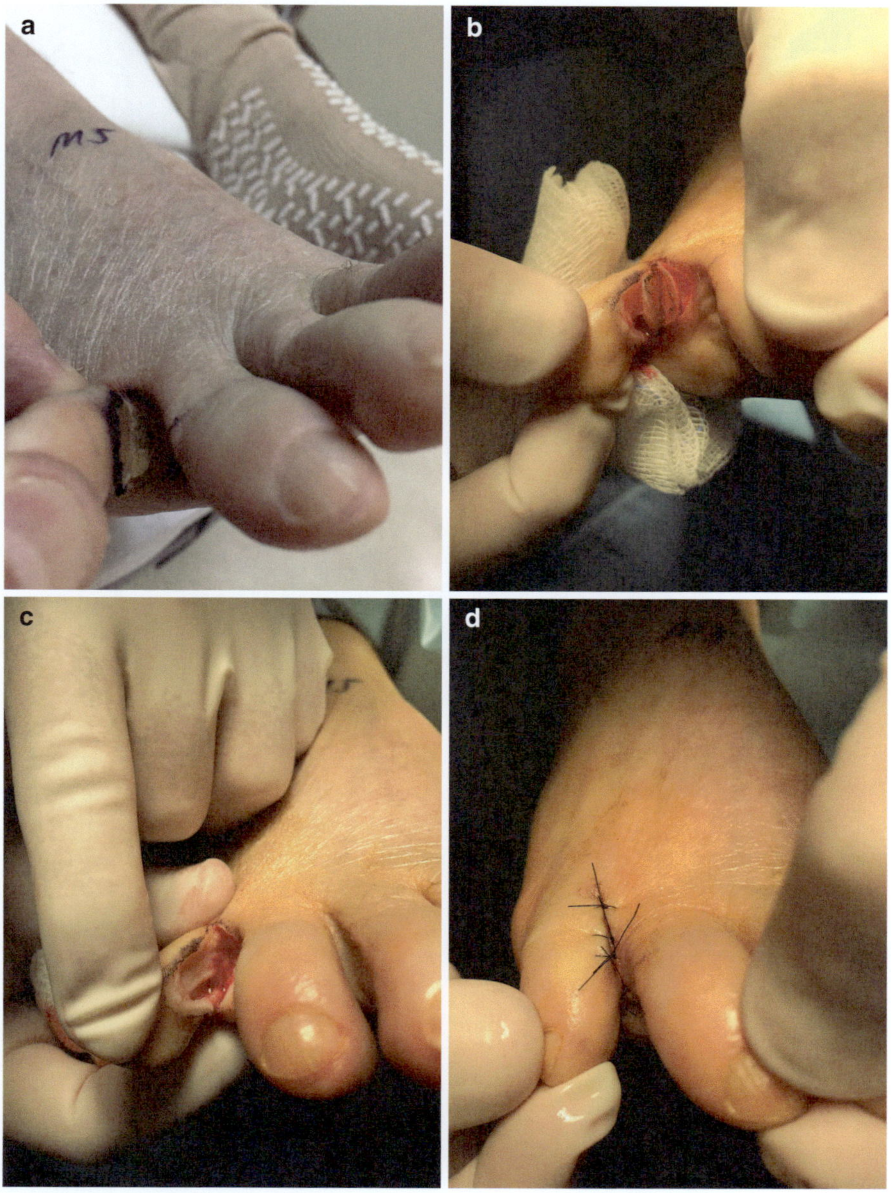

Fig. 20.17 (**a**) Preoperative heloma molle. (**b**) Excision of proximal web space for partial syndactylization. (**c**) Skin wedge removed. (**d**) Simple skin closure. (**e**) One week postoperatively

Fig. 20.17 (continued)

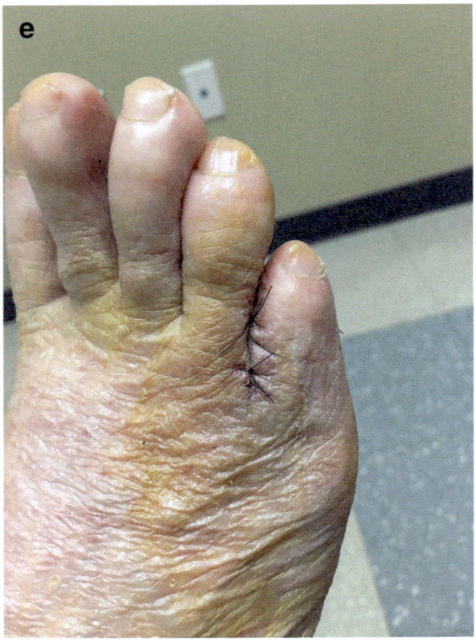

metatarsal. In this instance, a condylectomy of the involved prominent portion of bone would be performed with a partial syndactyly of the fourth and fifth toes.

Another simple procedure is for the lateral-based periungual hyperkeratotic lesion known as a Lister's corn or for the medial-based hyperkeratotic lesion at the DIPJ. When one of these isolated lesions is the only complaint, then a simple elliptical excision of the hyperkeratotic lesion with removal of the underlying prominent bone has proven to be very successful. The underlying bone can be removed with bone rongeurs, bone cutter, rasp, burr, or similar instrumentation (Figs. 20.18a–f and 20.19).

When the only hyperkeratotic lesion is at the fifth PIPJ, then location of the lesion and accompanying planal deformity will determine the appropriate selection of procedures. If the lesion is purely dorsal, as seen in a cavus foot or extensor substitution-type hammertoe, then an arthroplasty combined with a fifth MTPJ release would be appropriate. This may be performed through one longer incision or through two smaller incisions (Fig. 20.20). When the hyperkeratotic lesion is at the dorsolateral aspect of the fifth PIPJ, then an arthroplasty can be performed through a derotational skin plasty overlying the PIPJ (Fig. 20.21). If the dorsolateral lesion is present with dorsal contracture at the fifth MTPJ, then release of this contracture would be included with the derotational arthroplasty (Fig. 20.22a–b). This may be accomplished through a linear incision over the MTPJ or incorporating a V to Y skin plasty over the MTPJ, if skin contracture warrants (Wilson 1953).

If the isolated lesion is medial to the PIPJ, as seen in a transverse planal dominant deformity, then osseous procedures at the PIPJ and soft tissue procedures at the fifth

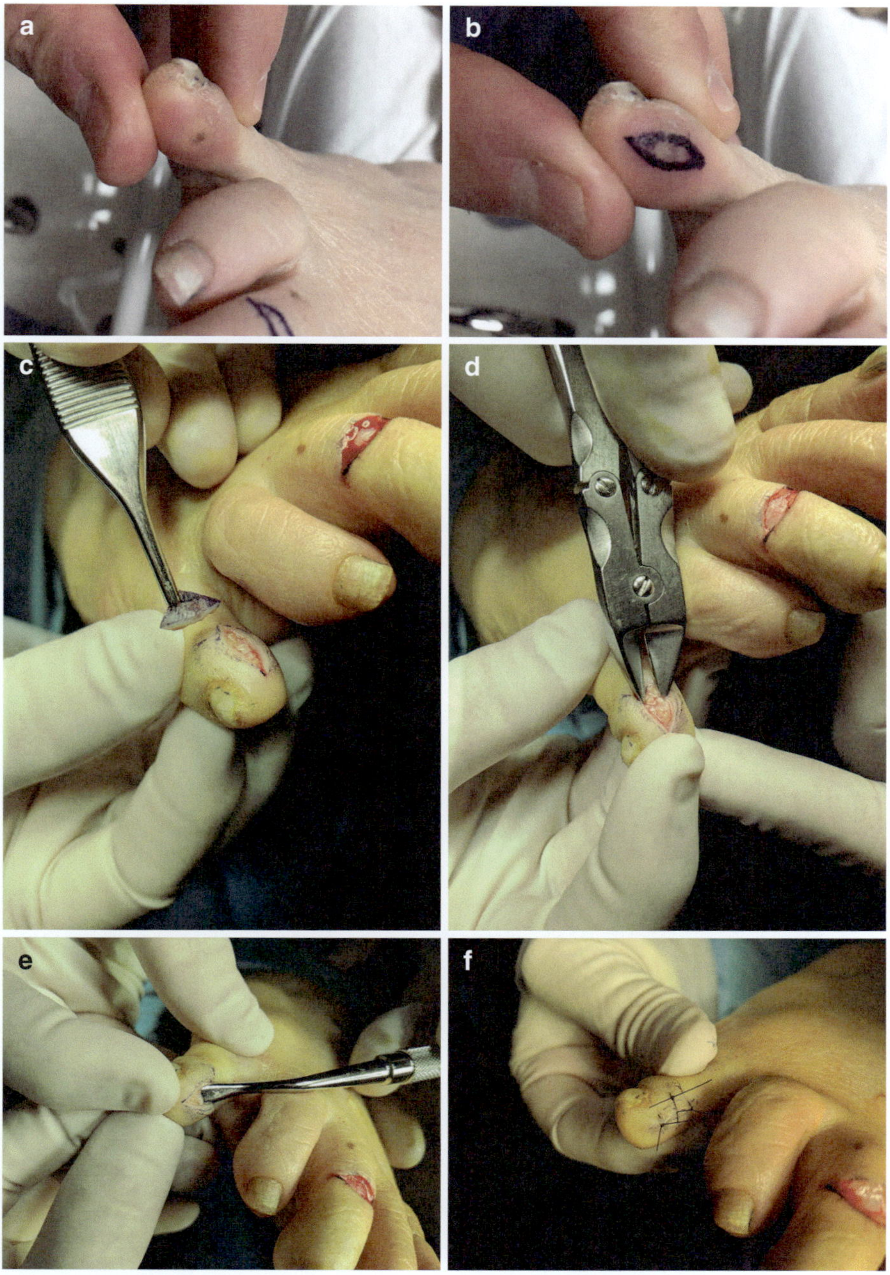

Fig. 20.18 (**a**) Preoperative medial DIPJ lesion. (**b**) Skin incision placement. (**c**) Skin ellipse of hyperkeratotic lesion. (**d**) Condylectomy of underlying bony prominence. (**e**) Smoothing of resected area of bone. (**f**) Simple skin closure

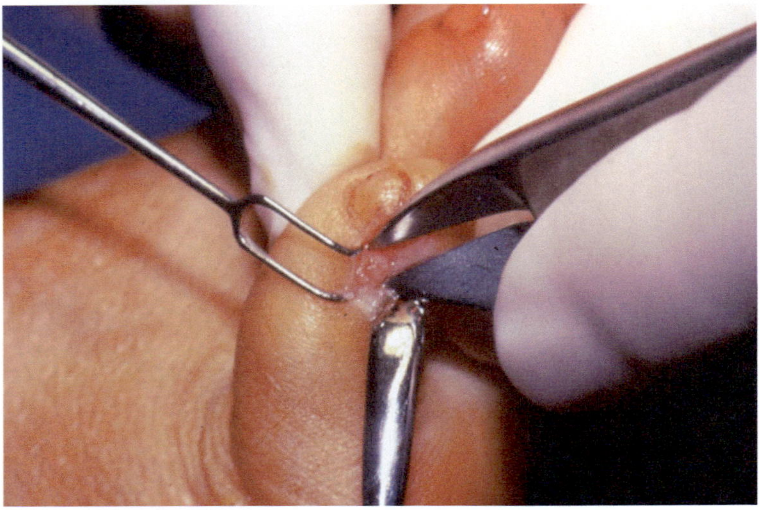

Fig. 20.19 Resection of prominent bone causing Lister's corn

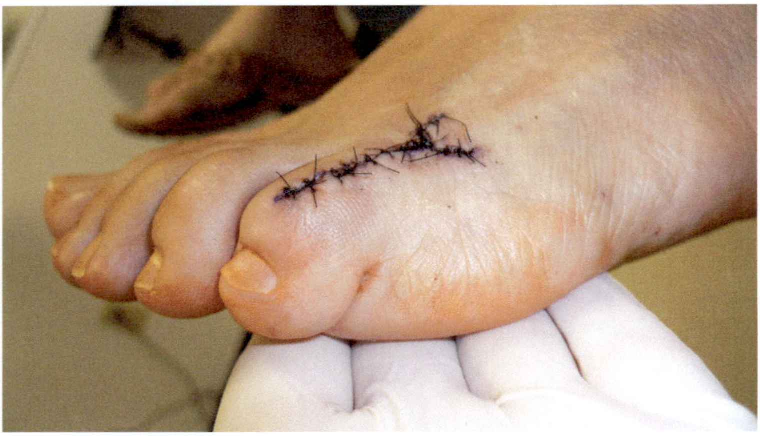

Fig. 20.20 Postoperative presentation of single long skin incision to address dorsal PIPJ lesion with MTPJ contracture. (Photo courtesy of Dr. William Fishco)

MTPJ with/without osseous surgery at the fifth MTPJ will need to be performed. The transverse planal deformity occurring at the MTPJ will be corrected with lateral release of the MTPJ with possible fifth metatarsal osteotomy if Tailor's bunion deformity present. For the medial PIPJ lesion, an arthroplasty of the PIPJ may be performed or simply a medial condylectomy of the head of the proximal phalanx of the fifth toe (Fig. 20.23).

When multiple lesions are present, careful surgical and incision planning will help prevent recurrence of lesions. For hyperkeratotic lesions on the fifth PIPJ and DIPJ, a PIPJ arthroplasty combined with a hemiphalangectomy of the middle pha-

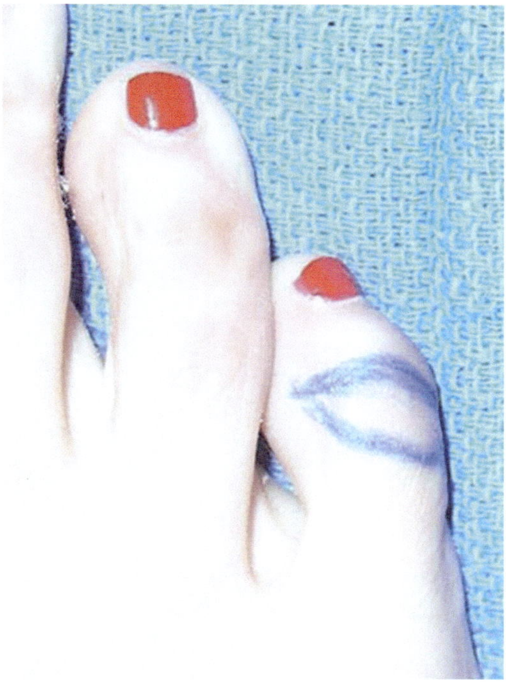

Fig. 20.21 Derotational skin plasty incision placement for dorsolateral PIPJ lesion without MTPJ contracture

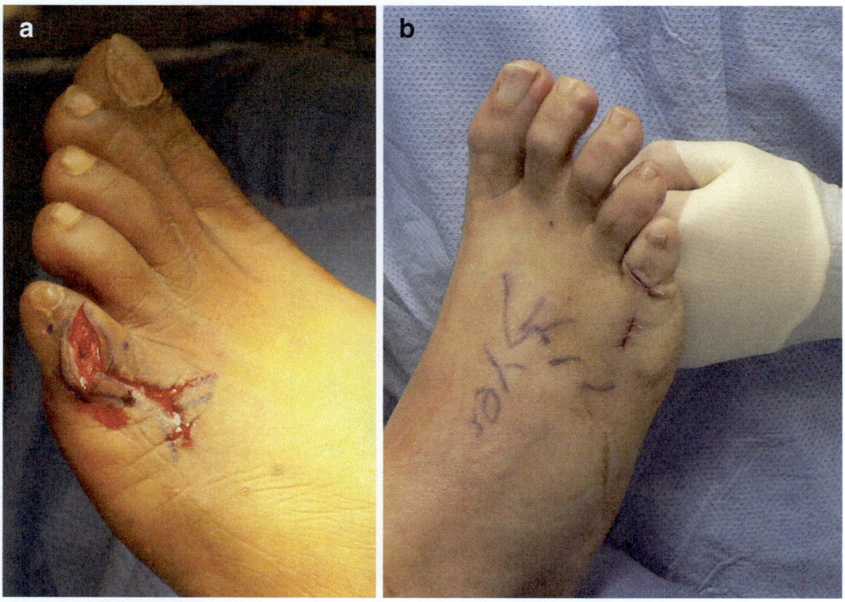

Fig. 20.22 (**a**) Intraoperative presentation of a combined derotational skin plasty with a V to Y skin plasty to release MTPJ contracture. (Photo courtesy of Dr. William Fishco). (**b**) Final closure of a combined derotational skin plasty with a separate linear incision to release MTPJ contracture. (Photo courtesy of Dr. Dave Alder)

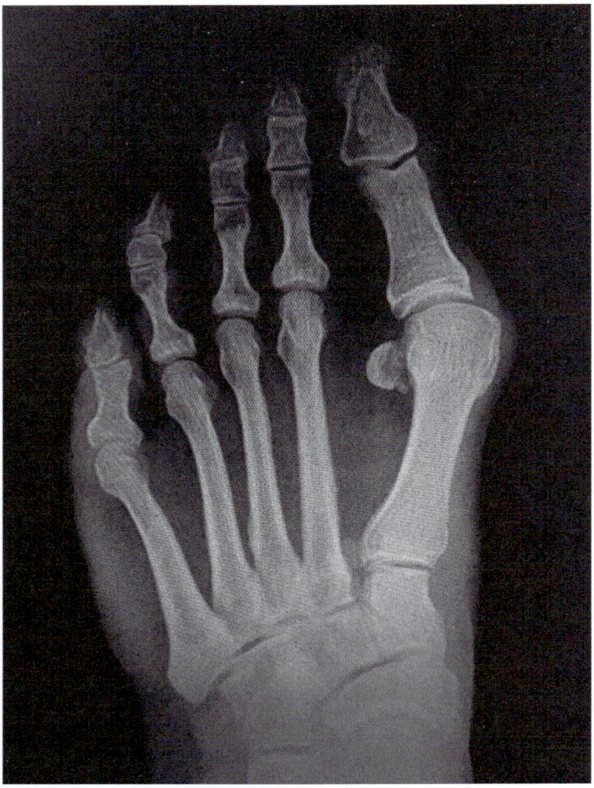

Fig. 20.23 Radiograph depicting a Tailor's bunion deformity with prominent medial PIPJ. Note the transverse planal dominant deformity and synostosis of the DIPJ

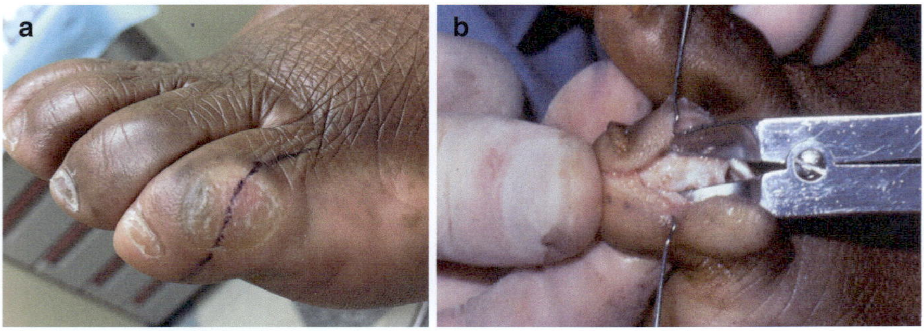

Fig. 20.24 (**a**) Photo depicting planned skin incision for arthroplasty and combined lateral hemiphalangectomy for lesion encompassing lateral PIPJ and DIPJ (Ruiz-Mora 1954). (**b**) Hemiphalangectomy performed through a laterally based curvilinear incision over the DIPJ extended from a midline PIPJ incision to perform the PIPJ arthroplasty

lanx will help ensure a successful outcome. Often times, this combination of lesions is due to an enlarged middle phalanx or possibly a DIPJ synostosis. Radiographs are evaluated prior to all cases of fifth toe surgery but especially important when multiple lesions are noted. If the lesion pattern is at the PIPJ and lateral aspect of the middle phalanx and/or DIPJ, then a midline arthroplasty incision is made over the

PIPJ and then curved laterally over the DIPJ toward the tip of the toe to obtain exposure of the lateral aspect of the middle phalanx and the DIPJ. A hemiphalangectomy or simple condylectomy at the DIPJ can then be performed (Fig. 20.24). If there are hyperkeratotic lesions on the PIPJ and medial aspect of the DIPJ, then a midline arthroplasty incision is made over the PIPJ and curved medially over the DIPJ toward the tip of the toe to obtain exposure of the medial aspect of the middle phalanx and the DIPJ. A hemiphalangectomy or simple condylectomy can then be performed at this side of the digit ensuring prominent area of bone is resected.

When a heloma molle is present with other lesions of the fifth toe, a partial syndactyly will not resolve all lesions. If a heloma molle is present with a medial-based PIPJ lesion, then a full syndactyly may resolve both lesions, but is not typically cosmetically accepted. In this instance, a small partial syndactyly and a medial condylectomy performed at the PIPJ will resolve both lesions and be more cosmetically accepted. When a heloma molle is combined with a classic PIPJ lesion dorsally or dorsolaterally, a partial syndactyly and arthroplasty with/without a derotational skin plasty will resolve both lesions (Fig. 20.25).

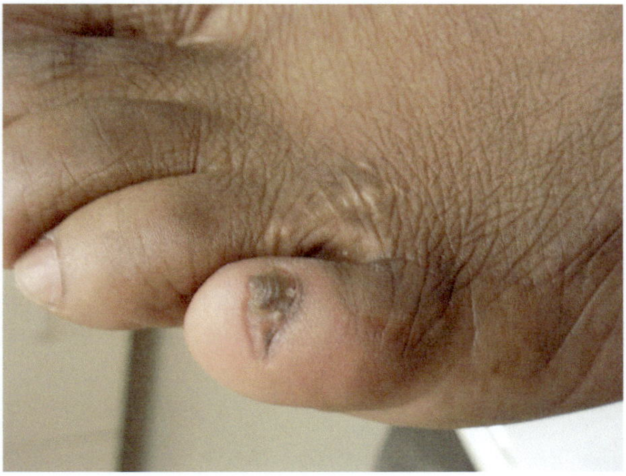

Fig. 20.25 Postoperative presentation after partial syndactylization and arthroplasty of PIPJ without derotational skin plasty

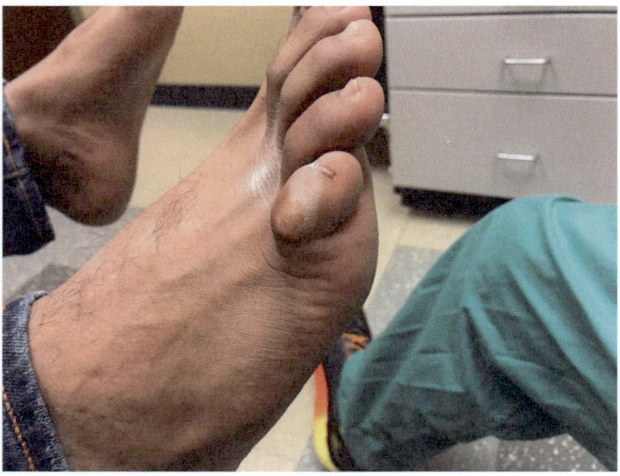

Fig. 20.26 Clinical presentation of congenital cock-up fifth toe

A cock-up fifth toe is a severe congenital hammertoe. Due to its typical familial component, the deformity is usually bilateral. It is best characterized by significant dorsiflexion of the digit with a subluxation of the proximal phalanx on the metatarsal head. This deformity commonly leads to pain and discomfort in the toe due to a prominence at the PIPJ with a subsequent large reactive hyperkeratotic lesion (Fig. 20.26). In some cases, there can be an overlapping component with the adjacent fourth digit. Conservative care often fails due the severity of the deformity. There are considerations of soft tissue and osseous structures that need to be addressed. Therefore, a surgical intervention at multiple levels is needed to correct the deformity.

A modified Ruiz-Mora procedure is the surgical option of choice for this severe congenital complex deformity [6, 7]. This procedure may also be utilized as a salvage procedure for failed previous surgical attempts of this congenital deformity or when a floating toe has developed as a complication of previous fifth toe surgery. This modified Ruiz-Mora procedure encompasses a combination of traditional hammertoe procedures, as well as a Z skin plasty to address the dorsal contracture of the skin and subcutaneous tissues. The procedure begins by marking a linear incision line over the dorsal fifth digit and proximally over the corresponding MTPJ. The Z skin plasty uses the planned central arm of the incision line but will be completed after release of the deeper underlying contracted tendon and joint structures. The contracted extensor tendon is identified and an open Z skin plasty performed on the tendon. Next, an arthroplasty at the PIPJ is performed followed by a MTPJ release. Note that the use of a McGlamry elevator may be necessary to release the plantar plate to achieve sufficient release of the deformity. Attention is then brought to the dorsal Z skin plasty. The arms of the Z skin plasty are incised with 60° angulations and liberated with the underlying subcutaneous tissues for transposition of the full-thickness flaps. Due to the amount of dorsal contracture release, a plantarly based elliptical wedge of skin may need to be excised from the proximal plantar sulcus of the digit to remove redundancy. This will also help prevent recurrence of deformity. Holding the foot with simulated weight bearing is advisable at this time to deter-

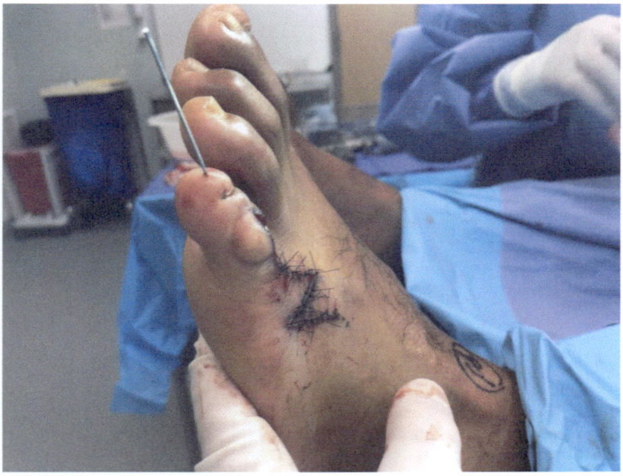

Fig. 20.27 Partial closure after transposition of full thickness flaps via Z skin plasty. Note K wire fixation and lack of need for plantar sulcus skin plasty

mine if any other intervention is needed to reduce the deformity. The toe in its corrected position should be held temporarily with a 0.045 K wire (Fig. 20.27). The K wire should be placed across the MTPJ for added stability and should be removed in 4 weeks.

Summary

Complications of fifth toe surgery are similar to any other open procedure of the foot and ankle. These include, but are not limited to, infection, prolonged swelling, nerve entrapment, slow healing, and painful scar. Special complications that are more unique to the fifth toe surgery include overcorrection from too aggressive bone resection resulting in floppy or unstable toe (Fig. 20.28), undercorrection causing lesion recurrence (Fig. 20.29), failure to address plane of deformity leading to recurrent deformity (Fig. 20.30), and failure to plan surgery accurately for the presenting lesion pattern.

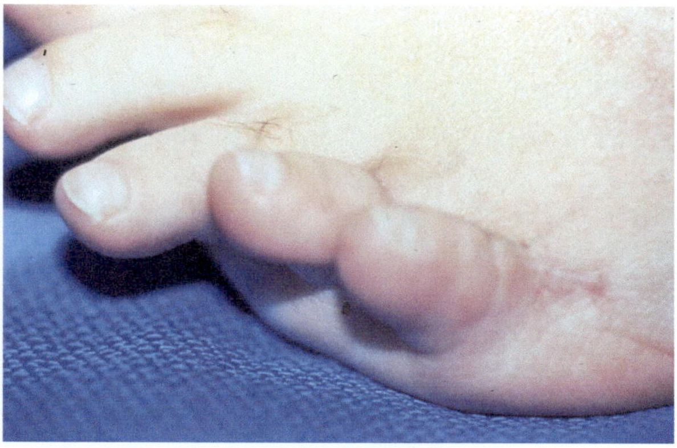

Fig. 20.28 Floating digital deformities resulting from overaggressive PIPJ arthroplasty in an attempt to address continued MTPJ contracture

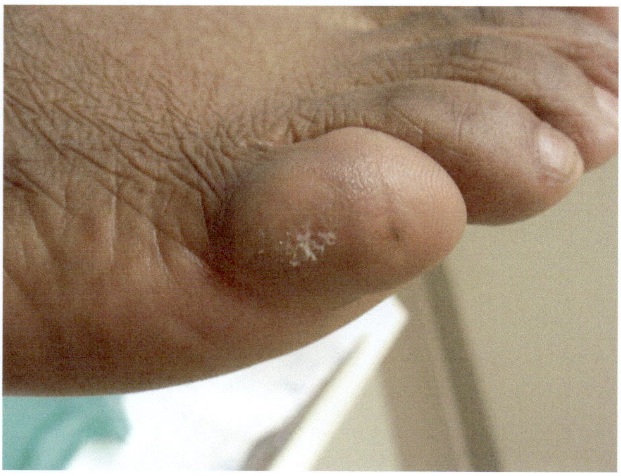

Fig. 20.29 Undercorrection of frontal planal deformity with recurrent lesion

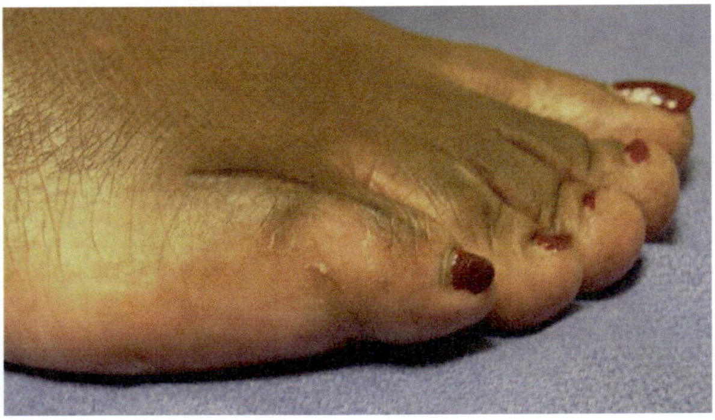

Fig. 20.30 Floating toe deformity from lack of adequate release of MTPJ contracture

Fifth toe surgery is common in foot and ankle surgical practices. The deformity must be evaluated clinically and radiographically. The deformity must be evaluated in all three planes. Special attention must be paid to the lesion pattern. The painful lesion or lesions associated with the deformity is typically the presenting complaint of the patient. If careful surgical planning is carried out, the risk of recurrent deformity and/or lesions will be greatly reduced.

References

1. Ellington JK. Hammertoes and clawtoes: proximal interphalangeal joint correction. Foot Ankle Clin. 2011;16(4):547–58.
2. Coughlin MJ, Kennedy MP. Operative repair of fourth and fifth toe corns. Foot Ankle Int. 2003;24(2):147–57.
3. Dereymaeker G, van der Broek c. Biphalangeal fifth toe. Foot Ankle Int. 2006;27(11):948–51.
4. George M. Biphalangeal fifth toe: an increasingly common variant? J Anat. 2001;198(Pt 2):251.
5. Wilson JN. V-Y correction for varus deformity of the fifth toe. Br J Surg. 1953;41(166):13–5.
6. Ruiz-Mora J. Plastic correction of overriding 5th toe. Orthop Lett Club. 1954;6:6.
7. Janecki CJ, Wilde AH. Results of phalangectomy of the fifth toe for hammertoe. The Ruiz-Mora procedure. J Bone Joint Surg Am. 1976;58(7):1005–7.

Chapter 21
Fifth Toe Proximal Interphalangeal Joint Arthrodesis

Thomas S. Roukis and Drew Davidson

Presentation/History

When considering correction of fifth toe proximal interphalangeal joint contracture, arthrodesis of the joint is often foregone in favor of arthroplasty, most likely secondary to concern over irritation within shoe gear following arthrodesis [1]. Although limited, fifth toe proximal interphalangeal joint arthrodesis is indicated when there is isolated rigid contracture of the fifth toe in isolation such as can occur following previous fracture (Fig. 21.1) or global lesser toe deformities such as can be seen with rheumatoid arthritis (Fig. 21.2). Fifth toe proximal interphalangeal arthrodesis is also indicated with neuromuscular conditions where the digital deformity is severe and arthroplasty would lead to deformity recurrence such as with Charcot-Marie-Tooth or following a cerebral vascular accident (Fig. 21.3) [2].

Diagnosis/Assessment

The diagnosis of a fifth toe proximal interphalangeal contracture involves clinical examination demonstrating extension of the proximal phalanx on the metatarsal head and flexion contracture of the intermediate and distal phalanges. The deformity may be rigid and non-reducible regardless of foot posture (i.e., in plantarflexion that relaxes the long flexor tendons or dorsiflexion that relaxes the long extensors)

T. S. Roukis (✉)
Orthopaedic Center, Gundersen Health System,
La Crosse, WI, USA
e-mail: tsroukis@gundersenhealth.org

D. Davidson
McFarland Clinic, Ames, IA, USA

E. A. Cook, J. J. Cook (eds.), *Hammertoes*,
https://doi.org/10.1007/978-3-319-16552-3_21

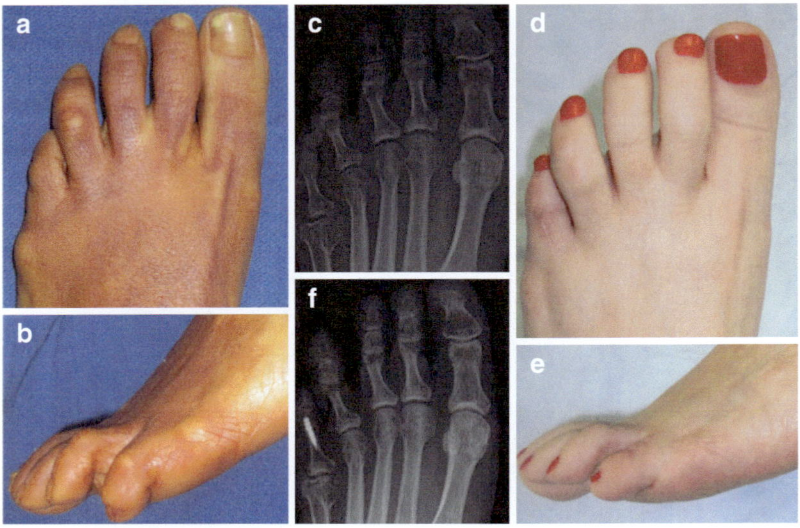

Fig. 21.1 Anterior-posterior (**a**) and lateral (**b**) intraoperative photographs, as well as weightbearing anterior-posterior radiograph (**c**) demonstrating a rigid fifth toe proximal interphalangeal joint contracture as a result of a prior stubbing injury. Clinical anterior-posterior (**d**) and lateral (**e**) photographs, as well as weightbearing anterior-posterior radiograph (**f**) demonstrating a well-aligned fifth toe proximal interphalangeal joint arthrodesis using an intramedullary fixation device

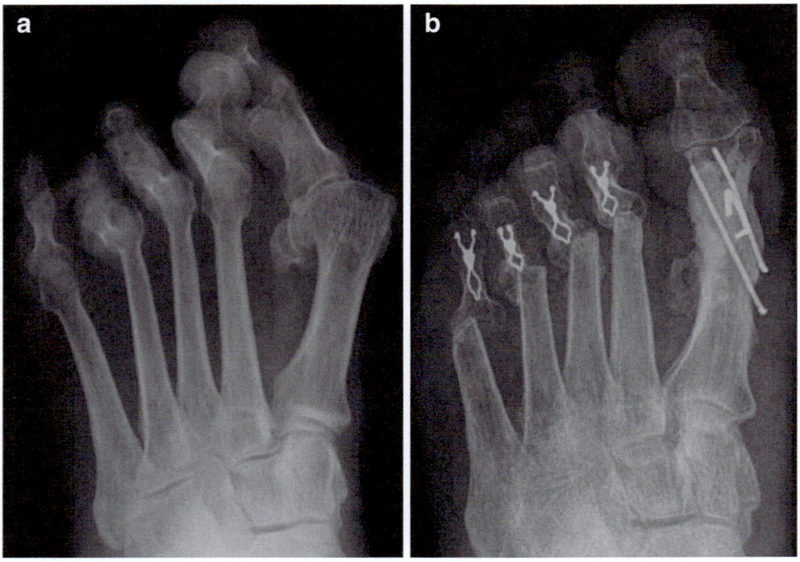

Fig. 21.2 Anterior-posterior weightbearing radiograph demonstrating a global forefoot deformity secondary to Rheumatoid arthritis prior to (**a**) and following (**b**) forefoot reconstruction with first metatarsal-phalangeal joint arthrodesis, lesser metatarsal head resection, and arthrodesis of the second through fifth toe proximal interphalangeal with intramedullary fixation devices

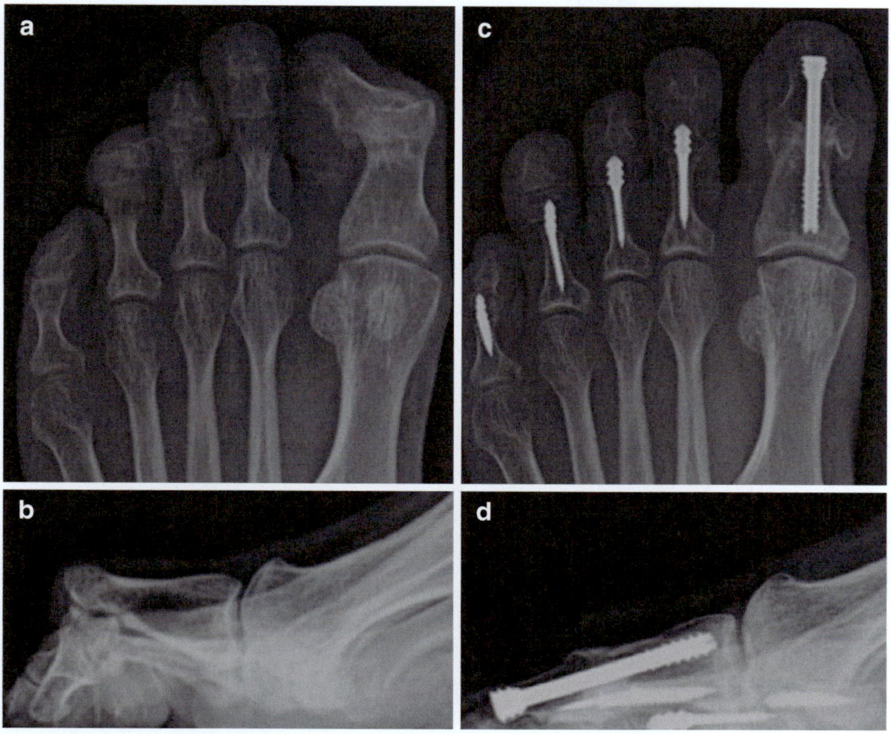

Fig. 21.3 Anterior-posterior (**a**) and lateral (**b**) weightbearing radiographs demonstrating global lesser toe contractures secondary to a cerebral vascular accident. Anterior-posterior (**c**) and lateral (**d**) weightbearing radiographs following hallux interphalangeal joint arthrodesis with a screw and arthrodesis of the second through fifth toe proximal interphalangeal joints with intramedullary fixation devices

or reducible, either partially or completely. Weightbearing radiographs of the foot are obtained to confirm the clinical examination findings with the oblique view being particularly beneficial.

Surgical Technique

We only have experience using intramedullary fixation devices for performing a fifth toe proximal interphalangeal joint arthrodesis [3, 4]. A dorsal linear incision, or converging semi-elliptical incision if a keratotic lesion is present, centered over the proximal interphalangeal joint is carried down through the extensor tendon complex to the level of the proximal interphalangeal joint. This is followed by release of the collateral ligaments, thereby allowing exposure of the proximal phalangeal head and base of the intermediate phalanx. The head of the proximal interphalangeal joint is resected at the metaphyseal-diaphyseal junction using a bone cutter or power instrumentation based on surgeon preference.

If the toe is severely contracted, additional soft tissue release will be required to both the long extensor and flexor tendons. First, the medial and lateral margins of the sling and wing components of the extensor digitorum longus tendon are incised vertically, parallel to the longitudinal axis of the proximal phalanx. The resultant extensor digitorum longus tendon flap is then grasped and underscored through a combination of sharp and blunt dissection to the level of the metatarsal head. A #66 Beaver mini-blade is then inserted deep to the extensor digitorum longus tendon flap, and the metatarsophalangeal joint capsule is penetrated, and the medial and lateral capsular and ligamentous structures are transected. This allows for lengthening of the extensor tendon complex and metatarsal-phalangeal joint capsulotomy through the same incision as employed to perform the fifth toe proximal interphalangeal joint arthrodesis [5]. Next, following lengthening of the extensor tendon complex and capsulotomy, attention is directed to the long flexor tendon. The shaft of the proximal phalanx is elevated which brings the plantar plate of the proximal interphalangeal joint into view. Upon longitudinal sectioning of the plantar plate, the flexor digitorum longus tendon is identified and grasped with a right-angle hemostat. A scissor or surgical knife is used to sever the flexor digitorum longus tendon [3]. This combination of osseous decompression through bone resection and soft tissue release with extensor tendon lengthening, metatarsal-phalangeal joint capsulotomy, and flexor tendon lengthening allows for global correction of the deformity.

The next step involves implantation of an axial cannulated mini-screw from the tip of the toe distally into the base of the proximal phalanx over a guidewire (Fig. 21.4) [3] or implantation of a one-piece intramedullary fixation device of the surgeon's preference [4]. All of the available one-piece intramedullary fixation device systems involve a similar sequence of steps. First, a small drill is inserted

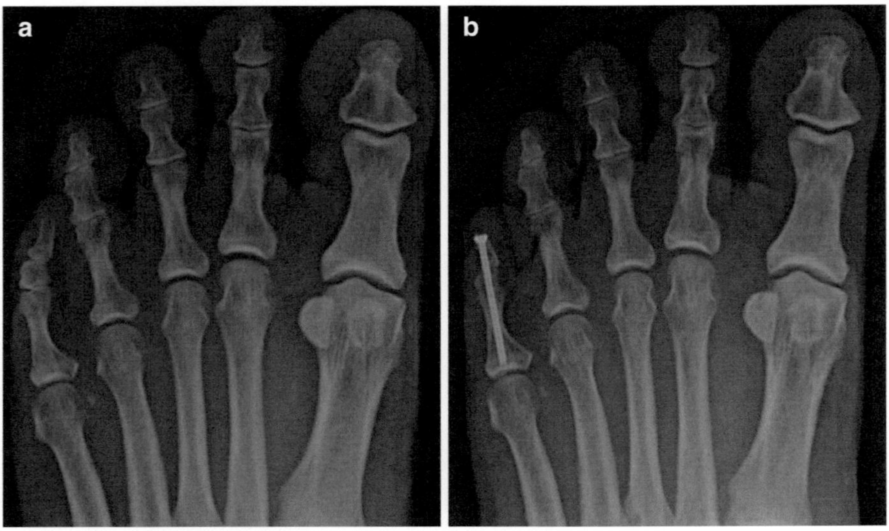

Fig. 21.4 Anterior-posterior weightbearing radiograph demonstrating a painful fifth toe contracture underlapping the fourth toe that failed prior exostectomy (**a**). Anterior-posterior weightbearing radiograph following fifth toe proximal interphalangeal joint arthrodesis with a cannulated mini-screw (**b**)

into the medullary canal of the proximal phalanx followed by insertion of a broach. Next, the same drill bit is then inserted through the center of the base of the intermediate phalanx. The articular surface is then resected with the use of a handheld reamer followed by insertion of a square-shaped broach. After irrigation of the surgical site the implant is inserted into the proximal phalanx side and then the intermediate phalanx is shish kebabed onto the exposed portion of the implant. Once proper seating is verified with intraoperative image intensification, the extensor tendon complex is approximated with absorbable suture followed by skin closure of the surgeon's preference.

Outcomes

Success rates for fifth toe proximal interphalangeal joint arthrodesis are not readily available in the literature; however, secondary to the small stature of the phalanges, it is likely that rates would be slightly lower than that of other digits and, therefore, the need for complications leading to revision greater (Fig. 21.5). Clearly, osseous

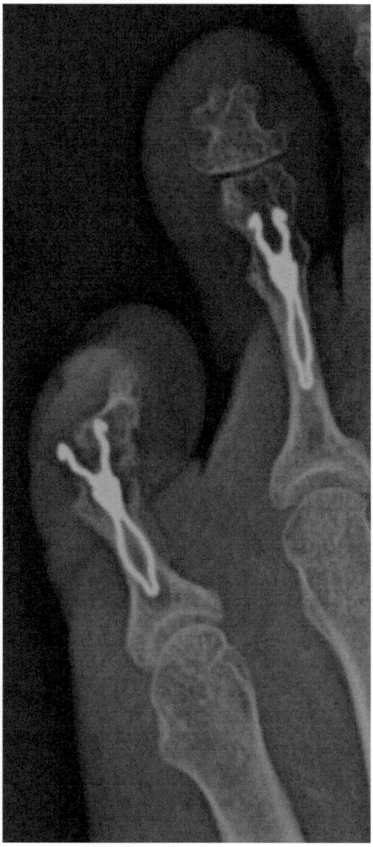

Fig. 21.5 Anterior-posterior weightbearing radiograph following fifth toe proximal interphalangeal joint arthrodesis with an intramedullary device demonstrating recurrence of the deformity and migration of the distal portion of the implant leading to pain that required removal

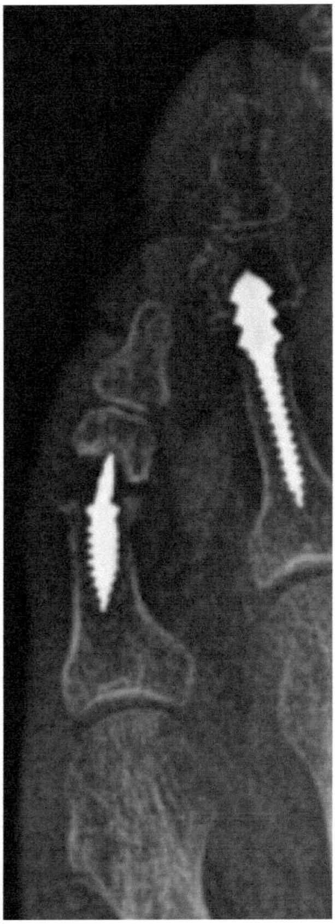

Fig. 21.6 Anterior-posterior weightbearing radiograph following fifth toe proximal interphalangeal joint arthrodesis with an intramedullary device demonstrating well-aligned toe with a stable fibrous union

union is the desired end result of arthrodesis, but it is not always required in order to obtain a successful outcome when performing proximal interphalangeal joint arthrodesis. In fact, patients often experience satisfaction when the final outcome results in a stable fibrous nonunion (i.e., soft fusion) (Fig. 21.6). Until published manuscripts are available, the outcomes associated with fifth toe proximal interphalangeal joint arthrodesis will remain a matter for conjecture.

Clinical Pearls/Pitfalls

- There are limited indications for performing fifth toe proximal interphalangeal joint arthrodesis.
- One must achieve muscular balance around the fifth toe proximal interphalangeal joint for successful maintenance of correction.
- Fifth toe proximal interphalangeal joint arthrodesis is technically demanding and likely has a higher incidence of complications than the other lesser toes.
- Consider fixation with a cannulated mini-screw or one-piece intramedullary fixation device.

References

1. Edwards WH, Beischer AD. Interphalangeal joint arthrodesis of the lesser toes. Foot Ankle Clin. 2002;7(1):43–8.
2. Fenton CF III, Schlefman BS, McGlamry ED. Surgical consideration in the presence of Charcot-Marie-Tooth Disease. J Am Podiatry Assoc. 1984;74(10):490–8.
3. Roukis TS. The use of a one-piece shape-metal nitinol intramedullary internal fixation device for arthrodesis of the proximal interphalangeal joint in neuropathic patients with diabetes. Foot Ankle Spec. 2009;2(3):130–4.
4. Roukis TS. Central metatarsal head-neck osteotomies: indications and operative techniques. Clin Podiatr Med Surg. 2005;22(2):197–222.
5. Roukis TS, Ringstrom JB. Lesser metatarsophalangeal release utilizing the #66 mini-blade. J Foot Ankle Surg. 1999;38(2):163–5.

Chapter 22
Congenital Overlapping Fifth Toe

Mark Gilheany

In this chapter congenital overlapping fifth toe is discussed.

As a clinical descriptor, the term overlapping fifth toe evokes a clear image of the presenting complaint. Anatomically the condition presents as a spectrum of malalignment about the fifth metatarsophalangeal joint characterised by adduction and rotation of the fifth digit. Based on this spectrum, the author prefers when describing this clinical entity to use another common descriptor of this condition digiti quinti varus (DQV). This anatomic descriptor encompasses the range of positional changes which may present when the fifth digit is adducted and rotated at the fifth metatarsophalangeal joint. Using an anatomic descriptor also potentially focusses therapy on addressing appropriate plane and level of deformity during treatment.

Presentation

DQV is a congenital condition presenting with various levels of severity. The exact occurrence rate is not known. Although there is no documented epidemiologic evidence of the condition occurring more frequently in females, typically a greater number of female patients will present with symptoms in relation to this condition. This gender imbalance is exampled by several surgical case series. Murgeir et al. [1] reported on 13 females and 3 males with an average age of 12.2 years. Abu Hassan et al. [2] in 1 case series reported on 27 females and 9 males and in another 25 females and 7 males [3]. Morris et al. [4] reported on a case series of 13 females and 5 males.

M. Gilheany (✉)
Foot and Ankle Specialists, Traralgon, VIC, Australia
e-mail: admin@fasa.net.au; https://www.eastmelbournepodiatry.com.au/about-us/

E. A. Cook, J. J. Cook (eds.), *Hammertoes*,
https://doi.org/10.1007/978-3-319-16552-3_22

The severity of DQV can worsen with age due to adaptation. These adaptive changes often lead to increased symptoms including development of pressure lesions when osseous and soft tissue maturity occurs.

DQV is described as a triplanar deformity of the fifth toe where the toe is rotated (externally), adducted and dorsiflexed relative to the fifth metatarsophalangeal joint. The clinical result is overriding of the fifth toe in relation to the fourth toe (Fig. 22.1).

Occasionally the condition is associated with lateral drift of the fifth metatarsal (Fig. 22.2) [1, 5].

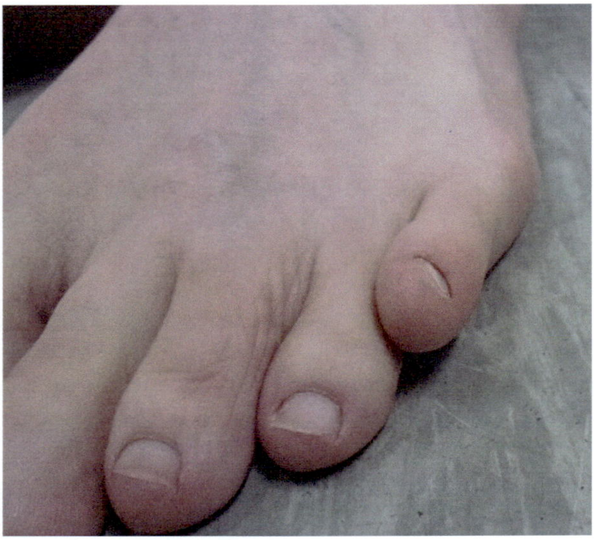

Fig. 22.1 Symptomatic DQV in a 24-year-old male athlete

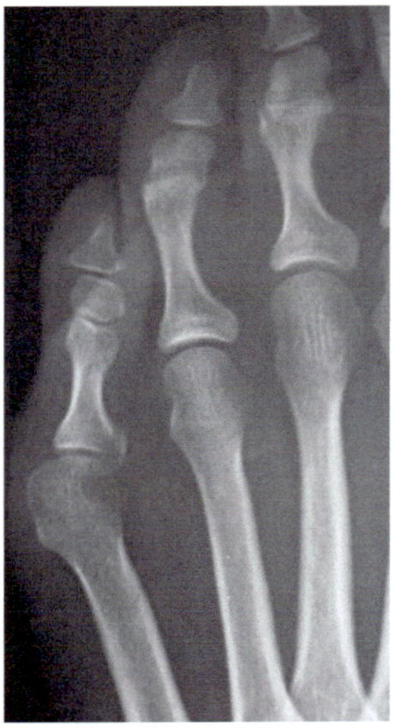

Fig. 22.2 Lateral splay of fifth metatarsal resulting in complex DQV and Tailor's bunionette

There are typically three patient demographics presenting to the clinician which can be allocated into the following categories.

- *Children*: Parents presenting with a young child concerned about the appearance of the small toes. They are generally concerned about the effect this might have upon function and shoe fit in the future. At this point in time, the condition is generally asymptomatic.
- *Adolescents*: The adolescent is becoming concerned about shoe fit issues. Cosmesis may be a concern at this stage.
- *Adults*: Having never been concerned about cosmetic appearance, the individual is now suffering with shoe fit issues and pain. The condition may be static or gradually worsening. There may also be blisters, chronic hyperkeratotic lesions or ulcerative lesions.

Assessment

Given the variability in severity, DQV requires individual assessment of both osseous and soft tissue contracture and adaptation. Such analysis will guide therapeutic intervention.

Although DQV is not associated with specific medical syndromes, routine general medical and physical assessment should be undertaken.

The author's management protocol is guided by an assessment both radiological and clinical against the following criteria:

Osseous

- Osseous maturity
- Alignment of the fifth metatarsal
- Presence of periarticular osteophytes
- Variation in the shape or number of phalanx bones

Soft tissue

- Location and severity of contracture. Specific assessment of joint capsule, flexor tendons, extensor tendons, ligament integrity and presence and location of hyperkeratotic lesions at either digital or metatarsophalangeal joint level

Lower limb mechanics

- Review of gait indices to identify any lower limb mechanical anomalies which may either be contributing to or are worsened by the DVQ

Outcome expectation

- In-depth discussion with the patient (and family) as to the nature and severity of the condition will facilitate the developement of realistic expectations of treatment.

Treatment

Management of an individual patient's expectations in the case of DQV is grounded in clinical assessment and appropriate education supporting the patient as a participant in the decision to undergo active treatment or monitoring. Should quality of life be adversely affected and nonsurgical measures fail to alleviate symptoms, surgical procedures can be considered.

Quality of life effects refer to measurement of various patient-centred domains, for example, foot pain, shoe fit, cosmesis and/or functional limitation. There are many quality of life measures commonly utilised in formal research assessing outcomes of treatment for foot pathology. A comprehensive summary of these measures is presented by Landorf and Burns [6].

Within the clinical setting, formal research protocols or use of validated measures although desirable is not always feasible. As a pragmatic alternative [7, 8], the author will commonly use an informal quality of life measurement activity which acts as a tool to encourage patients to become an active participant in the management of their health issue. This can be as simple as asking the patient to maintain a lifestyle diary to record impact on quality of life against such domains as listed above. The diary is maintained for a month and then repeated at a later date. This acts to provide a patient-focussed self-reflective assessment of the quality of life impact over time.

This approach is very useful as a guide to appropriate timing for intervention when dealing with non-acute foot pathology such as DQV.

Nonsurgical Management

Nonsurgical management techniques described for DQV include stretching and massage of contracted soft tissue in concert with taping or the use of splints [9, 10]. Footwear modification is also a suitable option in less severe cases. There is currently only limited evidence from clinical trials to support the effectiveness of such measures a trial of taping for toe deformity reported success rate of 90% in newborns [11]. It is appropriate to advise such treatments prior to surgery as any improvement in contracture may reduce the extent of surgical reduction required if surgical procedures are subsequently pursued (Fig. 22.3).

The period of nonsurgical care also allows time for the patient to self-assess quality of life impact as described above. This patient engagement enhances patient understanding and helps define expectations, both of which act as important elements of informed consent for surgery should it be required.

Additional physical therapy techniques such as splinting are generally required postoperatively to maintain correction (Fig. 22.3). If a patient is familiarised with these techniques preoperatively, compliance and effectiveness during the postoperative phase will be enhanced.

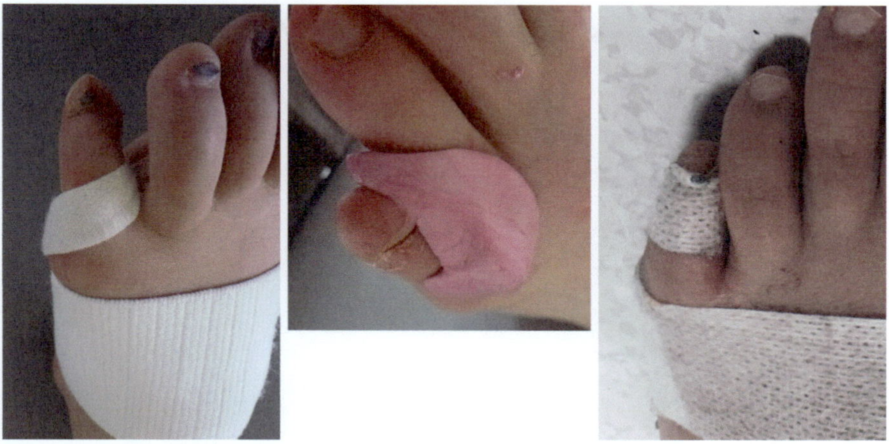

Fig. 22.3 Examples of splints and taping techniques commonly used pre- and postoperatively for DQV

Surgical Techniques

Historically a variety of surgical techniques have been described. These techniques have generally been conducted on small numbers and/or have not been subjected to valid outcome measures. As such it is not possible to identify the most universally accepted, most efficacious surgical approach for DQV.

Common to the majority of techniques is soft tissue release about the metatarsophalangeal joint including tendon lengthening and ligament release (Table 22.1). In addition skin plasty and osseous decompression or realignment procedures and postoperative splinting with either internal K-wires or external bandaging in various combinations are described in a number of case series and procedural descriptions. Concerns [1–4, 12, 13, 23–29] about scarring and tissue viability in association with skin plasty have been raised as a reason to consider avoiding extensive skin plasty [14].

Some reports described syndactyly of the fifth toe to the fourth toe and amputation or resection of the proximal phalanx of the fifth toes as means to treat DQV [15, 16, 30, 31]. In the author's view, these procedures should be reserved for failed reconstruction as cosmetically syndactyly is not acceptable to many patients and amputation has obvious cosmetic concern and can lead to functional overload and deformity in the remaining digits (Fig. 22.4).

Downey in 2002 [32] describes a consolidated approach to reduction of DQV which utilises aspects of all the reported techniques. This consolidated approach commits to extensive skin plasty. More recently a percutaneous technique suggests that skin plasty may not be necessary [1].

Table 22.1 Primary procedural elements as initially described in the literature for DQV [1, 4, 12–22]

Legend:
1. Metatarso phalangeal joint capsulotomy and ligament release
2. Extensor lengthening via tenotomy
3. Skin plasty: V-Y, Z(#) plantar ellipse (+)
4. Extensor tendon transfer to abductor digiti quinti
5. Syndactyly of the fifth to fourth toes
6. Amputation of the fifth toe
7. Phalanx or metatarsal osteotomy
8. Percutaneous approach as whole or part procedure

	1	2	3	4	5	6	7	8
Lapidus 1942	#	#		#				
McFarland 1950					#			
Wilson 1953	#		#	#				
Zanoli 1959	#	#		#				
Perkins 1961						#		
Hulman 1964	#	#	# +					#
Cockin 1968	#	#	#					
Morris 1982	#	#	#					
Weber 1982			#				#	
Leonard 1965					#			
Rosner 1978	#	#					#	
Lopez 2010		#					#	
Murgier etal 2013	#	#					#	#

This table highlights the acceptance of operative procedures to address soft tissue contracture

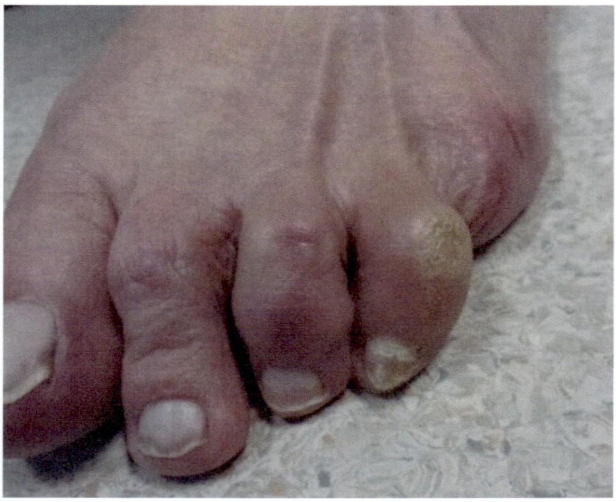

Fig. 22.4 An example of secondary overload that ultimately results from amputation of the fifth toe

The various procedural elements as described in the literature are presented in Table 1 to highlight the essential similarities with the technical approaches used. Release of soft tissue contracture is clearly demonstrated as a key component of the procedure.

The Author's Approach

The author employs the full range of procedures based upon the individual requirements of the case. The approach is sequential aiming to minimise trauma and subsequent risk to soft tissues. The focus is upon realigning the fifth ray as a functional unit using minimal incision techniques as a stand-alone approach or in combination with open techniques as required.

Technique

1. Percutaneous dorsomedial capsule, medial ligament and extensor tendon lengthening (tenotomy) is performed at the fifth MT joint using a 67 microblade.

> In many cases loading of the forefoot demonstrates reduction of deformity once this is performed. If this is the case, no further procedures are performed, and the toe is splinted in neutral.

2. Osseous procedures are performed sequentially if indicated and based on preoperative evaluation of x-rays. This will most commonly include percutaneous proximal phalanx osteotomy to plantar flex and abduct the digit with or without open chevron osteotomy of the fifth metatarsal.

> An alternative is decompression of the osseous components via arthrectomy of the proximal interphalangeal (PIP) joint. The author avoids arthrodesis of the PIP joint as the resultant rigidity in the fifth toe will often cause shoe irritation in the future.

3. Skin plasty is only performed if loading of the forefoot demonstrates persistent deformity once all soft tissue release and osseous work are complete. In the author's experience, this is rarely required.

> Dorsally "Z-plasty" or "V-Y plasty" is performed in the line of contracture incorporating the original percutaneous incision. Plantar transverse wedge can also be utilised.

Illustrative Cases

The following case histories illustrate the range of pathology and procedural variations that can be utilised for DQV. In each of these cases, the steps outlined above are the basis for sequential surgical reduction.

Case 1

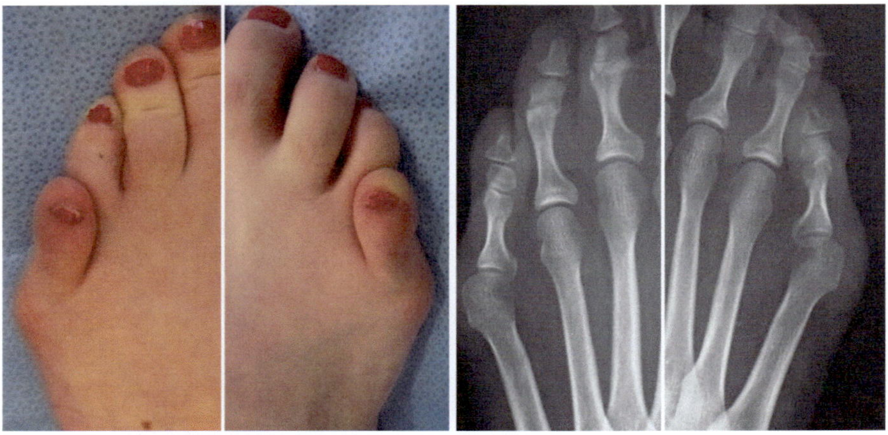

Deformity of the fifth toes in all three planes in a healthy 24-year-old female. Note fifth metatarsal involvement and contracture of medial ligament at MT joint.

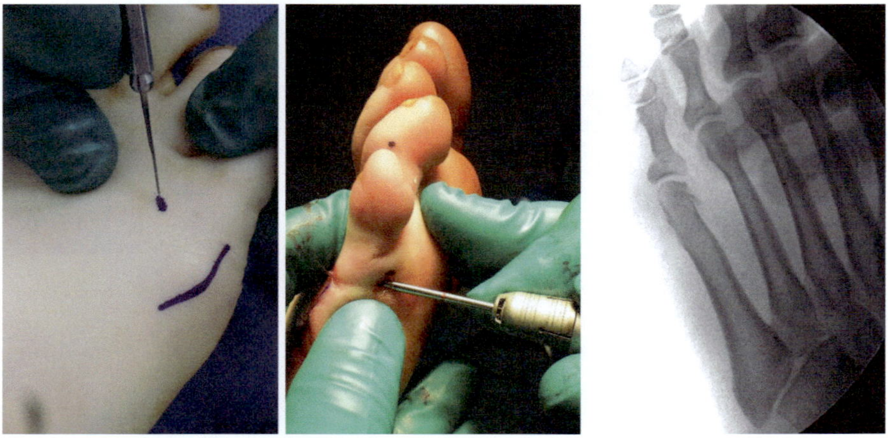

Surgical reduction required to achieve reduction of deformity:
Step 1 Percutaneous soft tissue relaxation: dorsal capsule, medial capsule including medial ligaments and extensor tenotomy via single portal

Step 2 Distal chevron style osteotomy of the fifth metatarsal via short lateral incision followed by percutaneous plantar flexor wedge osteotomy of the proximal phalanx

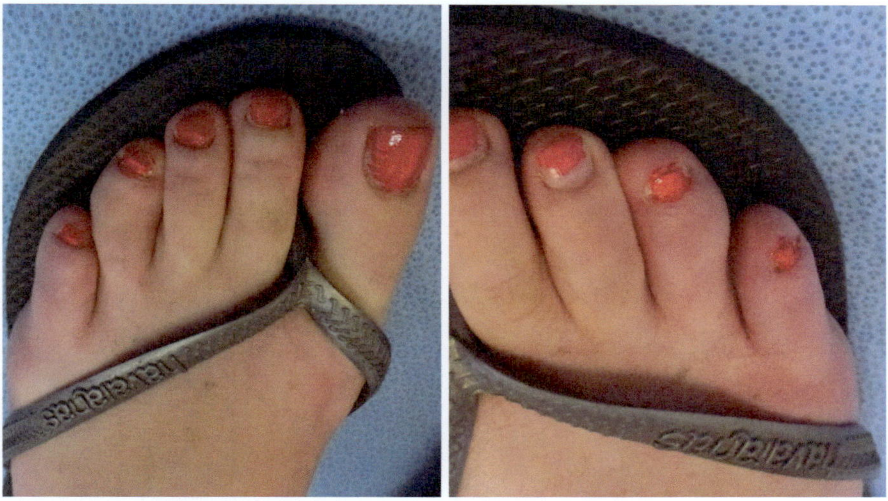

Postoperative appearance at 3 months

Case 2

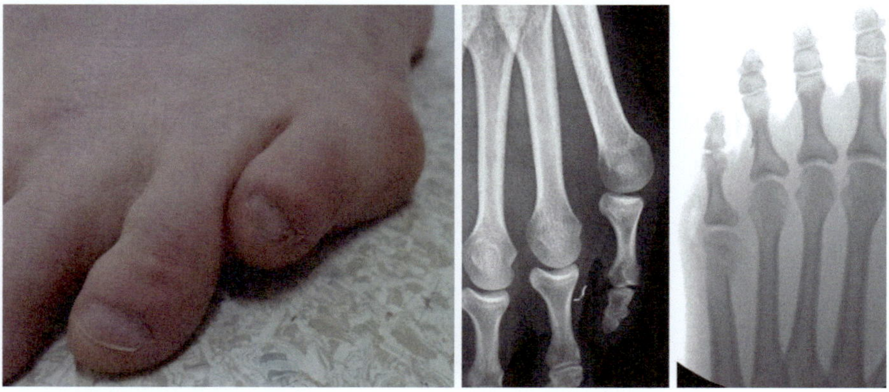

Deformity predominant in the transverse plane with mild sagittal plane elevation of the fifth toe in a healthy 27-year-old female. Note fifth metatarsal involvement and contracture of medial ligament at MT joint.

Case 3

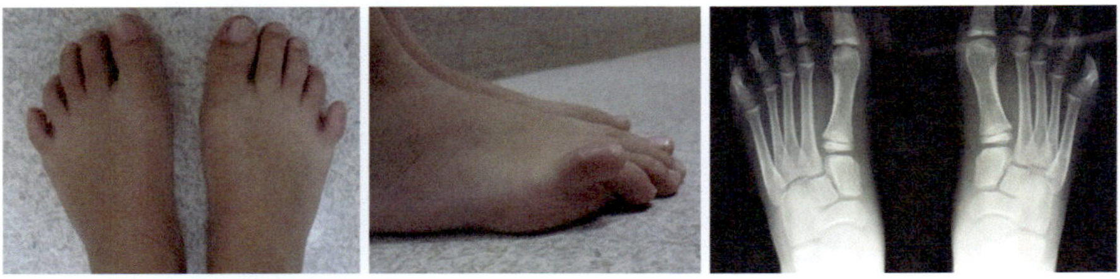

Surgical reduction required to achieve reduction of deformity:
Step 1 Percutaneous release of medial capsule and ligaments at MT level
Step 2 Open distal osteotomy fifth metatarsal

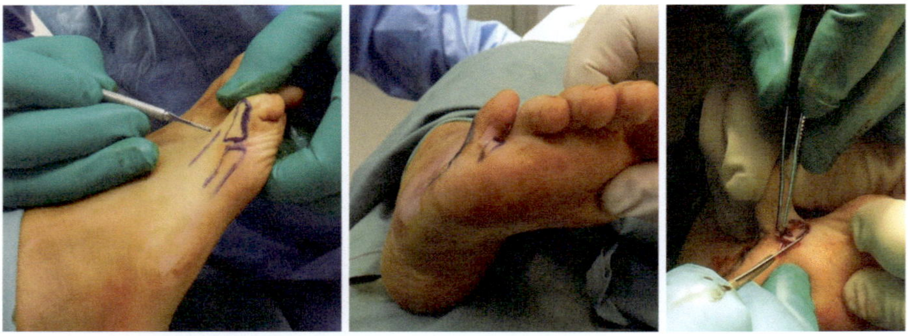

Severe deformity of the fifth toes in a healthy 10-year-old male. The contracture is predominant in the sagittal plane. Due to osseous immaturity, a decision to reduce the soft tissue deformity with potential for further reduction via osseous procedures at a later date was made.

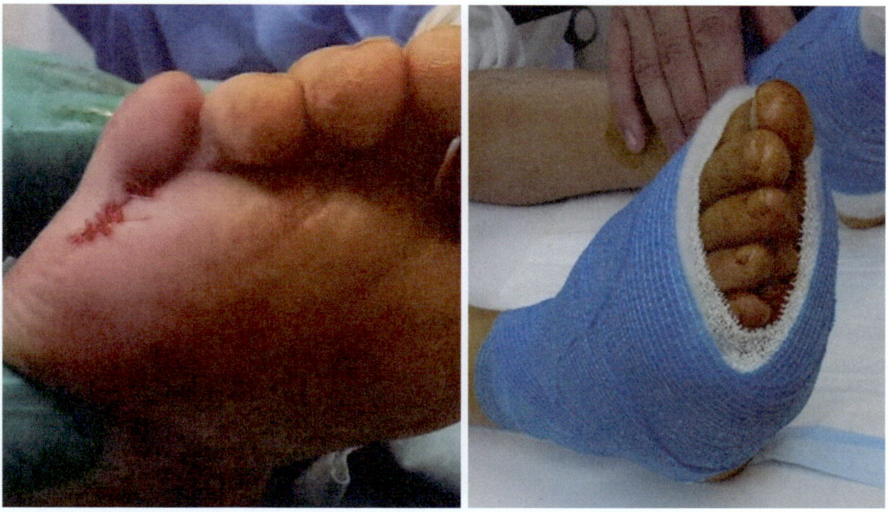

Surgical reduction required to achieve reduction of deformity:
Step 1 Percutaneous release of medial capsule and ligaments at MT level. Note that tension is placed on the contracted structures to facilitate release.

Step 2 On the right side, adequate reduction was not achieved. A plantar elliptical wedge of skin was removed to augment reduction of deformity. The toe and foot are protected post-surgery with a modified Jones bandage.

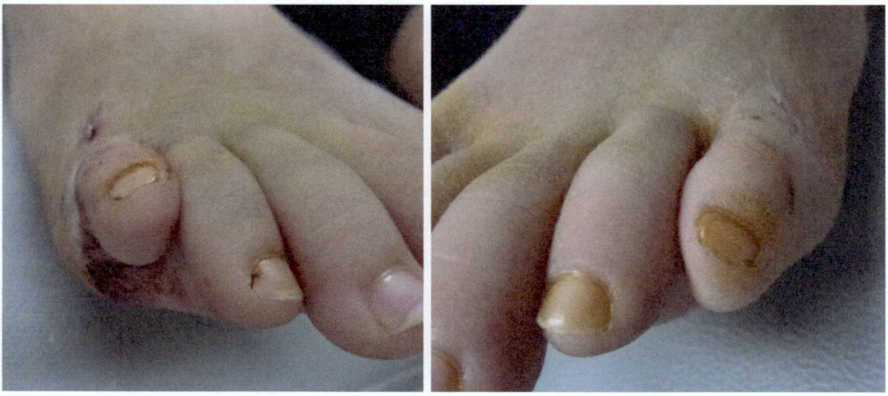

Postoperative progress:
At 1 week post procedure correction is noted.

At 6 weeks significant clinical improvement is maintained. Picture is weight-bearing with sling tape removed from fifth digits.

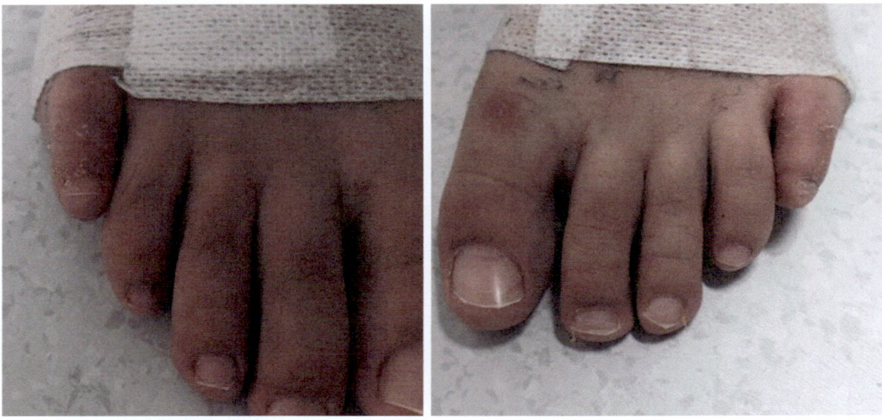

Deformity of the left fifth toe (adduction and dorsiflexion) in a healthy 26-year-old male athlete. Above left is preoperative image and above right 6 weeks postoperative image.

Surgical reduction required to achieve reduction of deformity:
Step 1 Percutaneous extensor tenotomy with release medial capsule and ligaments at MT level
Step 2 Percutaneous plantar flexor osteotomy of proximal phalanx

Case 4

Complications

The potential complications of DQV surgery are similar to all reconstructive procedures of the foot and ankle. These include neurovascular compromise, wound dehiscence, cosmesis in respect to scar tissue, under-correction and over-correction.

Complication rates of this type are not commonly reported in the literature in respect to DQV procedures. Minimally invasive procedures in general for digital deformity have been reported to be minimal [33].

The following case report does highlight that outcomes are adversely affected by procedures which do not pragmatically address the deformity.

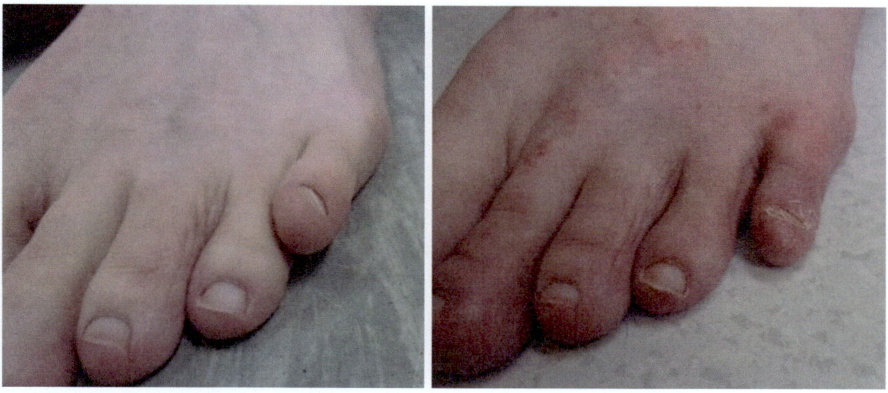

Pain and deformity about the fifth toe post failed reduction of DQV in a 61-year-old female. Previous surgery includes fifth metatarsal osteotomy and flexor tendon tenotomy. Neither procedure recognised the point of contracture and imbalance. Residual deformity of the fifth toe and increasing deformity of the fourth toe results.

Case 5

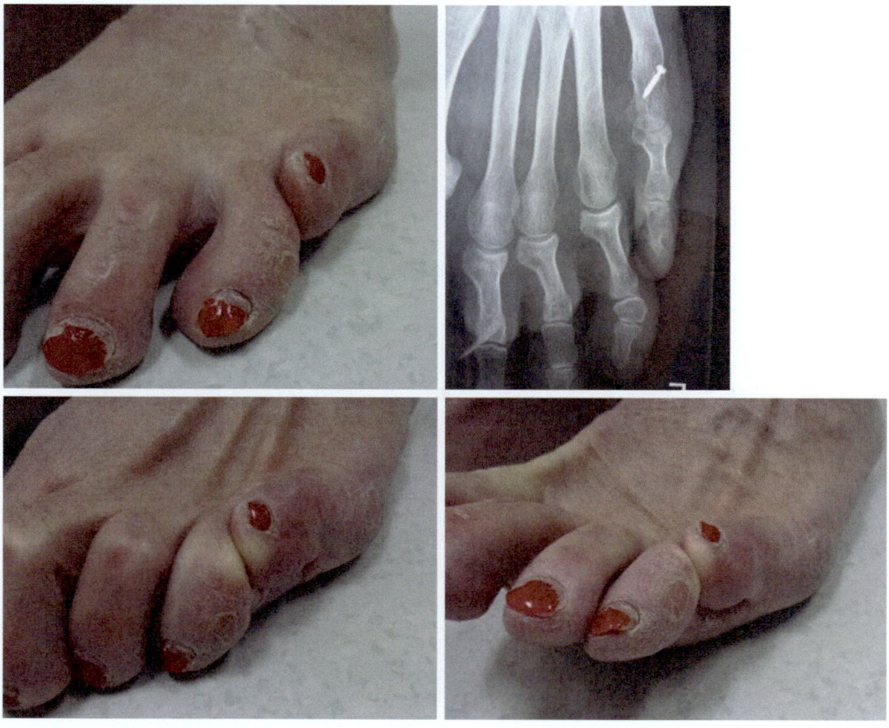

The digital balance test (chapter on tendon lengthening) is used to confirm imbalance.

When the patient actively contracts the flexors, the fifth toe remains deformed, whilst the extensor test confirms extensor overpowering. The preoperative planning in this case did not consider the plane and position of dominant soft tissue contracture. This adversely affecting outcome.

Postoperative Care

In all cases of surgical reduction for DQV, meticulous attention to postoperative splinting of the digit and all digits is required for a minimum of 8 weeks. This is sometimes achieved through the use of rigid internal fixation such as implantable pins or wires or percutaneous pins alternatively in the initial 3–6 weeks. The authors preference is to use nonallergenic tape as a splint. Such splinting will require regular changing often by an experienced clinician to reduce the possibility that correction is lost.

Taping can be followed with individually prepared prescribed splints (Fig. 22.3).

Clinical Pearls in Surgical Reduction of DQV

- Actively manage patient expectations.
- Consider using minimally invasive techniques.
- Plan to release soft tissue contracture and proceed to osseous and skin plasty techniques only if necessary.
- Lengthening of the extensor tendons can be performed via tenotomy at the level of the hood ligament (see chapter on tendon lengthening). Test to establish whether extensor or flexor lengthening is appopriate.
- Convert percutaneous incision approaches to open procedures where appropriate.
- Maintain postoperative splinting for a minimum of 2 months. This postoperative splinting can be achieved via external bandaging although many practitioners prefer to utilise percutaneous K-wire retrograded through the metatarsal head to maintain alignment for up to 6 weeks.
- If there is concurrent lateral splaying of the fifth metatarsal, this can be addressed through a small dorsal curvilinear incision and distal osteotomy to reposition the metatarsal fifth metatarsal head more medially.
- Throughout the performance of the procedure, loading of the forefoot in between surgical steps will demonstrate the level of correction obtained. Aim to have the fifth toe in a neutral position under forefoot load without the requirement of internal or external splinting.

- Postoperative splinting should be seen as a means of maintaining correction rather than creating correction.

Final Comments on Outcomes

Consistently excellent outcomes can be achieved in surgical reduction of DQV using the approaches described in the literature. Further research trials are encouraged to assist clinicians in choosing the most appropriate surgical techniques on a case-by-case basis.

Using a pragmatic approach including principles of minimally invasive surgey as outlined by the above case histories will yield consistently acceptable results.

This approach is consistent with literature reporting on the value of using percutaneous surgical techniques. Percutaneous approaches are amenable to a wide range of patients and are associated with minimal perioperative morbidity. Open techniques which involve extensive tissue dissection and percutaneous fixation could be considered as reserve procedures in situations of recalcitrance after less invasive approaches.

References

1. Murgier J, Knörr J, Soldado F, Bayle-Iniguez X, de Gauzy JS. Percutaneous correction of congenital overlapping fifth toe in paediatric patients. Orthop Traumatol Surg Res. 2013;99(6):737–40.
2. AbuHassan FO, Shannak A, McManus F. Butler's procedure for congenital varus 5th toe: evaluation with long-term follow-up. Foot. 2001;11(3):132–5.
3. AbuHassan FO, Shannak A, Stephens M. V-Y arthroplasty for congenital overriding fifth toe: a retrospective study of 34 operations between 1986 and 2000. Foot Ankle Surg. 2002;8(1):49–52.
4. Morris EW, Scullion JE, Mann TS. Varus fifth toe. J Bone Joint Surg Br. 1982;64(1):99–100.
5. Johnson CP, Hugar DW. A literature review of congenital digiti quinti varus: clinical description and treatment. J Foot Surg. 1983;22:116–20.
6. Landorf KB, Burns J. Chap. 4: Health outcomes assessment. In: Yates B, editor. Merriman's assessment of the lower limb. 3rd ed. London: Churchill Livingstone; 2012.
7. Landorf KB. In: Liamputtong P, editor. Research methods in health: foundations for evidence-based practice. South Melbourne: Oxford University Press; 2013). Clinical trials: the good, the bad and the ugly.
8. Higginson IJ, Carr AJ. Using quality of life measures in the clinical setting. BMJ. 2001;322:1297.
9. Goodwin F, Swisher F. The treatment of congenital hyperextension of the fifth toe. J Bone Joint Surg Am. 1943;25:193–6.
10. Black GB, Grogan DP, Bobechko WP. Butler arthroplasty for correction of the adducted fifth toe: a retrospective study of 36 operations between 1968 and 1982. J Pediatr Orthop. 1985;5:439–41.
11. Smith WG, Seki J, Smith RW. Prospective study of a noninvasive treatment for two common congenital toe abnormalities (curly/varus/underlapping toes and overlapping toes). Paediatr Child Health. 2007;12(9):755–9.

12. Rosner M, Knudsen HA, Sharon SM. Overlapping fifth toe: a new surgical approach. J Foot Surg. 1978;17(2):67–9.
13. López EG, Parra PT, Burgos RP, Vázquez JE. Clinical course of the quintus varus supraductus osteotomy in postoperative patients subjected to the LP-INR surgical approach. Acta Ortop Mex. 2010;24(4):235–41.
14. Cockin J. Butler's operation for an overriding fifth toe. J Bone Joint Surg Br. 1968;50-B:78.
15. Leonard MH, Rising EE. Syndactylization to maintain correction of overlapping 5th toe. Clin Orthop Relat Res. 1965;43:241–3.
16. Hulman S. Simple operation for the overlapping fifth toe. Br Med J. 1964;2:1506–7.
17. Lapidus P. Transplantation of the extensor tendon for correction of the overlapping fifth toe. J Bone Joint Surg Am. 1942;24:555–9.
18. McFarland B. In: Platt H, editor. In modern trends in orthopaedics. London: Butterworth; 1950. p. 107.
19. Wilson JN. V-Y correction for varus deformity of the fifth toe. Br J Surg. 1953;41:133–5.
20. Zanoli R, Negri L. Correzione chirurgica del quinto dito varo. Chir Org Mov. 1959;47(4):345–50.
21. Perkins G. Orthopaedics. London: Athlone Press; 1961. p. 662.
22. Weber RB. Surgical criteria for correcting the overlapping fifth toe. J Foot Surg. 1982;21:30–6.
23. Gerrand CH, Sammon DJ. Z-plasty for correction of overriding fifth toe. Foot. 1997;7(1):11–3.
24. De Boeck H. Butler's operation for congenital overriding of the fifth toe: retrospective 1–7-year study of 23 cases. Acta Orthop Scand. 1993;64(3):343–4.
25. Gollamudi S, Turnbull JT. Butler's procedure for correction of overriding fifth toe: a retrospective study. Foot Ankle Surg. 2007;13(2):67–8.
26. Talusan PG, Milewski MD, Reach JS Jr. Fifth toe deformities: overlapping and underlapping toe. Foot Ankle Spec. 2013;6:145–9.
27. Simsek T, Yosma E, Abdullayev A, Demir B, Aksakal II. Correction of overlapping fifth toe deformity with combination of Z-Plasty and transposition skin flap. Surg Curr Res. 2015;5:222.
28. Thordarson DB. Congenital crossover fifth toe correction with soft tissue release and cutaneous Z-plasty. Foot Ankle Int. 2001;22(6):511–2.
29. de Palma L, Zanoli G. Zanoli's procedure for overlapping fifth toe: retrospective study of 18 cases followed for 4–17 years. Acta Orthop Scandinavica. 1998;69:505–7.
30. Marek L, Giacopelli J, Granoff D. Syndactylization for the treatment of fifth toe deformities. J Am Podiatr Med Assoc. 1991;81:248–52.
31. Janecki CJ. Results of phalangectomy of the fifth toe for hammertoe. The Ruiz Mora procedure. JBJS. 1976;58(7):1005–7.
32. Downey M. Chap. 2: Congenital overlapping fifth toe deformity: a consolidated surgical approach. Atlanta: Podiatry Institute Update; 2002. p. 4–16.
33. Gilheany M, Baarini O, Samaras D. Minimally invasive surgery for pedal digital deformity: an audit of complications using national benchmark indicators. J Foot Ankle Res. 2015;8:17. https://doi.org/10.1186/s13047-015-0073-x.

Chapter 23
Chapter: Primary Mallet Toe Correction

Simon E. Smith and Nicholas D. Ryan

Introduction

Mallet toe describes a flexion deformity of the distal interphalangeal joint (DIPJ) of a lesser digit, with preservation of the alignment of the proximal interphalangeal joint (PIPJ) [1–4]. Mallet toe deformity can present as an isolated digital pathology [5] or in multiple digits [6, 7].

In a study investigating the risk factors for falls and balance in an elderly population, the incidence of mallet toe pathology was found in 4.3% in 255 subjects [8]. In a retrospective case series involving operative repair of mallet toe deformity, Coughlin [7] reported a ratio of 1:9 for mallet to hammer toe deformity. He observed equal frequency of occurrence of mallet toe in the second, third and fourth toes (with the longer toe affected in 73% of cases). It has been reported to affect females in up to 84% of case series [2, 7, 9–11]. This highly significant gender difference has been attributed to constrictive footwear choices in the female population [2]. Indeed, constrictive footwear has been proposed as a primary cause of the mallet toe pathology by several authors [2–4, 7, 9, 10, 12].

In addition to constrictive footwear, other factors, such as inflammatory arthropathy and motor neuropathy, have been associated with mallet toe deformity [2]. Biomechanical causes have also been reported as a primary cause of the deformity [2–4, 7, 9, 10, 12]. McGlamry et al. [3] describe mallet toe pathology occurring when the mechanical advantage of the long flexor over the intrinsic stabilizers occurs in isolation, such as in pes planovalgus foot type.

S. E. Smith (✉)
Australasian College of Podiatric Surgeons, Melbourne, VIC, Australia
e-mail: simon@smithfootsurgeon.com.au

N. D. Ryan
Footlab+, Ringwood, VIC, Australia

E. A. Cook, J. J. Cook (eds.), *Hammertoes*,
https://doi.org/10.1007/978-3-319-16552-3_23

Presentation and Diagnosis

A general history and lower-extremity physical examination is prudent before attention is drawn to the clinical evaluation of mallet toe deformity. Lower extremity neurovascular examination and assessment of neuromuscular function is prudent. Indeed, there is a higher likelihood of pressure ulceration at the apex of a digit in patients with mallet toe deformity and loss of protective sensation [2–4, 13–16]. It is imperative to assess the fit of patient shoe gear, especially with respect to appraisal of the length of the affected digit. This also has importance with consideration to the length of the affected digit following surgical correction.

Patients with mallet toe deformity will present with flexion deformity of the DIPJ of a single digit or multiple lesser digits (Fig. 23.1a). There may be a history of pain at the apex of the digit(s) secondary to weight-bearing pressure. Ulceration of the apex of the digit or hyperkeratosis with extravasation may be present, particularly in cases of loss of protective sensation. Nail deformity such as onychauxis or clubbing of the nail and subungual extravasation may also be present secondary to microtrauma (Fig. 23.1b).

Determining whether the flexion deformity is reducible helps to determine success of conservative and surgical intervention [2, 4]. Therefore, clinical evaluation must include an attempt to passively reduce the deformity. In addition to assessment of the primary mallet toe deformity, it is important to determine whether mallet toe or claw toe deformity is present in the adjacent digits. The presence of adjacent lesser digital deformities may worsen following surgical management of an isolated mallet toe deformity, particularly in cases where a long flexor tenotomy is performed, secondary to increased tension of the adjacent long digital flexor tendons (termed flexor transfer deformity).

The severity of the mallet toe pathology may be worsened upon weight-bearing examination. Indeed, in severe cases, a patient may be observed to weight bear on

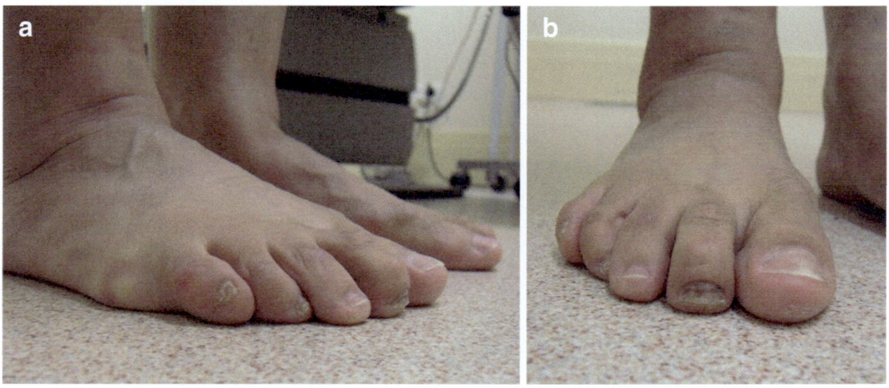

Fig. 23.1 (**a**) Clinical photo (lateral view) of mallet toe deformity affecting the second toe. Note the flexion contracture of the distal interphalangeal joint. (**b**) Clinical photo (anterior view) of onychauxis second toenail with subungual extravasation secondary to microtrauma

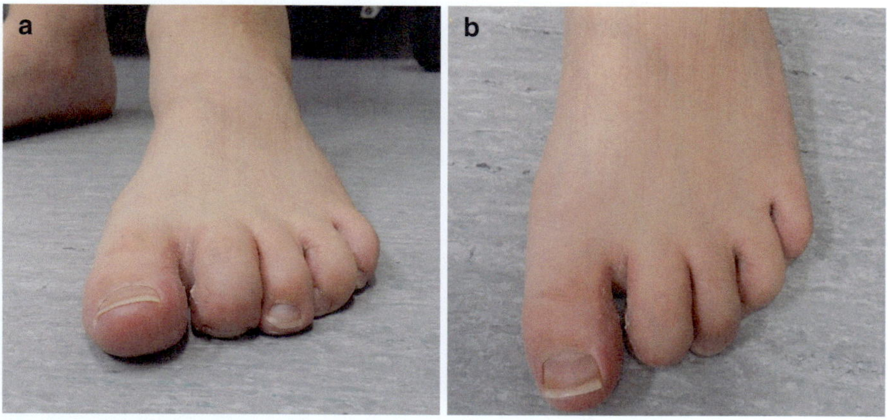

Fig. 23.2 (**a**) Clinical photo (anterior view) of severe second mallet toe deformity. Note the patient is weight-bearing on the dorsal aspect of the nail plate. (**b**) Clinical photo (superior view) of patient from Fig. 23.2a. The nail plate cannot be visualized from the superior view

the dorsal surface of the nail plate (Fig. 23.2). In addition, determination of the presence of transverse plane deformity or isolated sagittal plane deformity may become more apparent with weight-bearing examination [2, 3]. Transverse plane deformity needs to be taken into account when determining additional surgical tactics and discussing expectations following surgical management with the patient.

One should observe for pes planovalgus foot type or function in patients with mallet toe deformity. Consideration to the flexor digitorum longus providing an inversion moment at the rearfoot is important in people with pes planovalgus. In people with adult-acquired flatfoot deformity or tibialis posterior tendinopathy, flexor tenotomy to multiple digits for the management of mallet toe deformity may cause increased strain on the tibialis posterior tendon or induce worsening of the adult-acquired flatfoot deformity. Attention should also be paid to determining if patients have an unsteady gait at risk of falls or balance problems. Release of the long flexor tendon to multiple digits for the management of multiple mallet toe deformity has the potential to exacerbate existing balance problems, as a patient may lose their ability to maintain firm ground purchase with the lesser digits.

Radiographic assessment should include plain film x-rays. In cases of moderate or severe mallet toe pathology, superimposition of the distal phalanx on the middle phalanx may be observed on the AP view (Fig. 23.3). Isolated flexion contracture of the distal phalanx on the intermediate phalanx on the lateral view is also observed (Fig. 23.4) [2, 3]. Plain film x-rays are helpful to assess for any congenital morphological abnormalities of the intermediate or distal phalanx, such as a truncated phalanx, that may contribute to the presentation of abducted mallet toe deformity (Fig. 23.5). This will help with surgical planning and patient expectation following less invasive procedures, such as flexor tenotomy. Plain film x-rays are necessary in cases of persistent ulceration, to rule out osteomyelitis of the terminal phalanx versus mechanical osteolysis (Fig. 23.6a). In addition, an MRI scan may be required to aid in assessment of osteolysis versus osteomyelitis (Fig. 23.6b).

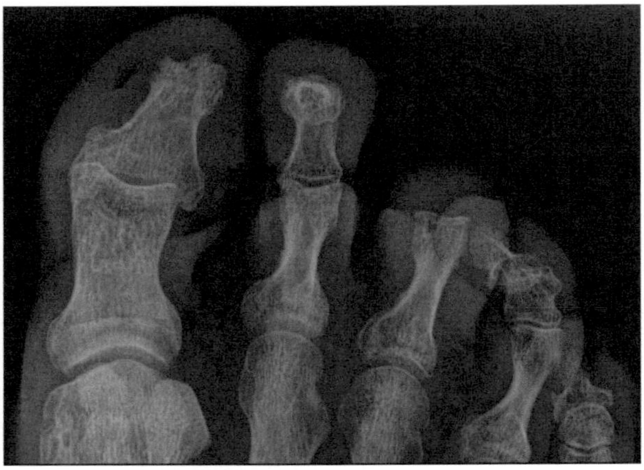

Fig. 23.3 Plain film radiograph (AP view) demonstrating superimposition of the distal phalanx on the middle phalanx of the second toe

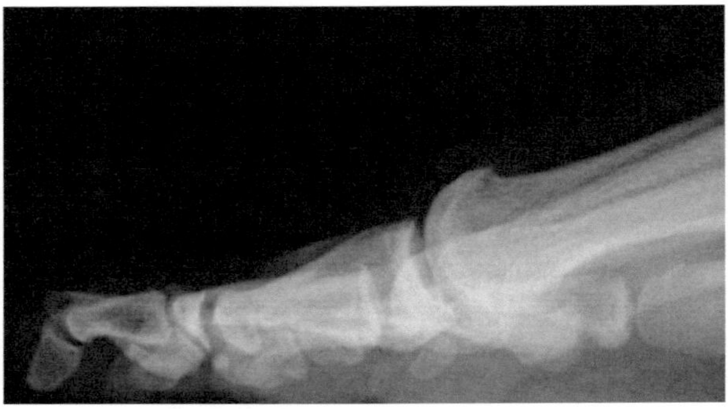

Fig. 23.4 Plain film radiograph (lateral view) demonstrating flexion of the distal phalanx on the intermediate phalanx of the second toe

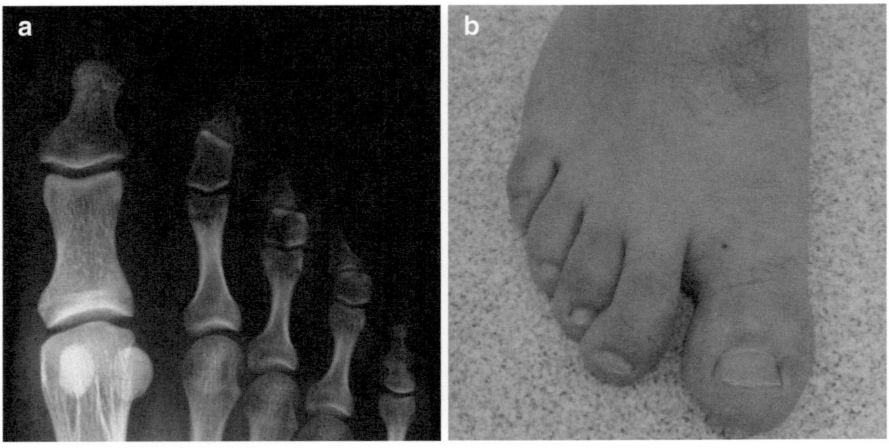

Fig. 23.5 (**a**) Plain film radiograph (AP view) demonstrating truncated intermediate phalanx contributing to abduction of the distal interphalangeal joint. (**b**) Clinical photo (superior view) demonstrating abducted mallet toe from Fig. 23.5a

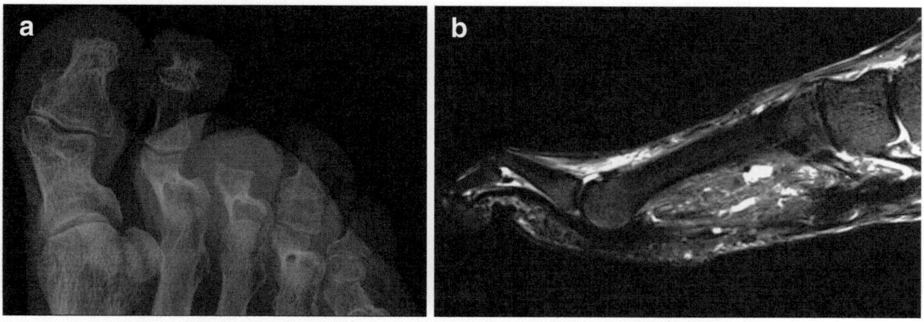

Fig. 23.6 (**a**) Plain film radiograph (oblique view) of a patient with peripheral sensory neuropathy and mallet toe deformity with persistent ulceration at the apex of the second toe. Note the erosion of the terminal aspect of the distal phalanx. This patient has previously undergone partial third toe amputation for osteomyelitis. (**b**) T2-weighted MRI of patient from Fig. 23.6a (sagittal view). There is no marrow oedema of the distal phalanx or evidence suggesting osteomyelitis. This patient was determined to have mechanical osteolysis secondary to mallet toe deformity and erosion of the distal phalanx from abutment with the weight-bearing surface

Treatment

Conservative

Management of mallet toe deformity may be treated in an escalating manner depending on symptoms and response to conservative care. Conservative management typically consists of pressure reduction strategies to offload the apex of the affected toe. This involves a combination of footwear changes to reduce crowding of the digits and splinting of the toe with felt offloading versus toe props or wedges, cushioned toe sleeves and palliative reduction of hyperkeratotic lesions [2–4, 12]

Surgical

Several different surgical techniques have been described for the management of mallet toe deformity, including percutaneous or open flexor digitorum longus tenotomy, flexor-to-extensor tendon transfer, arthroplasty versus arthrodesis of the DIPJ and distal phalangectomy versus terminal Syme amputation [2–4, 6, 7, 12–19]. While there are several retrospective studies describing the surgical management of mallet toe deformity, there are no prospective studies reporting on outcomes of surgical management for primary mallet toe deformity. Historically, procedure selection for the management of mallet toe deformity is based on whether the pathology is fixed or reducible.

Flexor Tenotomy

The percutaneous long flexor tenotomy has been described in instances when mallet toe deformity is reducible [2–4, 7, 12, 15, 16]. Several studies support the effectiveness of isolated long flexor tenotomy for the management of apical toe ulceration [13–16, 18, 19]. These studies report high patient satisfaction and demonstrate expedited healing of apical toe ulcerations. Unfortunately, these studies do not make a distinction between mallet toe deformity and claw or hammertoe deformity. Percutaneous long flexor tenotomy for correction of flexible and rigid primary mallet toe pathology is performed with a mini blade (no. 61, 64 or 67). A simplified technique for the flexor tenotomy, reported by Stapp and Camasta [20], describes the use of an 18-gauge needle. Flexor tenotomy can be performed under local anaesthesia in the office or outpatient setting. Percutaneous flexor tenotomy is the author's preference to address primary flexible mallet toe deformity. While the long flexor tenotomy is effective at reducing apical toe pressure in cases of rigid mallet toe deformity, isolated flexor tenotomy is not a predictable procedure for rigid mallet deformity *correction*. In cases where rigid mallet toe deformity correction is desirable, the flexor tenotomy is an effective adjunct procedure in combination with an osseous procedure, such as arthroplasty or arthrodesis.

Technique

A digital field block is performed to provide anaesthesia of the respective digit. The forefoot is prepped with 10% povidone-iodine solution or 0.5% tinted chlorhexidine solution. The forefoot is draped with a sterile field and shutout draping. The respective digit is held in extension or rectus position, and the patient is then asked to flex or "claw" their toe, while the surgeon provides resistance with their contralateral hand. This places the flexor apparatus under tension. If the patient is under sedation or general anaesthesia, then the tenotomy is performed while the toe and ankle are held in extension. This places the flexor apparatus under tension. The tip of the 18-gauge needle is then inserted just proximal to the distal flexor crease. Using the sharp bevelled edge of the needle, a slow and controlled sweeping motion is carried out to transect the tendon (Figs. 23.7 and 23.8). Sound release of the long flexor tendon is observed with loss of flexor power to the DIPJ. Care needs to be taken if using a mini blade no. 64 or 67, as these blades have a side cutting edge that may cause inadvertent skin laceration beyond the intended percutaneous stab incision. In cases of fixed flexion contracture of the DIPJ, the tip of the needle can also be employed to perform a capsulotomy of the joint capsule of the DIPJ. The tip of the needle is propagated deeper to contact with the inferior aspect of the DIPJ. The bevelled tip of the needle is carefully swept back and forth to transect the capsule, while the terminal phalanx is placed under extension force. Release of the capsule is noted with loss of resistance of the contracture and straightening of the terminal phalanx.

The toe is splinted in a rectus position with a half-inch Steri-Strip (Fig. 23.8d). If a beaver blade has been used, a single 5–0 nylon simple interrupted suture may be used to appose the stab incision. The percutaneous needle or stab incision site

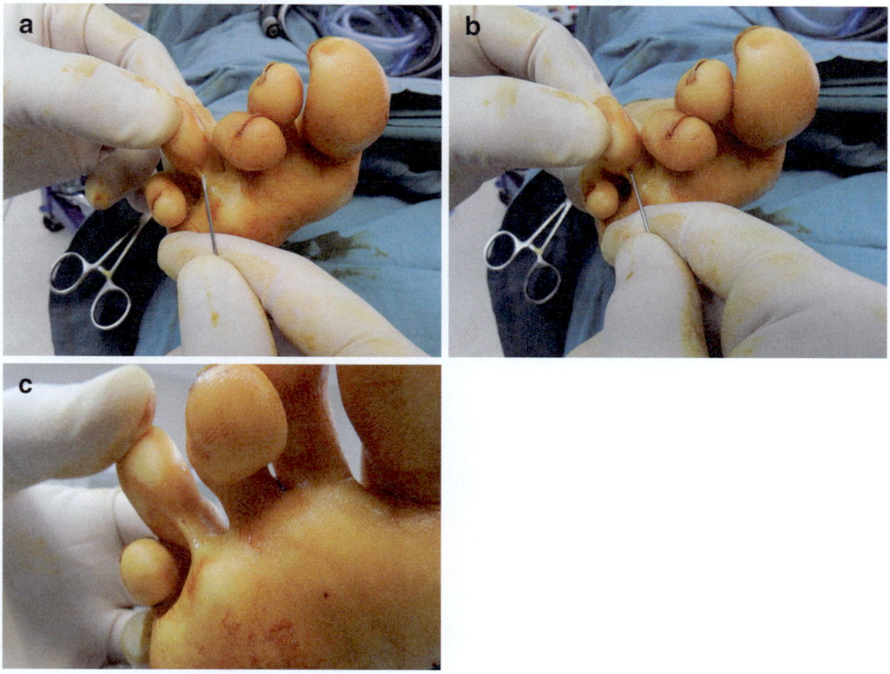

Fig. 23.7 (**a**) Percutaneous tenotomy for adductovarus mallet toe deformity affecting the right fourth digit. An 18-gauge needle is used in this instance. (**b**) The fourth digit is held in maximum extension and the no. 18-gauge needle is inserted at – or just proximal to – the distal flexor crease. The cutting tip of the needle is then carefully translated, side to side, in a transverse sweeping motion to transect the flexor digitorum longus. Loss of flexor resistance is noted following completion of flexor tenotomy. (**c**) Following removal of the 18-gauge needle. Note the small needle hole at the tenotomy site

is dressed with an antispetic solution, such as 10% povidone iodine, and sterile foam dressing. The site is kept dry and the initial dressing is maintained for 3–7 days. The patient is reviewed at this time and the percutaneous needle site inspected. The needle site will typically be healed by this time (Fig. 23.9). The correction of the digit(s) is then assessed (Figs. 23.10 and 23.11). If a suture has been used, this is removed at 10-day post procedure. Any concurrent ulceration can be dressed at the time of procedure and then managed accordingly following the first post procedure review.

In some instances, patients may experience mild discomfort and soft tissue prominence to the plantar and proximal aspect of the 2nd digit, as the long flexor retracts and can become scarified to the short flexor apparatus. Additionally, in cases where mallet toe deformity affects a long 2nd digit, 2nd metatarsophalangeal joint overload pain may be observed following long flexor tenotomy. While this is generally transient, care should be taken to ensure appropriate footwear, mechanical offloading and digital strapping in people who report pain underlying the 2nd metatarsophalangeal joint in the short- to midterm following flexor tenotomy to prevent 2nd metatarsophalangeal pre-dislocation syndrome.

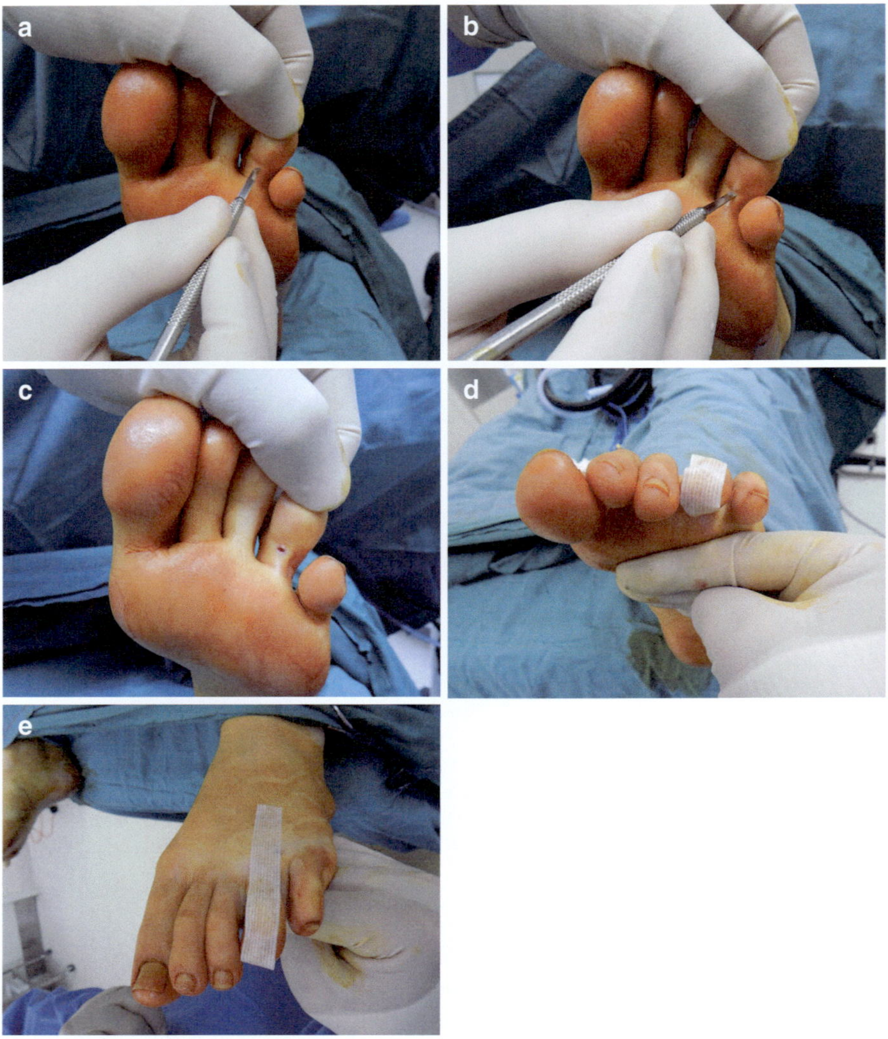

Fig. 23.8 (**a**) Percutaneous tenotomy for adductovarus mallet toe deformity affecting the left fourth digit. A no. 67 mini blade is used in this instance. (**b**) The fourth digit is held in maximum extension and the no. 67 blade is inserted via stab incision at – or just proximal to – the distal flexor crease. The blade is advanced to bone and then carefully translated in a transverse direction to transect the flexor digitorum longus. Loss of flexor resistance is noted following completion of flexor tenotomy. (**c**) Following removal of the no. 67 blade. Note a slightly larger stab incision hole at the tenotomy site. The stab incision is then flushed with saline and dressed. Alternatively, a single interrupted 5–0 nylon suture may be used to close the stab incision before dressing the toe. (**d**) The digit is then splinted with a sterile 1/2 inch Steri-Strip in a rectus position (anterior view). The percutaneous needle or stab incision is then dressed with an antiseptic solution, such as 10% povidone iodine, and sterile foam dressing (i.e., Biatain® or Allevyn®). (**e**) Superior view of foot following application of 1/4 inch Steri-Strip to splint toe

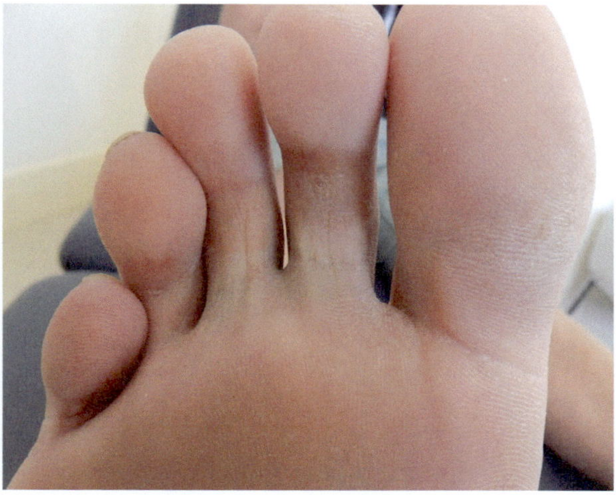

Fig. 23.9 Post-operative clinical photo of patient who underwent right second to fourth percutaneous long flexor tenotomies at 7 days. This patient underwent percutaneous long flexor tenotomy using an 18-gauge needle. Note the percutaneous needle sites (proximal to distal flexor crease) are well healed

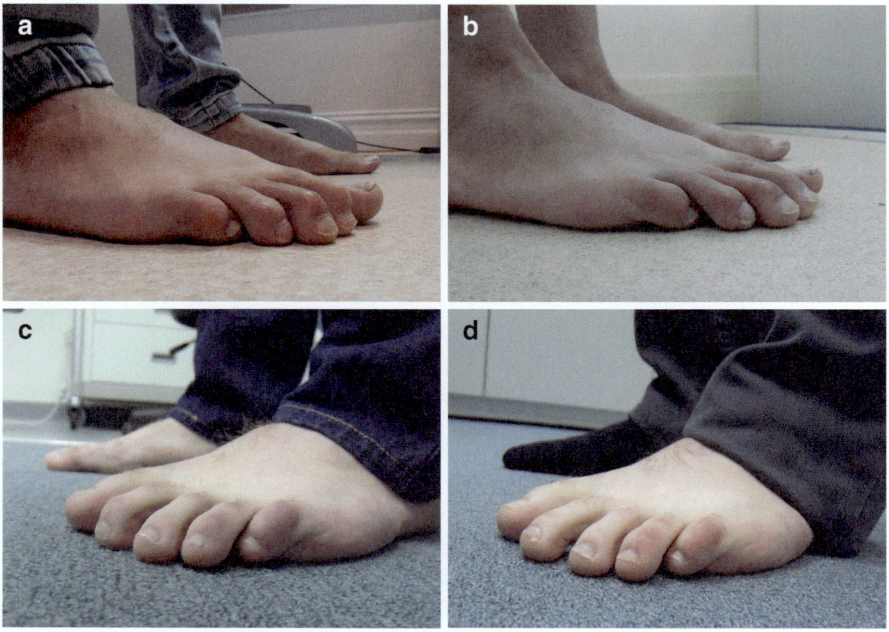

Fig. 23.10 (**a**) Preoperative clinical photo (lateral view) of patient from Fig. 23.9. Moderate mallet toe deformity affecting the right second to fourth digits is demonstrated. (**b**) Post-operative clinical photo (lateral view) of patient from Figs. 23.9 and 23.10a, 7 days following flexor tenotomy. Correction of mallet toe deformity is observed. (**c**) Preoperative clinical photo (lateral view) of moderate mallet toe deformity affecting the left second digit. (**d**) Post-operative clinical photo (lateral view) of patient from Fig. 23.10c 2 weeks following flexor tenotomy. This patient underwent percutaneous long flexor tenotomy using an 18-gauge needle

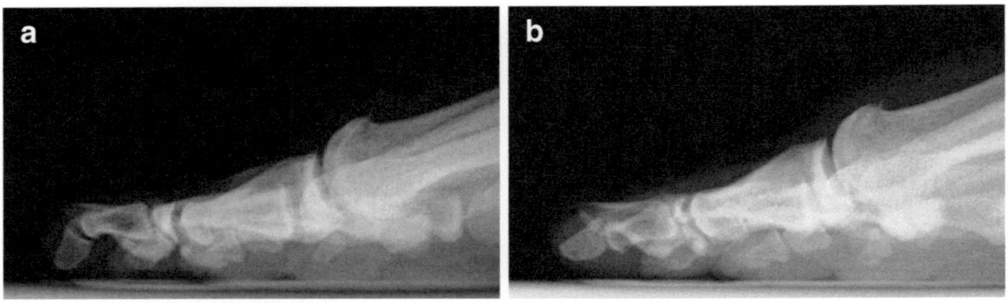

Fig. 23.11 (**a**) Preoperative plain film radiograph (lateral view) of a patient with symptomatic second mallet toe deformity. Note the flexion of the distal phalanx on the intermediate phalanx. (**b**) Post-operative radiograph (lateral view) of patient from Fig. 23.11a following long flexor percutaneous tenotomy. Not the improved position of the distal phalanx

Distal Interphalangeal Joint Arthrodesis

In circumstances where flexor tenotomy fails or in cases with morphological abnormality of the intermediate or distal phalanx, arthrodesis may be performed. In addition, in cases where mallet toe deformity affects an exceptionally long toe, shortening of the toe through DIPJ may be considered. Coughlin reported on DIPJ arthrodesis via temporary intramedullary Kirschner wire fixation in combination with flexor tenotomy [7]. Pain relief was noted in up to 97% of cases. Successful fusion was only noted in 72% of cases, and there was an 8% incidence of recurrent deformity. Arthrodesis of the DIPJ may be performed via Kirschner wire fixation, an intramedullary implant or buried screw fixation.

Joint Preparation Technique

A transverse 3–5 mm fusiform elliptical incision is made over the dorsal aspect of the respective DIPJ (Fig. 23.12). The width of the incision is made to approximate the width of the digit. The DIPJ is exposed through a "U-type" incision, releasing the collateral ligaments and transecting the long extensor. The head of the intermediate phalanx is exposed using the tip of a no. 15 scalpel blade (Fig. 23.13). Rongeurs are used to resect the cartilage and subchondral bone plate of the head of the intermediate phalanx (Fig. 23.14), and a combination of rongeur and curette is employed to resect the corresponding cartilage and subchondral bone plate of the base of the distal phalanx. A small power burr may also be used to prepare the base of the distal phalanx. One should observe for the "paprika" sign or bleeding cancellous bone (Fig. 23.15).

If a flexor tenotomy is to be performed in conjunction with the DIPJ arthrodesis, then a transverse incision is made through the plantar plate of the DIPJ using a no. 15 scalpel blade, from dorsal to plantar, and through the flexor digitorum longus

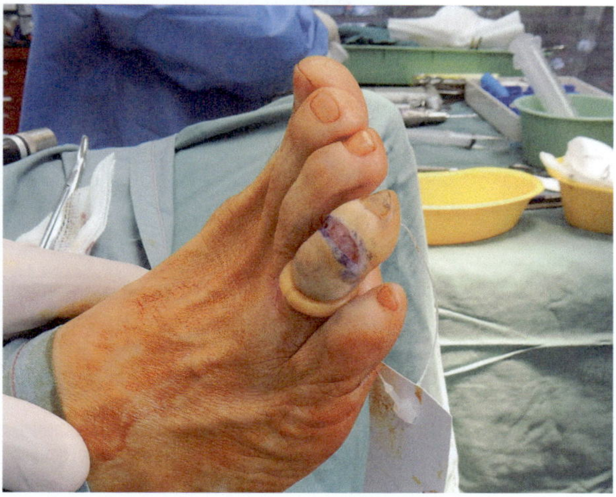

Fig. 23.12 A transverse 5 mm fusiform elliptical incision has been made over the dorsal aspect of the right fourth DIPJ

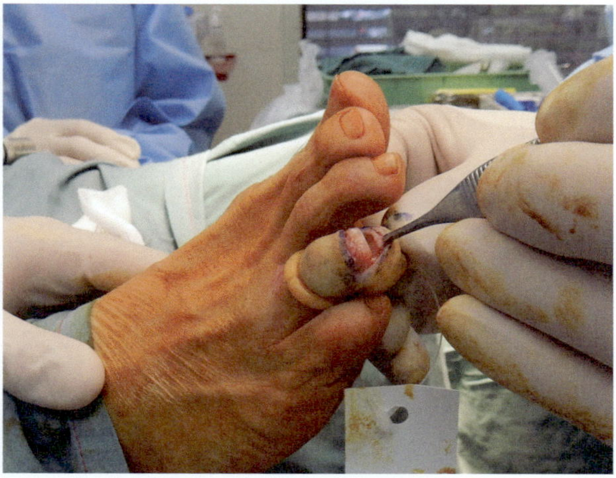

Fig. 23.13 A DIPJ capsulotomy is performed, and the head of the intermediate phalanx has been exposed

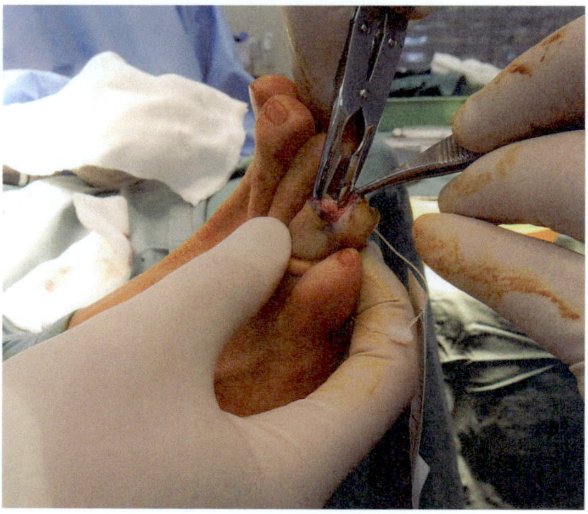

Fig. 23.14 Rongeurs are used to resect the cartilage and subchondral bone plate of the head of the intermediate phalanx

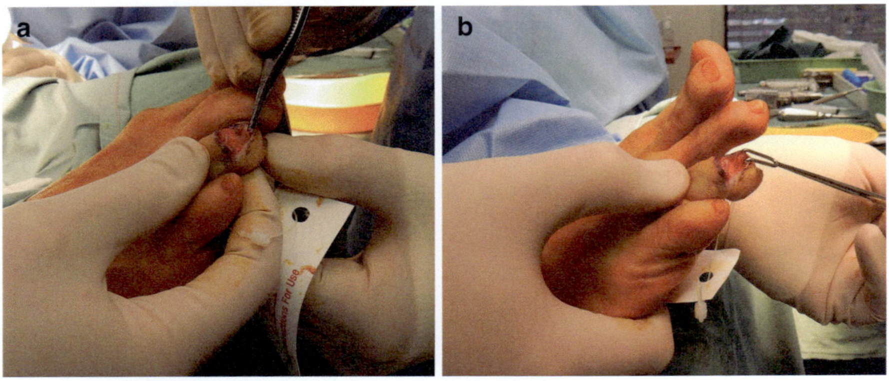

Fig. 23.15 (**a**) The cancellous bone of the head of the intermediate phalanx is observed following resection of the cartilage and subchondral bone plate. (**b**) The cancellous bone of the base of the distal phalanx is observed following resection of the cartilage and subchondral bone plate

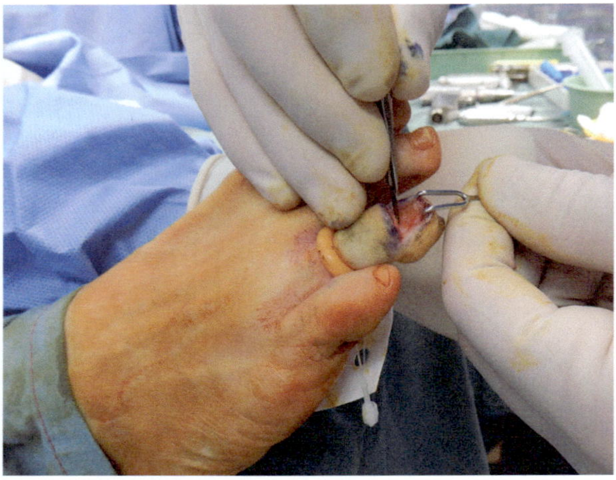

Fig. 23.16 A no. 15 blade is used to perform an intra-articular plantar DIPJ capsulotomy and then flexor tenotomy

(Fig. 23.16). In the author's experience, there is a higher non-union rate when a long flexor tenotomy is not performed. This is consistent with previous findings by Coughlin [2].The wound is flushed with copious amounts of sterile saline.

Fixation Technique: Temporary Intramedullary Kirschner Wire Fixation

When using temporary intramedullary Kirschner wire fixation, a 1.25 mm Kirschner wire is drilled through the centre of the distal phalanx, from proximal to distal, and antegraded out of the apex of the digit, approximately 2–3 mm inferior to the hyponychium of the nail plate. The DIPJ arthrodesis site is then approximated in a rectus

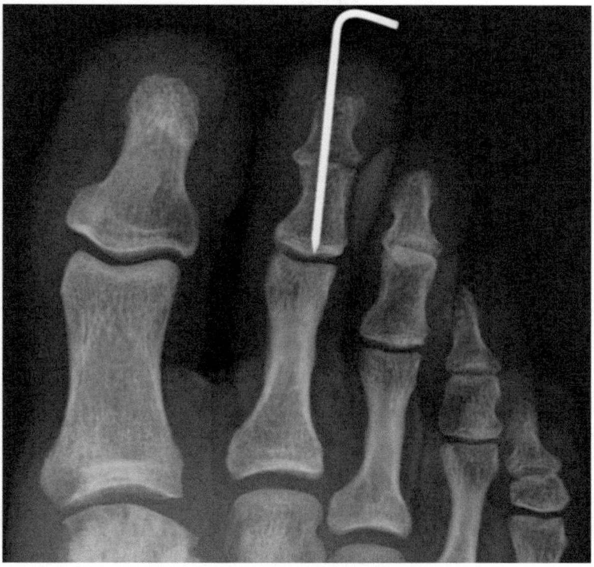

Fig. 23.17 Immediate post-operative radiograph (AP view) following arthrodesis procedure of the right second DIPJ for mallet toe deformity. A 1.25 mm Kirschner wire has been used for temporary percutaneous fixation. In this case, the Kirschner wire is embedded within the base of the intermediate phalanx. The Kirschner wire is removed at 6 weeks post-operation

position, and the joint is brought together. It is important to ensure that no soft tissue interposes between the joint surfaces. The Kirschner wire is then driven proximally through the intramedullary canal of the intermediate phalanx (Fig. 23.17). It is the author's preference to drive the wire across the proximal interphalangeal joint and seat the wire into the base of the proximal phalanx. This tends to afford more stability to the arthrodesis site by preventing flexion at the proximal interphalangeal joint and prevent migration of the wire out of the toe during the post-operative course.

Fixation Technique: Intramedullary Implant

An alternative to percutaneous Kirschner wire fixation is via an intramedullary implant that maintains stability of the DIPJ arthrodesis site with the benefit of no percutaneous Kirschner wire fixation or the potential complications associated with this, such as contiguous infection and trauma to the wire.

The author's preference is to use the Stryker Smart Toe® II DIPJ Intramedullary Implant. The implant is made of a body temperature activated alloy of nickel and titanium. When considering using a Smart Toe® implant, ot is important to ensure that there is a freezer within the surgical facility. The implant is required to be stored in a freezer, under 0 °C (32 °F) for a minimum of 2 h before implantation into a patient. The Smart Toe® is designed to recover its original shape, via expansion of the implant arms, progressively after implantation. Specific hand instrumentation is required for utilization of the Smart Toe® implant. The implant is available in sizes 11 mm and 13 mm. The surgeon needs to determine the size of the implant based on the patient morphology.

Following joint preparation, a 1.25 mm Kirschner wire is employed to drill a pilot hole in the intermediate and distal phalanx. A stop drill is then used to create a guide hole in the respective phalanges (Fig. 23.18). The drill is antegraded into the intermediate phalanx until the stop contacts the intermediate phalanx. The drill is then antegraded into the distal phalanx (Fig. 23.19). In cases with small or short phalanges, the surgeon can cease drilling prior to the stop engaging the base of the distal phalanx. Care must be taken to ensure that the trajectory of the pilot and guide holes is rectus or straight. Following this, a middle phalanx broach is employed to create a rectangular trough in the intermediate phalanx in preparation to receive the Smart Toe® implant. The broach is pushed into the intermediate phalangeal guide hole up to the laser mark on the broach (Fig. 23.20). The Smart Toe® implant is then removed from the freezer.

Implant forceps are used to remove the implant from its support package. The forceps are used to grip the implant at its triangular base. At this point, it is impor-

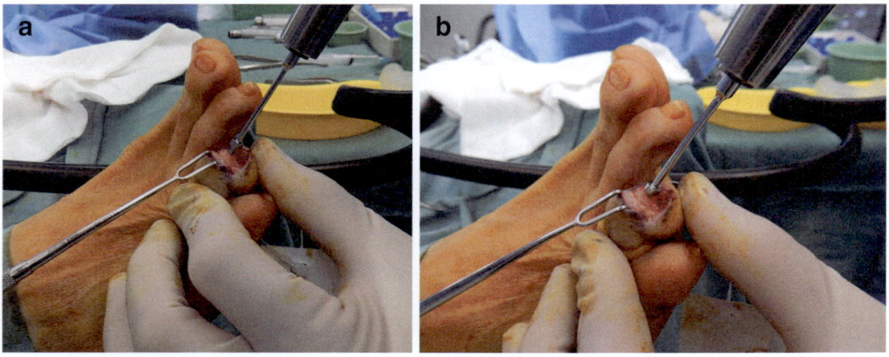

Fig. 23.18 (**a**) A Smart Toe® stop drill is used to create a guide hole in the intermediate phalanx. (**b**) The stop drill is antegraded until the stop contacts the intermediate phalanx

Fig. 23.19 The stop drill is antegraded into the distal phalanx

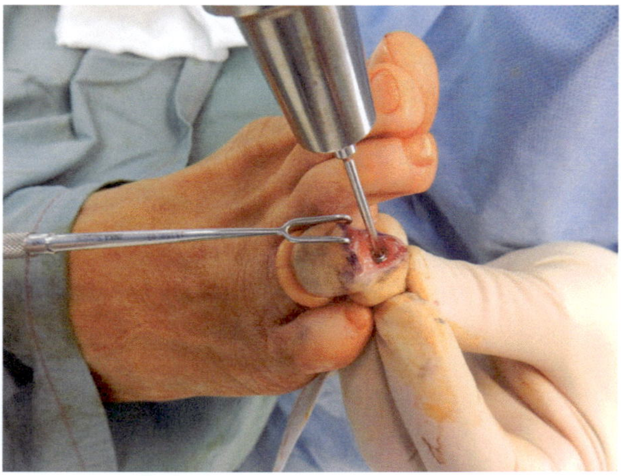

tant to ensure the correct orientation of the Smart Toe® for implantation (Fig. 23.21). The distal portion of the implant is inserted into the guide hole of the distal phalanx (Fig. 23.22). The forceps are maintained on the implant as the distal portion of the toe, and the implant is then carefully manipulated to deliver the proximal portion of the implant partially into the broach hole of the intermediate phalanx. The forceps are then removed, and the DIPJ arthrodesis site is manually compressed for 1–2 min (Fig. 23.23). During this time the arms of the implant diverge or expand to "bite" into the phalanges and maintain stability of the arthrodesis site. Bathing the site with warm saline can facilitate this process. Intraoperative imaging may be used to ensure adequate apposition of the arthrodesis site.

Following completion of the procedure, the extensor apparatus is apposed with 4–0 Vicryl simple interrupted sutures and the skin apposed with 5–0 simple interrupted nylon sutures (Fig. 23.24). The wound is dressed with an antiseptic

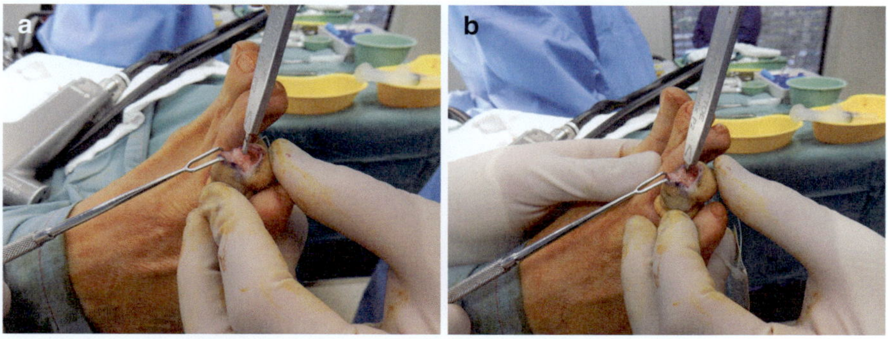

Fig. 23.20 (**a**) The Smart Toe® broach is used to create a rectangular receiving hole in the intermediate phalanx. (**b**) The broach is pushed into the intermediate phalangeal guide hole up to the laser mark on the broach

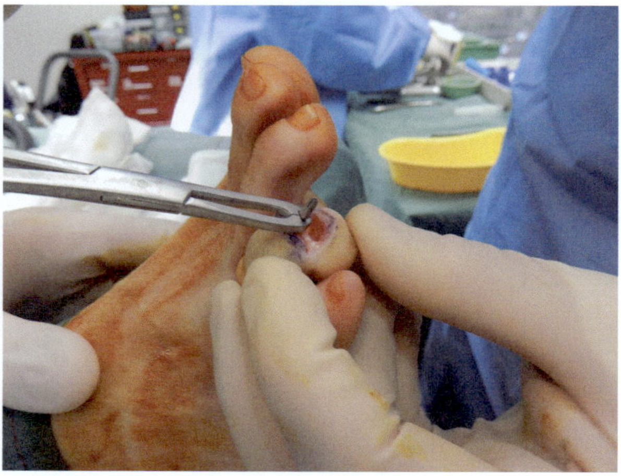

Fig. 23.21 Smart Toe® forceps are used to grip the implant at its triangular base. It is important to ensure the correct orientation of the implant

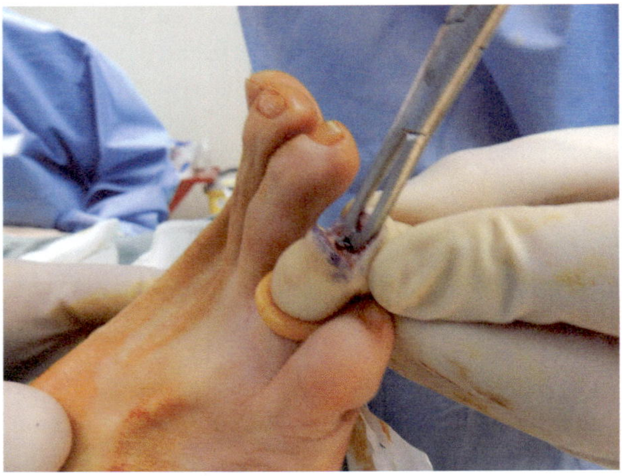

Fig. 23.22 The distal portion of the implant is inserted into the guide hole of the distal phalanx

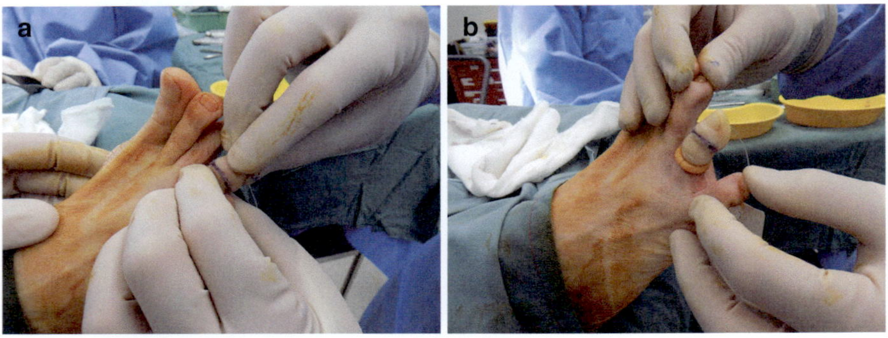

Fig. 23.23 (**a**) The DIPJ arthrodesis site is manually compressed for 1–2 min. (**b**) The DIPJ maintains its corrected position

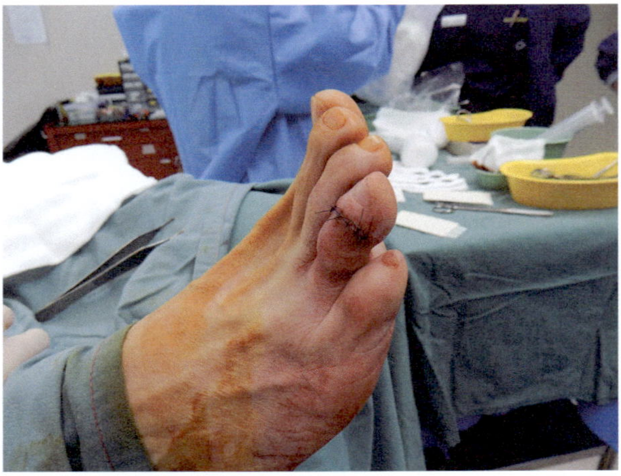

Fig. 23.24 The skin apposed with 5–0 simple interrupted nylon sutures

solution, such as 10% povidone-iodine solution or chlorhexidine impregnated paraffin gauze. In cases of intramedullary implant fixation, several Steri-Strips are employed to help splint the toe in a corrected position (Fig. 23.8d, e). The wound is dressed with saline-soaked gauze, sterile dry gauze and a Jones compression bandage to the ankle. In cases where percutaneous Kirschner wire fixation has been employed, betadine ointment may be applied to the percutaneous wire site, and a malleable metal splint is applied to protect the percutaneous wire. In these cases, additional padding is often required under the metatarsal head level to ensure the wire and metal splint do not contact the post-operative shoe during ambulation. The dressing is changed at 7 days post-surgery, and an x-ray is taken at this time (Fig. 23.25). Stiches are removed at 14–21 days post-surgery.

For intramedullary implant fixation, the patient is instructed to wear the post-operative shoe for 6 weeks, including in bed to reduce the risk of complication during sleep. For percutaneous wire fixation, the foot is required to be dressed for 6 weeks, and it is the author's preference to remove the percutaneous wire 6 weeks post-surgery.

An alternative method of fixation for DIPJ arthrodesis is via screw fixation. Small calibre headless compression screws enable them to be buried within the distal phalanx and provide compression and stability across the arthrodesis site (Fig. 23.26). While non-union following DIPJ arthrodesis has been reported as high as 28%, it is the author's experience that these generally progress to a painless fibrous non-union (Fig. 23.27) or malunion in the mid-long term (Fig. 23.28). However, Coughlin noted a lower patient satisfaction rate (75%) with fibrous non-union versus a higher satisfaction rate in patients with successful arthrodesis (89%) [7].

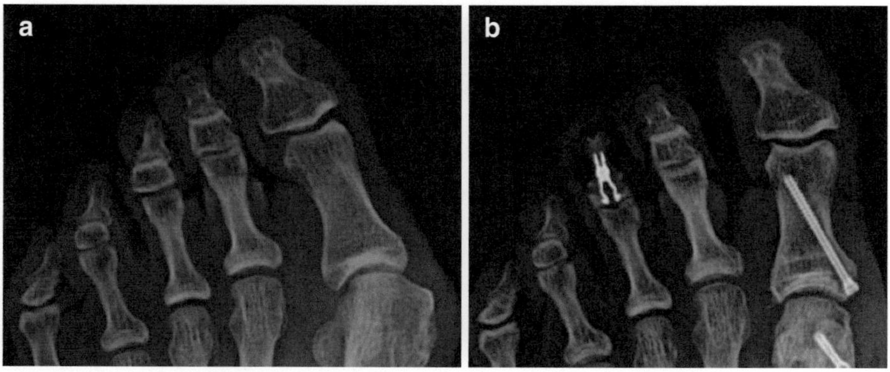

Fig. 23.25 (**a**) Preoperative radiograph (AP) of patient with symptomatic left third mallet toe deformity. (Image courtesy of Thomas S. Roukis PhD, DPM). (**b**) Post-operative radiograph (AP) of patient from Fig. 23.25a. (Image courtesy of Thomas S. Roukis PhD, DPM)

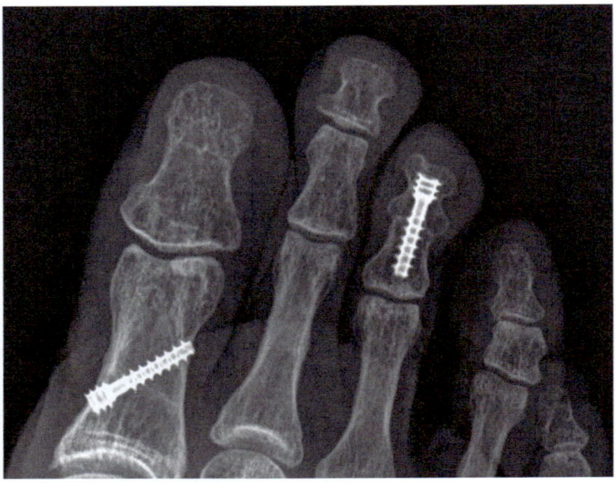

Fig. 23.26 Post-operative radiograph (AP) of a buried headless compression screw employed to fixate a distal interphalangeal arthrodesis site

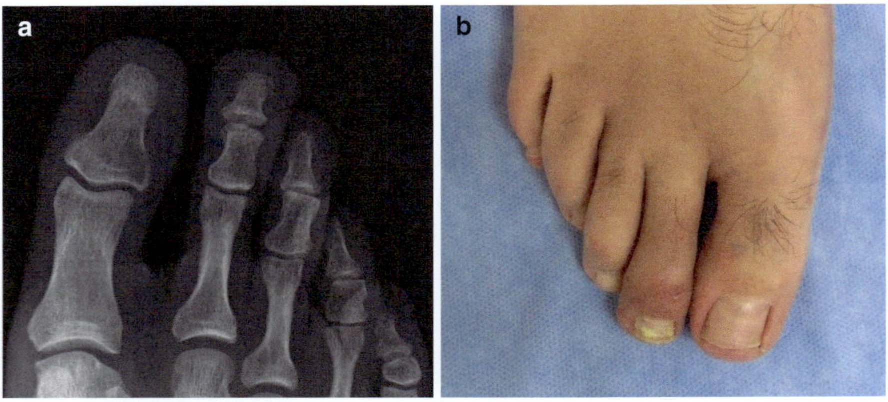

Fig. 23.27 (**a**) Plain film radiograph (AP view) of patient who underwent distal interphalangeal arthrodesis procedure with percutaneous Kirschner wire fixation for symptomatic second mallet toe deformity at 3 months post-surgery. The patient developed a painless fibrous non-union. Correction of deformity was maintained. (**b**) Clinical photo (superior view) of patient from Fig. 23.27a. Mild erythema is noted at the non-union site at 3 months post-operation

Terminal Syme Versus Distal Phalangectomy

While the terminal Syme has been described for the management of mallet toe deformity, the author's preference is for distal phalangectomy [4, 6, 12]. Up to 97% patient satisfaction has been reported following terminal Syme. Raja et al. [6] describe terminal Syme technique is often suited to an older, sedentary population where onychodystrophy, such as onychauxis or onychogryphosis, is present. Both terminal Syme and distal phalangectomy shorten the affected toe, and this must be taken into consideration when discussing cosmetic expectations with a patient prior

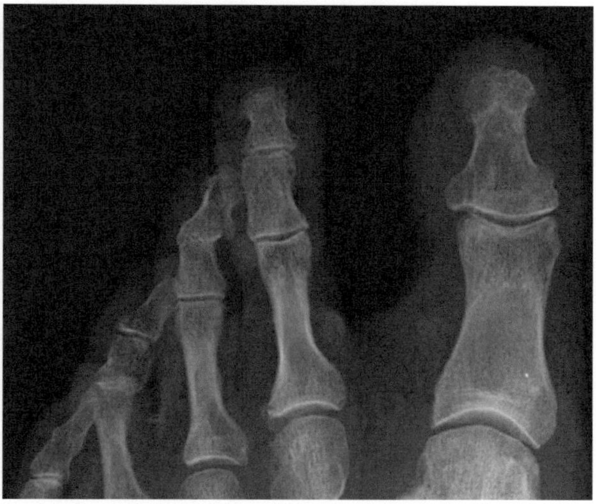

Fig. 23.28 Plain film radiograph (AP view) of a patient that developed a mal-union of a right third distal interphalangeal joint arthrodesis site. In this instance, a flexor tenotomy was not performed. Following removal of percutaneous Kirschner wire, the long flexor tendon caused movement of the distal phalanx and recurrence of adductovarus mallet toe deformity

to surgery. It is the author's preference to perform this procedure (with or without partial resection of the intermediate phalanx) in cases involving ulceration to the apex of the toe with associated osteomyelitis affecting the distal phalanx.

Technique

For distal phalangectomy a dorsal transverse incision is made overlying the DIPJ (Fig. 23.29). The medial and lateral borders of the dorsal incision are tapered proximally, to avoid dog ears upon closure. A fishmouth incision is then performed at the apex of the toe, slightly inferior to the midline of the apex of the toe. The incisions are carried to bone using a no. 15 scalpel blade. The inferior surface of the distal phalanx is then carefully dissected from the plantar fat pad of the toe (Fig. 23.30). The DIPJ is exposed through a "U-type" incision, releasing the collateral ligaments, transecting the long extensor, plantar plate and long flexor tendon. The distal phalanx and apex of the toe is then excised in toto (Figs. 23.31 and 23.32). At this point the cartilage of the head of the intermediate phalanx may be resected with a rongeur. The wound is flushed with copious amounts of sterile saline. An attempt is then made to advance the DIPJ plantar pate/inferior joint capsule to the extensor apparatus dorsally. This is apposed with 4–0 Vicryl simple interrupted sutures. The skin is closed with 5–0 simple interrupted nylon sutures (Fig. 23.33).

The toe is dressed with 10% povidone-iodine to the incision site. The wound is dressed with chlorhexidine-impregnated paraffin gauze, saline-soaked gauze, sterile dry gauze and Jones compression bandage to the ankle. The dressing is changed at 7 days post-surgery, and the stitches are removed at 21 days post-surgery (Fig. 23.34).

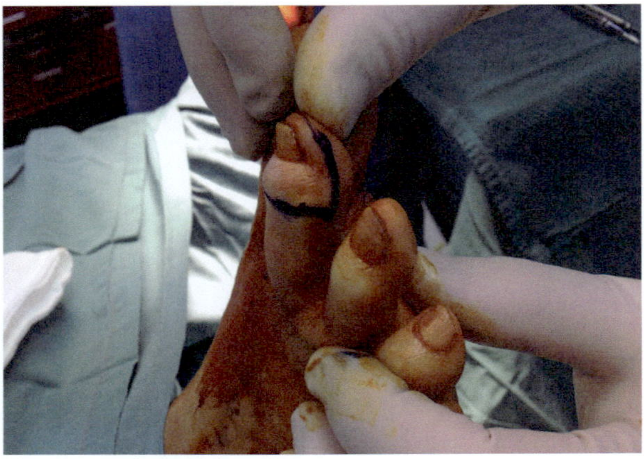

Fig. 23.29 The incision to perform a disarticulation amputation through the distal interphalangeal joint is drawn preoperatively. Care is taken to ensure the plantar flap is adequate to provide closure without tension

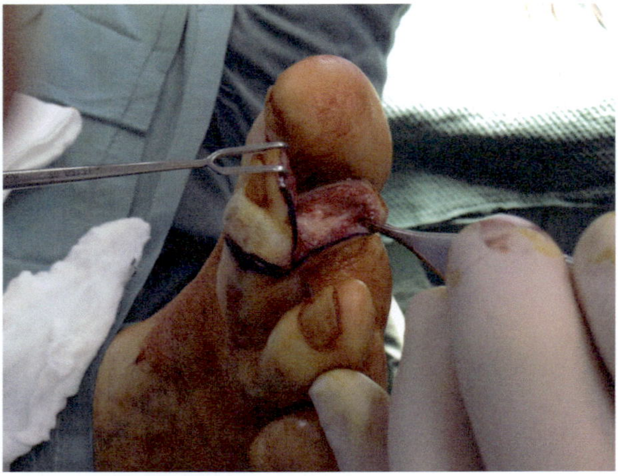

Fig. 23.30 Following performance of the dorsal incision (to bone), care is taken to reflect the plantar flap from the distal and inferior aspect of the distal phalanx

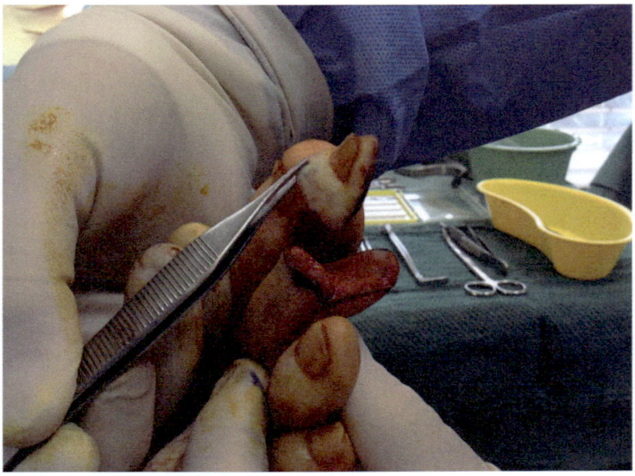

Fig. 23.31 The distal phalanx and apex of the toe is then excised in toto following disarticulation of the distal phalanx from the intermediate phalanx at the distal interphalangeal joint

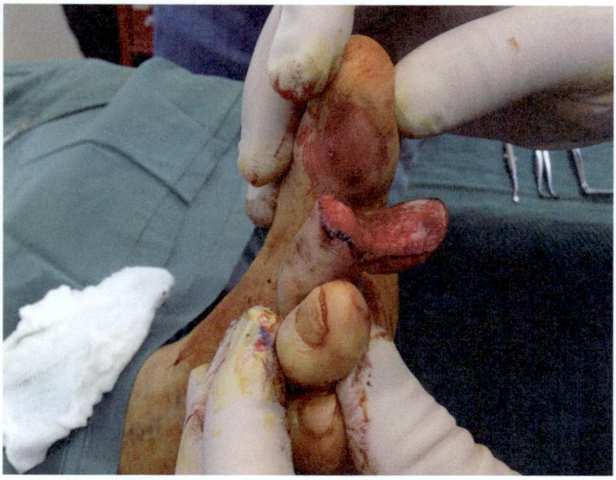

Fig. 23.32 A robust plantar flap is created to close over the residuum of the second digit

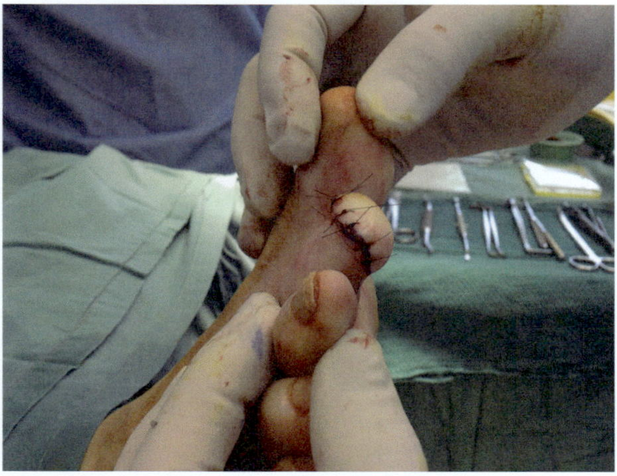

Fig. 23.33 The plantar skin flap is brought superiorly to appose the proximal dorsal skin margin with simple interrupted 5–0 nylon sutures

Distal Interphalangeal Joint Arthroplasty

The DIPJ arthroplasty has been reported as a common procedure for the management of mallet toe deformity [10]. However, this procedure can result in post-operative instability of the DIPJ and allow for iatrogenic transverse plane deviation of the distal phalanx and patient dissatisfaction associated with this. This commonly occurs in cases of adjacent transverse plane toe deformity, such as hallux valgus deformity, whereupon abutment of the hallux can cause lateralisation of a 2nd DIPJ arthroplasty site; or secondary to pressure from shoes with a narrow toe box, causing medialisation of a 3rd or 4th DIPJ arthroplasty site. Arthroplasty of the DIPJ involves resection of the head, or distal articular surface, of the intermediate phalanx [10]. The approach to this procedure is performed in a similar manner as for arthrodesis of the DIPJ (Figs. 23.12, 23.13 and 23.14), without resection of the cartilage and subchondral bone plate of the distal

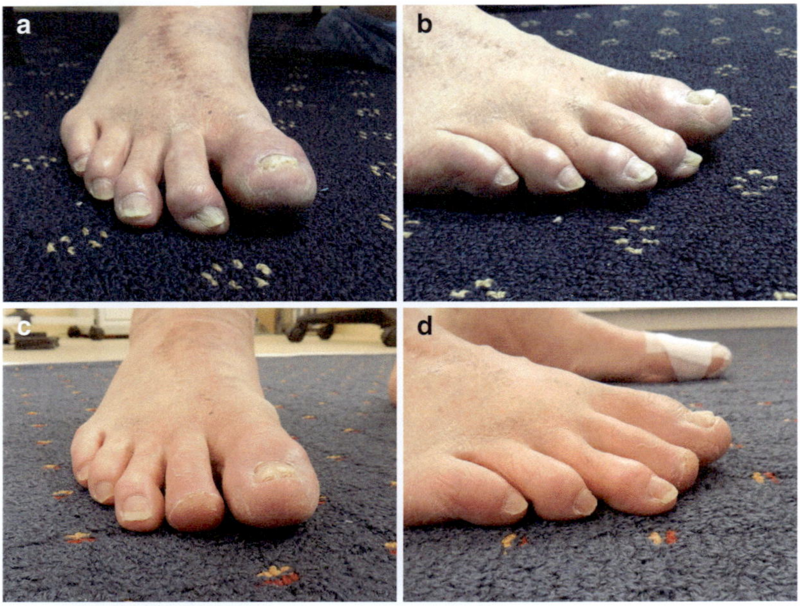

Fig. 23.34 (**a**) Preoperative clinical photo (anterior view) of patient with rigid second mallet toe deformity (with adduction and varus rotation of the distal phalanx). (**b**) Preoperative clinical photo (lateral view) of patient from Fig. 23.34a. (**c**) Post-operative clinical photo at 6 weeks post-operation (anterior view). A distal phalangectomy has been performed. The incision line is well healed. (**d**) Post-operative clinical photo of patient from Fig. 23.34c (lateral view)

Clinical Pearls

- The percutaneous long flexor tenotomy is a simple and effective procedure to address flexible mallet toe deformity and can be performed in the outpatient setting. The flexor tenotomy has excellent utility in the management of apical toe ulceration in high-risk patients, in the presence of flexible or rigid mallet toe deformity.
- Global long flexor tenotomy has the potential to worsen foot posture or symptoms in tibialis posterior tendon dysfunction or increase falls and balance issues. Thorough clinical assessment and patient education are paramount to help manage patient expectation associated with mallet toe correction.
- A long flexor tenotomy performed in conjunction with DIPJ arthrodesis increases the success rate of osseous union of the arthrodesis site.
- Flexor tenotomy performed in conjunction with DIPJ arthrodesis also reduces the risks of malposition in cases of delayed or non-union.
- When using a percutaneous Kirschner wire to stabilize DIPJ arthrodesis, enhanced stability of is attained when the wire crosses the proximal interphalangeal joint and is seated in the base of the proximal phalanx (rather than the intermediate phalanx).
- While non-union of DIPJ arthrodesis has been associated with lower patient satisfaction rates, the authors find that these generally go on to painless fibrous unions in the midterm, without the need for revision surgery.

phalanx. Although not necessary, percutaneous Kirschner wire fixation may be employed for added stability of the arthroplasty site, which is then removed at 4-weeks post-surgery. A flexor tenotomy can be performed in conjunction with this procedure, and this has been recommended in cases with flexion contracture of greater than 45° [10]. Concomitant flexor tenotomy can also reduce the risk of recurrent flexor contracture or mallet toe deformity at the arthroplasty site.

References

1. Barakat MJ, Buckingham R, Gargan MF. Curly toe, hammer toe, claw toe and mallet toe: are they good descriptive terms of the associated deformities of the lesser toes? Eur J Orthop Surg Traumatol. 2005;15:226–8.
2. Coughlin MJ. Lesser toe deformities. In: Coughlin MJ, Mann RA, Saltzmann CL, editors. Surgery of the foot and ankle. Volume 1. 8th ed. Philadelphia: Mosby; 2007. p. 363–464.
3. McGlamry E, Jimenez A, Green D. Lesser ray deformities. In: Banks A, Downey M, Martin D, Miller S, editors. McGlamry's comprehensive textbook of foot and ankle surgery. Volume 1. 3rd ed. Philadelphia: Lippincott Williams & Wilkins; 2001. p. 253–304.
4. Murphy G. Mallet toe deformity. Foot Ankle Clin. 1998;3:279–92.
5. Brahms M. The small toes. In: Jahss M, editor. Disorders of the foot and ankle. Philadelphia: WB Saunders; 1991. p. 1187.
6. Raja S, Barrie JL, Henderson AA. Distal phalangectomy for mallet toe. Foot Ankle Surg. 2003;9:215–6.
7. Coughlin MJ. Operative repair of the mallet toe deformity. Foot Ankle Int. 1995;16:109–16.
8. Turhanoglu AD, Guler H, Kalici A, Inanoglu D, Ozer C. Can foot pain and musculoskeletal disorders be counted as risk factors for falls in the elderly? Turk Geriatri Dergisi. 2010;13:225–30.
9. Coughlin MJ. Lesser toe abnormalities. J Bone Joint Surg (Am Vol). 2002;84:1446–69.
10. Coughlin MJ. Common causes of pain in the forefoot in adults. J Bone Joint Surg Br. 2000;82:781–90.
11. Coughlin MJ. Second metatarsophalangeal joint instability in the athlete. Foot Ankle Int. 1993;14:309–19.
12. Shirzad K, Kiesau CD, DeOrio JK, Parekh SG. Lesser toe deformities. J Am Acad Orthop Surg. 2011;19:505–14.
13. Kearney TP, Hunt NA, Lavery LA. Safety and effectiveness of flexor tenotomies to heal toe ulcers in persons with diabetes. Diabetes Res Clin Pract. 2010;89:224–6.
14. Laborde JM. Neuropathic toe ulcers treated with toe flexor tenotomies. Foot Ankle Int. 2007;28:1160–4.
15. Rasmussen A, Bjerre-Christensen U, Almdal TP, Holstein P. Percutaneous flexor tenotomy for preventing and treating toe ulcers in people with diabetes mellitus. J Tissue Viability. 2013;22:68–73.
16. Roukis TS, Schade VL. Percutaneous flexor Tenotomy for treatment of neuropathic toe ulceration secondary to toe contracture in persons with diabetes: a systematic review. J Foot Ankle Surg. 2009;48:684–9.
17. Good J, Fiala K. Digital surgery: current trends and techniques. Clin Podiatr Med Surg. 2010;27:583–99.
18. Kearney TP, Hunt NA, Lavery LA. Safety and effectiveness of flexor tenotomies to heal toe ulcers in persons with diabetes. Diabetes Res Clin Pract. 2010;89:224–6.
19. Tamir E, McLaren AM, Gadgil A, Daniels TR. Outpatient percutaneous flexor tenotomies for management of diabetic claw toe deformities with ulcers: a preliminary report. Can J Surg. 2008;51:41–4.
20. Stapp M, Camasta C. Flexor tenotomy: a simplified technique. In: The podiatry institute update. Dekalb: The Podiatry Institute; 2008. p. 1–3.

Chapter 24
Hammertoe Correction in the Neuropathic Patient

Barry Rosenblum and Christopher P. Tveter

Hammertoe deformities in the presence of sensory neuropathy have the potential to cause increased skin irritation and ulcer formation. If not diagnosed and treated properly, this can become complicated by infection, need for antibiotics, inpatient admission, and/or amputation. Goals of surgery in these types of patients are to reduce bony prominences at risk for ulceration, restore alignment and stability to the digit, and allow for functional ambulation [1–3].

Diagnosis/Assessment

A thorough history and physical examination are essential in determining the etiology of hammertoe deformity and underlying neuropathy. Reviewing the patient's comorbidities, medications, activity level, and history of digital deformity will aid in diagnosis and eventual treatment plan. In addition, collaboration with the primary care physician or other specialists may be required prior to surgery if the patient's medical history warrants further workup.

Clinical assessment of digital deformities will largely dictate what surgical options are available. Evaluation of the patient's vascular status is imperative prior to any surgical procedure. Absence of a palpable pulse should prompt further work up in the form of noninvasive vascular studies and consultation with vascular surgery. Neuropathy can manifest as a sensory, motor, autonomic, or combination of all three. They may predispose the patient to skin breakdown, callus formation, and ulcer formation. The locations of these lesions vary depending on the type of digital deformity but are most frequently seen at the distal aspect of the toe or dorsally at

B. Rosenblum · C. P. Tveter (✉)
Beth Israel Deaconess Medical Center, Division of Podiatry, Department of Surgery, Harvard Medical School, Boston, MA, USA
e-mail: brosenbl@bidmc.harvard.edu; ctveter@bidmc.harvard.edu

E. A. Cook, J. J. Cook (eds.), *Hammertoes*,
https://doi.org/10.1007/978-3-319-16552-3_24

the level of the proximal or distal IPJ (Fig. 24.1a). It is important to determine whether the hammertoe deformity is reducible or rigid in nature, as it will establish the need for soft tissue or bony correction (Fig. 24.1b). The Kelikian push-up test can aid in this and determine whether surgical work is required at the MTPJ level or more proximally. Flexible deformities on the other hand can be treated by a combination of soft tissue releases and/or bony work. Rigid deformities cannot be corrected with tendon or capsule release and typically require joint destructive procedures in the form of an arthroplasty or arthrodesis [4, 6]. If an ulcer is present, it is important to note the depth of tissue involvement and the presence of infection (Fig. 24.2a). Fissures may also be seen on the plantar sulci of the toe (Fig. 24.2b).

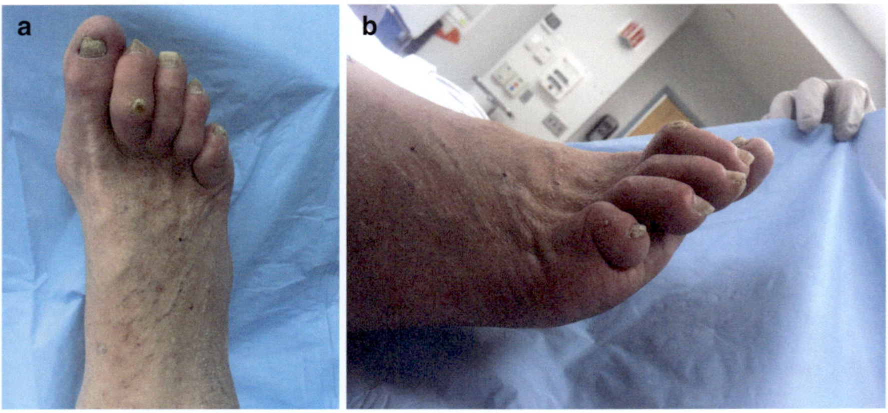

Fig. 24.1 (**a**) Chronic lesion overlying dorsum of the second digit PIPJ, (**b**) Note MTPJ contractures of all lesser digits

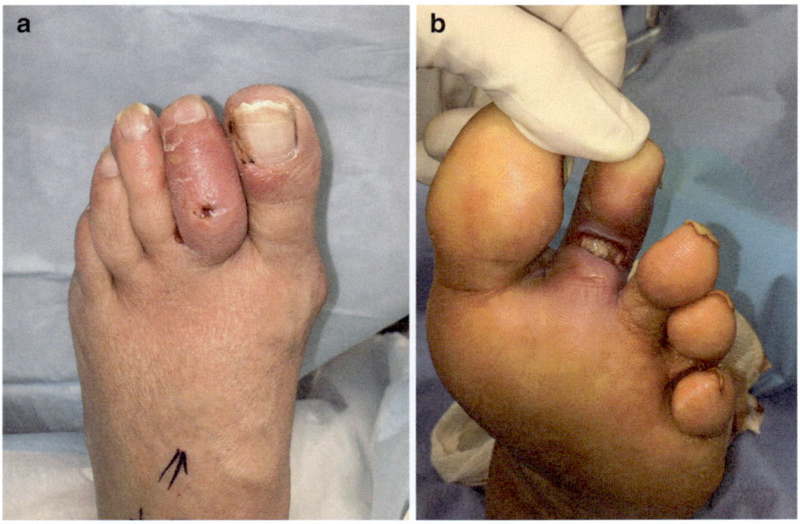

Fig. 24.2 (**a**) Second digit PIPJ ulceration that probes to bone with associated cellulitis. (**b**) Plantar sulcus ulceration at the level of the PIPJ

Treatment/Surgical Technique

Percutaneous Tenotomy of the Flexor Hallucis Longus Tendon

Indications Flexion contracture noted to the distal interphalangeal joint that is reducible in nature. Patients may also present with a hyperkeratotic lesion or ulceration to the distal aspect of the digit. Release of the FHL tendon will prevent excessive plantarflexion at the DIPJ and decrease pressure to this area [5].

Surgical Technique A #15 blade can be utilized to make a stab incision on either the medial or lateral aspect of the distal interphalangeal joint. Care should be taken to avoid lacerating neurovascular structures as they course to the distal aspect of the digit. Holding the distal interphalangeal joint in extension will increase tension across the FHL tendon and allow for easier transection. This can also be performed with use of the beveled edge of an 18 gauge needle, minimizing the need for suture closure. Once performed, the digit should be maintained in a corrected position with use of a Betadine splint or taping technique. If an ulcer is present, this may be excised and closed primarily or left to heal by secondary intention (Figs. 24.3a–f).

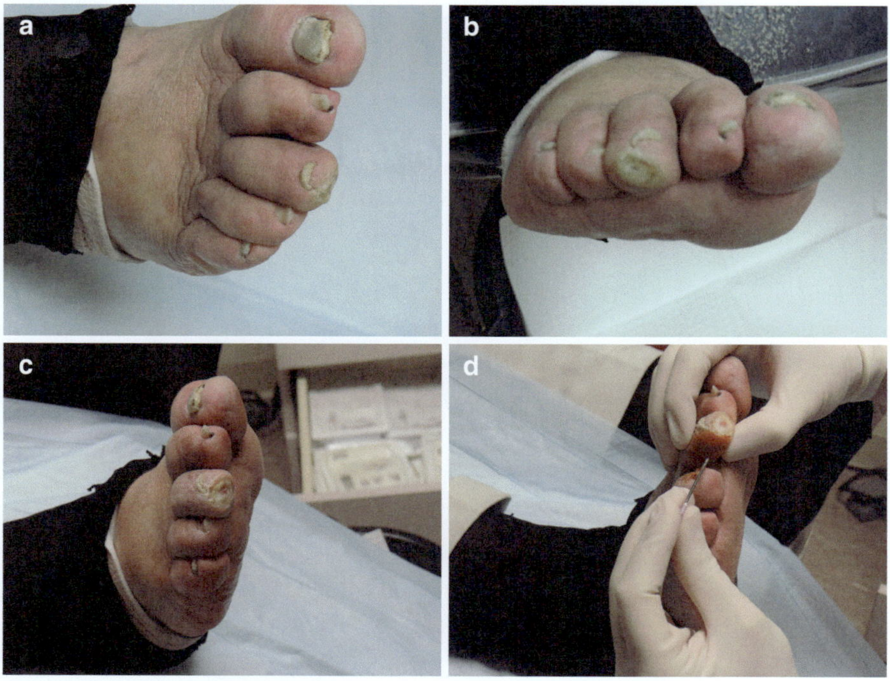

Fig. 24.3 (**a**) Pre-op appearance hammertoe with distal ulcer, third toe. (**b**) Pre-op appearance distal view, third toe. (**c**) Distal callus has been debrided, third toe. (**d**) Procedure with 18 gauge needle performing flexor tenotomy. (**e**) Toe straightened as procedure proceeds. (**f**) Toe is straighter following procedure

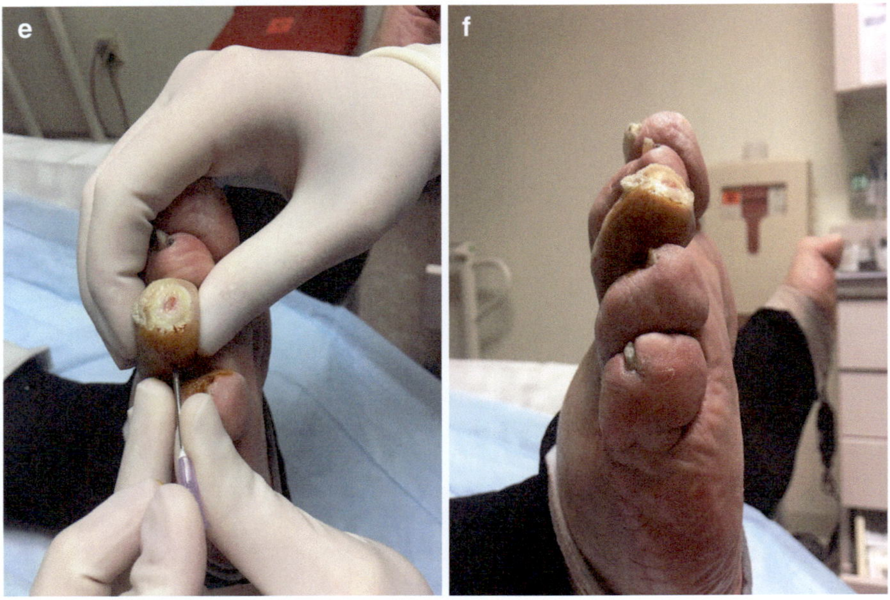

Fig. 24.3 (continued)

Interphalangeal Joint Arthroplasty

Indications Dorsal skin lesions or ulcerations to either the proximal interphalangeal joint or distal interphalangeal joint would benefit from an IPJ arthroplasty. Resection of the proximal or middle phalanx head decreases dorsal skin tension, decreasing the chance for recurrence [6]. Similarly, this procedure can be performed in hammertoe deformities that cannot be manually reduced.

Surgical Technique A dorsal linear incision is made over the DIPJ or PIPJ, depending on the area of concern. If an ulcer is present, it can be excised using two semielliptical incisions, either longitudinally or transversely. If transverse, this can be extended proximally with a linear incision if needed, creating a "T"-type incision (Fig. 24.4). Dissection is carried down to the level of the extensor tendon, which is transversely cut to expose the interphalangeal joint. Collateral ligaments are resected using a J-stroke maneuver to isolate the head of the phalanx. A sagittal saw or bone cutter is used to resect the phalanx head, reducing the deformity. Maintaining correction of the deformity can be performed with use of K-wires or splinting (Figs. 24.5a,b). Hardware should be avoided if there is a question of infection or osteomyelitis.

Terminal Syme Amputation

Indications Indications for a Syme amputation include chronic, non-healing distal tip ulcerations of the lesser digit with underlying hammertoe deformity. This proce-

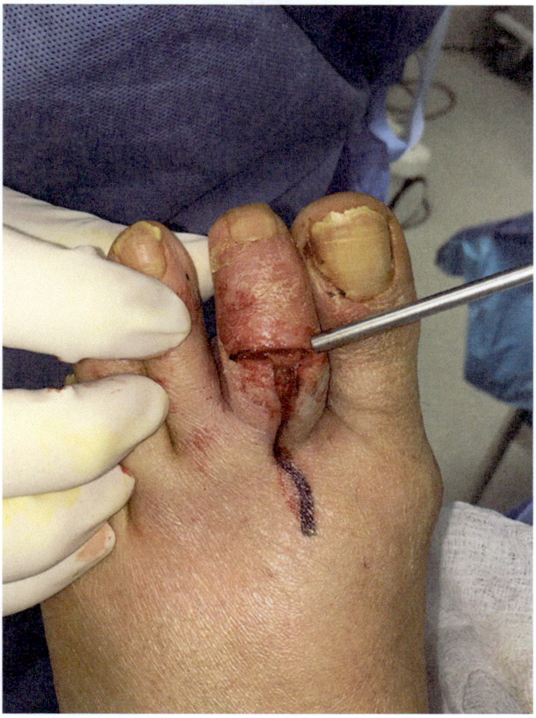

Fig. 24.4 Transverse elliptical incision made to excise ulcer. This is then extended proximally to create a "T" incision

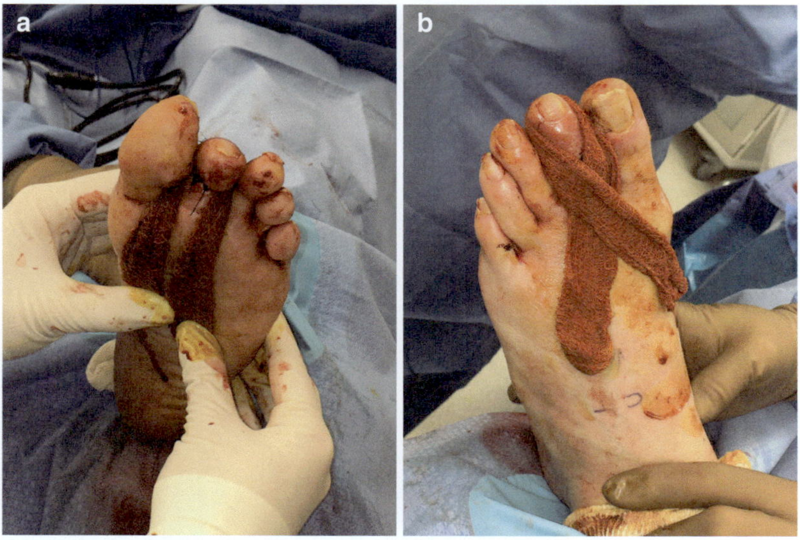

Fig. 24.5 (**a**) Splinting of the second toe with Betadine-soaked gauze, keeping the MTPJ in a rectus position. (**b**) Splinting distal aspect of toe with Betadine-soaked gauze, maintaining IPJs in a straightened manner

dure allows for correction of deformity, as well as excision of wound and/or underlying infection [7] (Figs. 24.6 and 24.7).

Surgical Technique A fishmouth-type incision is made with apex at the level of the DIPJ, ideally with a small dorsal flap and larger plantar flap. This should allow for full excision of ulceration, along with the distal phalanx and nail complex. If

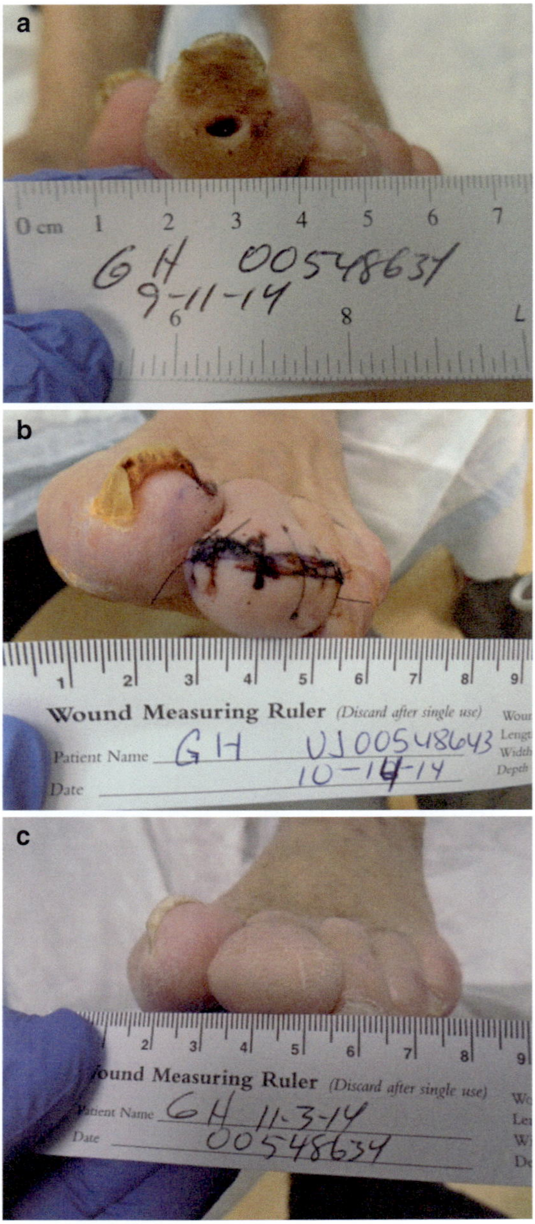

Fig. 24.6 (**a**) Distal second toe ulceration that probes to bone. (**b**) One-month status post second digit distal phalangectomy. (**c**) Two-month status post second digit distal phalangectomy

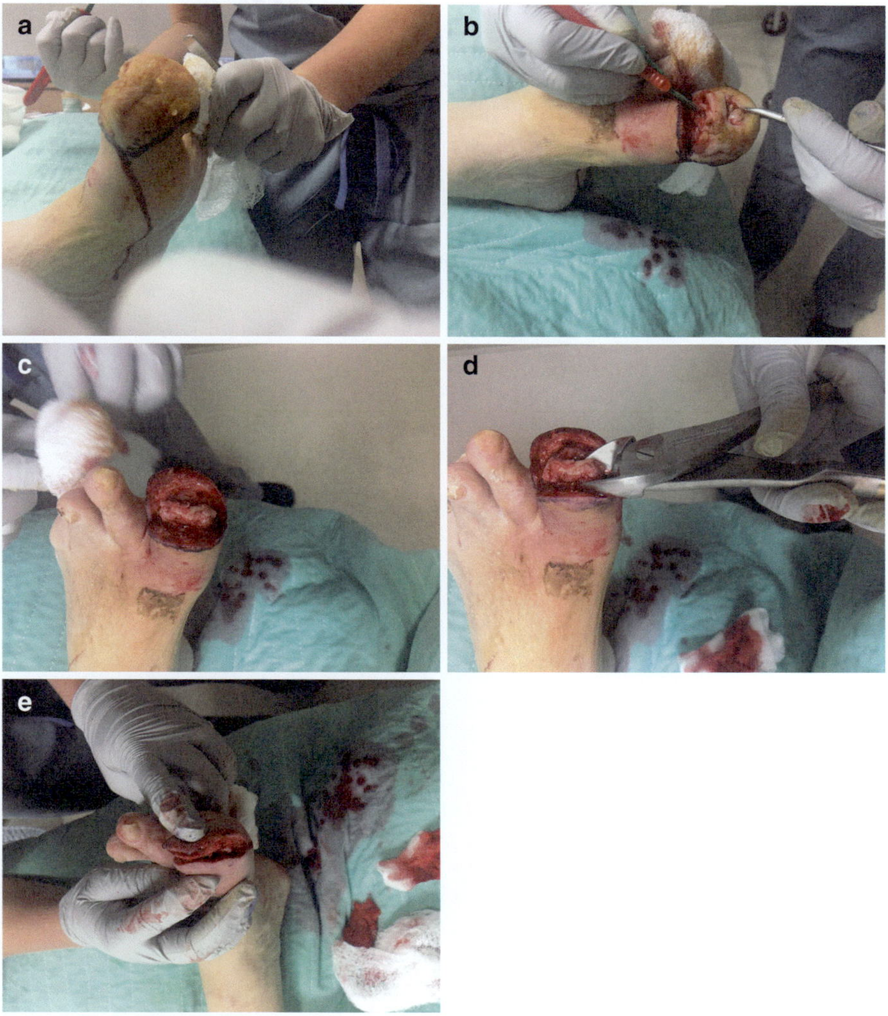

Fig. 24.7 (**a**) Large plantar flap for Syme's amputation. (**b**) Smaller dorsal flap for Syme's amputation. (**c**) The distal phalanx and nail complex excised. (**d**) The proximal phalanx head may be resected to allow for closure under minimal tension. (**e**) Approximation of dorsal and plantar skin flaps

required, the head of the middle phalanx can be resected as a clean margin or to allow for approximation of skin edges. The dorsal and plantar flaps are subsequently brought together using nonabsorbable 4–0 suture.

Postoperative Management

Postoperative dressings should be used to splint the toes in a corrected position. If not stabilized with a K-wire, this can be accomplished with a combination of taping techniques or Betadine-soaked gauze. Weightbearing is generally allowed in the form of a surgical shoe or CAM walker. Felt padding may be incorporated to off-load the toes if K-wires are used. K-wires are typically removed in 4–6 weeks, depending on surgeon preference.

Clinical Pearls/Pitfalls

- In the case that continued contracture is noted proximally at the MTPJ, further soft tissue release in the form of capsulotomies or tendon release/ lengthenings may be performed. One may also perform EDL tendon lengthenings of the lesser toes through one incision along the midfoot if multiple toes are involved, minimizing multiple incisions (Fig. 24.8).

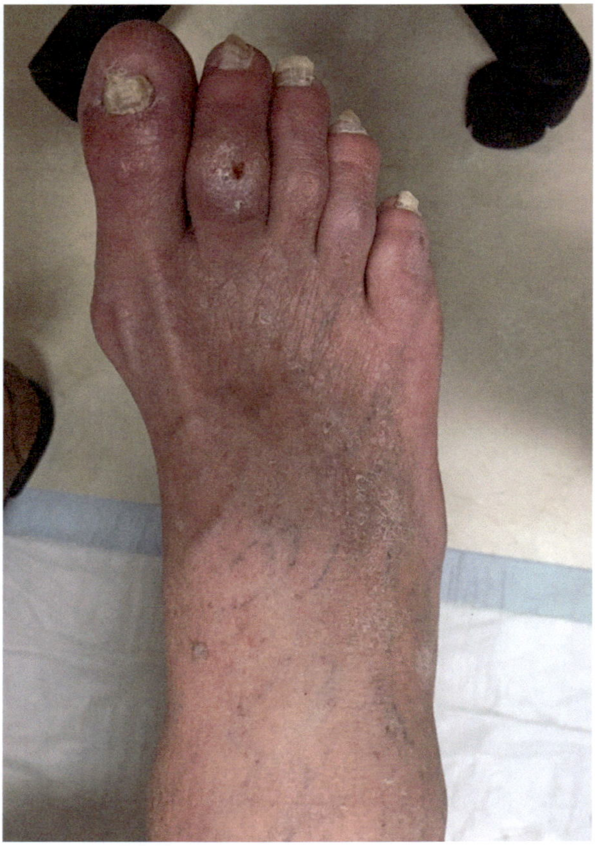

Fig. 24.8 Postoperative clinical photo 3-week s/p second digit PIPJ arthroplasty, EDL lengthenings 2–5 (single midfoot incision)

References

1. Armstrong DG, Lavery LA, Stern S, Harkless LB. Is prophylactic diabetic foot surgery dangerous? J Foot Ankle Surg. 1996;35(6):585–9.
2. Giurini JM, Rosenblum BI. The role of foot surgery in patients with diabetes. Clin Podiatr Med Surg. 1995;12:119–27.
3. Bus SA, Maas M, de Lange A, et al. Elevated plantar pressures in neuropathic diabetic patients with claw/hammer toe deformity. J Biomech. 2005;38(9):1918–25.
4. Roukis TS. A 1-piece shape-metal nitinol intramedullary internal fixation device for arthrodesis of the proximal interphalangeal joint in neuropathic patients with diabetes. Foot Ankle Spec. 2009;2(3):130–4.
5. Tamir E, Vigler M, Avisar E, Finestone AS. Percutaneous tenotomy for the treatment of diabetic toe ulcers. Foot Ankle Int. 2014;35(1):38–43.
6. Kim JY, Kim TW, Park YE, Lee YJ. Modified resection arthroplasty for infected non-healing ulcers with toe deformity in diabetic patients. Foot Ankle Int. 2008;29(5):493–7.
7. Boffeli TJ, Abben KW, Hyllengren SB. In-office distal Symes lesser toe amputation: a safe, reliable, and cost-effective treatment of diabetes-related tip of toe ulcers complicated by osteomyelitis. J Foot Ankle Surg. 2014;53(6):720–6.

Chapter 25
Percutaneous Tenotomies and Capsulotomies in Neuropathic Claw Toes

Rachel Baisch Kang and Thomas S. Roukis

Presentation/History

The most common forefoot deformity noted among patients with diabetes for >10 years is a claw toe [1–3], with incidence of 3% in patients with diabetes [4]. Traditionally, the mechanical etiology for claw toes in diabetic motor neuropathy is thought to be secondary to dysfunction of the interossei and lumbricals with overpowering of the long extensors and flexors that consequently lead to extension at the metatarsophalangeal joints and flexion contractures at the distal and proximal interphalangeal joints [5]. Consequently, ulcers frequently develop in areas of increased pressure and concentrated mechanical stress such as the distal tuft and dorsal proximal interphalangeal joint (Fig. 25.1) [6]. It is well known that a pre-existing ulceration can serve as a direct portal for bacteria to seed into the foot, which results in infection [7–12]. The direct and indirect costs associated with foot ulcerations, infections, and amputations as a result of diabetes are immense. Thus, the goal in diabetic ulcerations with flexible claw toes would be to heal them but also decrease the rate of ulceration development. Although traditional methods of offloading ulcers with accommodative inserts and extra-depth shoe gear can temporarily relieve pressure and heal forefoot ulcers, they are not a permanent solution. Conversely, open surgical approaches can be technically demanding with unnecessary soft tissue and osseous trauma in patients with diabetes. Thus, it seems reasonable that percutaneous procedures can be of great benefit in diabetics with flexible claw toes.

R. B. Kang
The Foot and Ankle Center of Kirkland PLLC, Kirkland, WA, USA

T. S. Roukis (✉)
Orthopaedic Center, Gundersen Health System, La Crosse, WI, USA
e-mail: tsroukis@gundersenhealth.org

E. A. Cook, J. J. Cook (eds.), *Hammertoes*,
https://doi.org/10.1007/978-3-319-16552-3_25

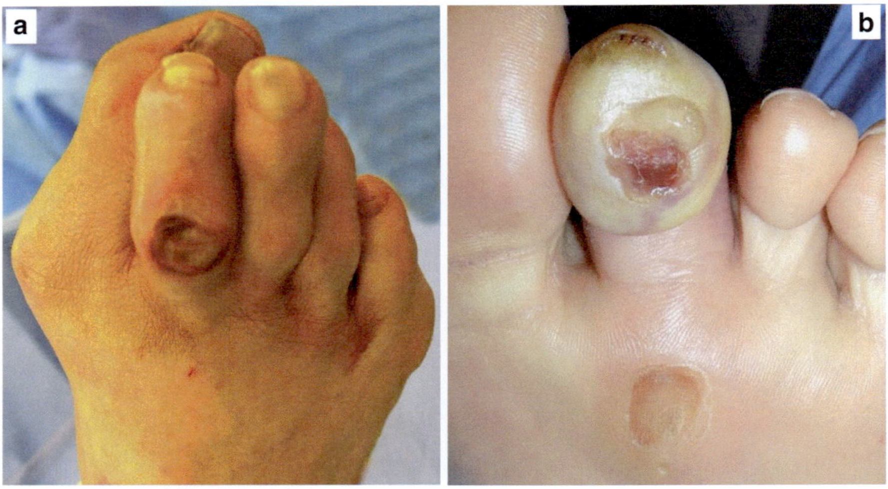

Fig. 25.1 Clinical photograph demonstrating a global forefoot deformity with combined rigid and flexible toe deformities. Note the dorsal contracture of the second toe that has ulcerated at the proximal interphalangeal joint (**a**). Clinical photograph of an infected ulceration at the distal tip of the second toe associated with combined flexible and rigid toe contracture (**b**)

Diagnosis/Assessment

During the initial assessment of claw toes, it is important to distinguish between flexible and rigid deformities. The diagnosis of flexible claw toe can be made when the contractures are reduced with plantar flexion of the ankle or manually reducible to neutral at the interphalangeal joints when loading the forefoot [13]. In addition, it is useful to note whether or not ulceration is present, and when present, the location of the ulceration should be noted. For example, is the ulcer located at the distal tuft or dorsal interphalangeal joint?

Surgical Technique

The surgical technique begins with the patient positioned in a supine position. A tourniquet is not required as blood loss is minimal. Patients with diabetes and dense peripheral neuropathy will not require anesthesia, but in sensate patients a regional infiltration of local anesthesia can be performed. A 2- to 3-mm incision is drawn on the plantar aspect of the toe at the apex of the deformity, which is usually at the level of the proximal or distal interphalangeal joint. The incision is made in-line with the longitudinal axis of the toe (i.e., perpendicular to the course of the tendon) through the skin and carried down to the underlying flexor digitorum longus tendon. This tendon is transected under tension, which is created by the surgeon's nondominant hand simultaneously extending of the tip of the toe with their index finger and extending the proximal interphalangeal joint with their thumb. Alternatively, the incision can be placed at the plantar aspect of the base of the proximal phalanx, which will release both the flexor digitorum longus and flexor digitorum brevis tendons. This technique should be reserved for severe contractures as it will result in a nonfunctional albeit straightened toe. Following transection of the flexor digitorum longus tendon, the toe is manipulated to release any remaining tendon fibers and disrupt the plantar plates to the proximal and distal interphalangeal joints (i.e., phalangeal set procedure) [14, 15]. Once correction is achieved, the surgical site is closed with a single metallic staple or nylon suture if deemed appropriate; otherwise it can be left open to heal via secondary intent (Fig. 25.2).

If the toe contracture is fully corrected but the metatarsal-phalangeal joint remains contracted, a percutaneous extensor tenotomy with or without capsulotomy can be performed. The toe is grasped in the surgeon's nondominant hand and simultaneously distracted and plantarflexed at the metatarsal-phalangeal joint which places the extensor tendon and capsule under tension as well as makes them more superficial. A No. 11 blade, No. 64 Beaver blade, or the bevel of an 18-gauge needle is then inserted through the skin overlying the metatarsal-phalangeal joint, and the tip of the blade is deepened a few millimeters and in a lateral direction. The tip of the blade is then rotated medially with care taken not to further incise the skin, which releases the extensor tendon. The toe is manipulated in plantar flexion at the metatarsal-phalangeal joint level, and the degree of correction is ascertained by loading the forefoot. If the release was complete, the toe will lie in a rectus position at the metatarsal-phalangeal joint; however, if the correction was not adequate, the blade can be reinserted into the incision and deepened to the metatarsal-phalangeal joint capsule which is then incised using the same technique. Once correction is achieved, the surgical site is closed with a single metallic staple or nylon suture if deemed appropriate; otherwise it can be left open to heal via secondary intent (Fig. 25.3).

Following completion of these procedures, a specialized dressing is applied. This dressing consists of gauze padding placed over the dorsal aspect of metatarsal-phalangeal joints as well as at the plantar aspect of the toes, which maintains reduction of the deformities [16, 17]. The patient is allowed guarded full weightbearing in a postoperative shoe. The initial surgical dressings are removed in 3–5 days unless a wound is present that requires closer monitoring and then every 7–10 days thereafter until full healing has occurred. Once healed the diabetic patient is returned to extra-depth shoe gear with accommodative multi-density insoles for life.

Outcomes

A systematic review [18] evaluated complications associated with percutaneous flexor tenotomies for treating diabetic neuropathic toe ulcerations secondary to contracture deformities. The first compilation of studies included in the systematic review was by Laborde [19–23] with 18 toe ulcerations and a mean follow-up of

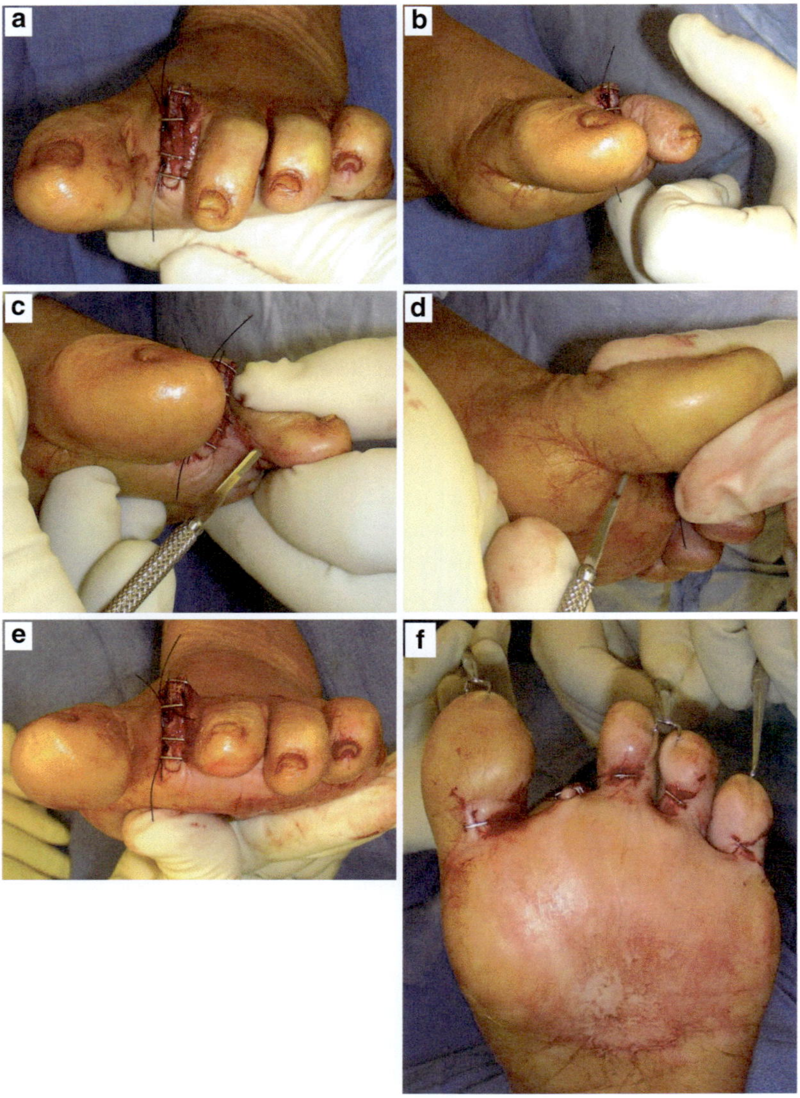

Fig. 25.2 Intraoperative photograph of a patient following amputation of the second toe for osteomyelitis due to a chronic neuropathic distal tuft ulceration (**a**). The forefoot has been loaded in a dorsal direction to simulate weightbearing, and this reveals flexion contractures of the remaining toes at the interphalangeal joints and metatarsal-phalangeal joints. Intraoperative photograph demonstrating the proper approach to grasp the lesser toe (**b**) as described in the text, as well as the incision location to perform percutaneous flexor tenotomy of the lesser toes (**c**) and hallux (**d**). Intraoperative photograph following percutaneous flexor tenotomy of the hallux and third toe with the forefoot loaded in a dorsal direction (**e**). Note the resting extended position of the hallux and third toe compared with the adjacent toes and with Fig. 25.2a. Plantar view following percutaneous tenotomy of all remaining toes demonstrating the incision placement and closure technique as discussed in the text (**f**)

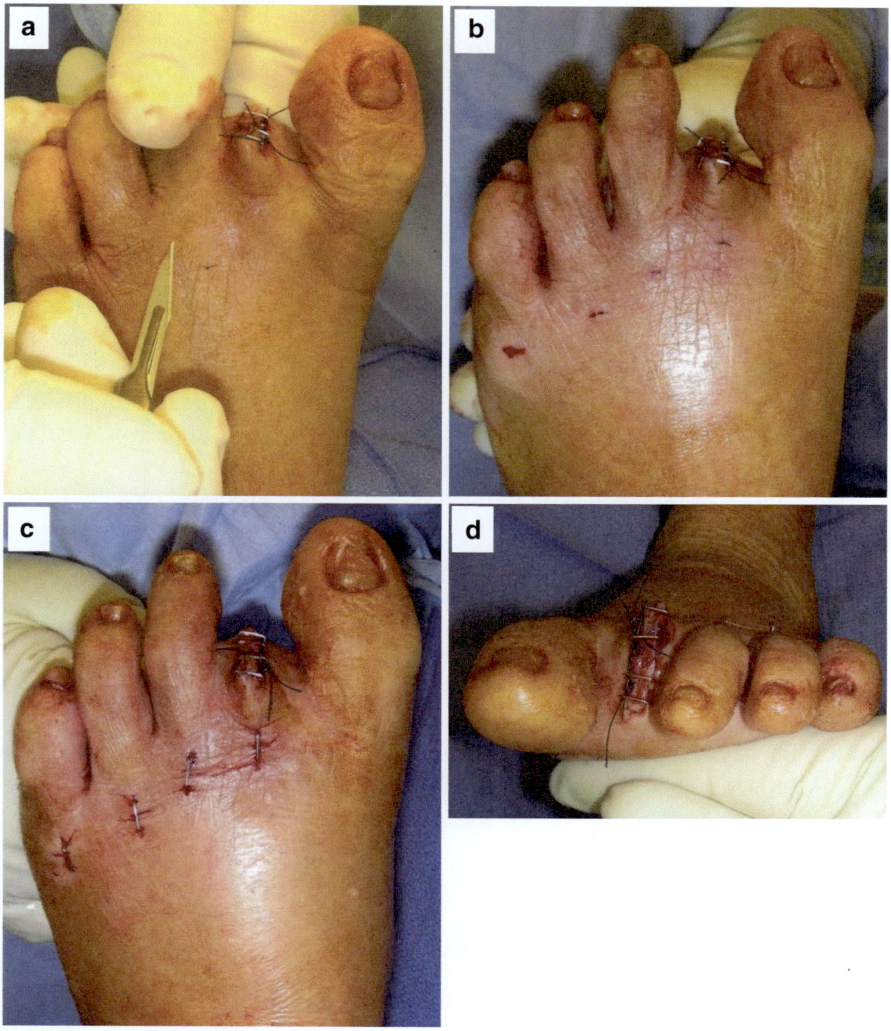

Fig. 25.3 Intraoperative photograph of the same patient shown in Fig. 25.2 demonstrating plantar flexion of the third toe with slight distal traction along with a No. 11 blade that is employed to transect the extensor tendon and perform a capsulotomy of the metatarsal-phalangeal joint as discussed in the text (**a**). Photograph following completion of the extensor tenotomy and metatarsal-phalangeal joint capsulotomy as discussed in the text prior to (**b**) and following skin closure (**c**). Photograph of the foot with the forefoot loaded in a dorsal direction demonstrating the final result achieved following percutaneous flexor tenotomy and extensor tenotomy with metatarsal-phalangeal joint capsulotomy to all remaining toes (**d**). Note the reduction of the deformities when compared with Fig. 25.2a

35.3 months. After percutaneous tenotomies, all incisions healed primarily without any infections, but transfer ulcerations developed in 5 [27.8%] toes. The second study by Tamir et al. [24] included 24 toes that had ulcerations at the distal tuft. After a mean follow-up of 13 months, no complications were reported, and all patients with ulcers healed. Since this systematic review, more recent studies have been published supporting percutaneous tenotomies in diabetic toe ulcerations with claw toe deformity. Schepers et al. [25] included 43 toe ulcerations, and after a mean follow-up of 11 months, only one complication was noted consisting of a volar plate injury that led to digital amputation and one recurrence of ulceration. Tamir et al. [6] published a larger retrospective review in 2013, in which tenotomies were performed for ulcerations located in four different regions in diabetic claw toe deformities. For purposes of this chapter, only the tenotomies performed for distal tuft ulcerations were included in the chart [Table 25.1]. Of the 103 distal tuft ulcerations, there were 14 minor complications, but no major complication such as recurrence, infection, or vascular compromise.

Interestingly, Rasmussen et al. [26] not only looked at distal tuft ulcerations but also preventative tenotomies in those who had claw toes but no open ulceration. In the 38 toes where prophylactic percutaneous flexor tenotomies were performed, none developed toe ulcerations at a mean of 31-month follow-up. Finally, van Netten et al. [27] performed percutaneous flexor tenotomies in 47 toes, 38 of which had distal tuft ulcerations and 9 without open ulceration. Recurrence of ulceration was noted in seven toes; however, no ulceration developed in the prophylactic group at a mean follow-up of 23 months.

Overall, percutaneous flexor tenotomies have been demonstrated to be beneficial in neuropathic diabetic claw toes with distal tuft ulcerations. Moreover, more recent data supports the benefits of prophylactic percutaneous flexor tenotomy in preventing recurrence of diabetic claw toe ulcerations (Fig. 25.4). Unfortunately, thus far, there is very sparse literature on percutaneous capsulotomy for neuropathic claw toes in the diabetic population. However, as research continues to support percutaneous flexor tenotomy as prophylactic measures, prospective research for percutaneous capsulotomy is also anticipated.

Clinical Pearls/Pitfalls

- Identifying rigid versus flexible claw toe deformity in the diabetic patient with neuropathy is critical as an initial assessment.
- Percutaneous tenotomy can be performed in an outpatient setting with early ambulation.
- Results in less soft tissue and osseous trauma with low incidence of wound healing and minimal complications.
- Percutaneous flexor tenotomy can assist with healing recalcitrant distal tuft ulcerations in diabetic claw toe ulcers as well as serving a prophylactic function in preventing ulcerations.
- Ultimately, decrease incidence of diabetic foot infections and amputations.

Table 25.1 Summary of available data for percutaneous toe tenotomy to treat claw toe deformity associated with neuropathic ulceration

Authors (citation)	Year	Source	Level of clinical evidence	Toes 1	Toes 2	Toes 3	Toes 4	Toes 5	Toes Total	Follow-up (months) [mean (range)]	Age (years) [mean (range)]	Indications (duration) (mean [range])	Recurrence (count [%])	Complications (count [%])
Laborde [19–23]	2007	Peer-reviewed journal	4	8	7	2	0	1	18	35.3 (27–64)	59.6 (48–81)	Toe ulceration at distal tip that has failed to heal with decreased weightbearing, debridement, shoe modification; (9.2 [1–60])	None	Transfer ulceration to adjacent digit (5 [27.8%])
Tamir et al. [24]	2008	Peer-reviewed journal	4	4	8	7	5	0	24	13 (3–27)	58 (37–79)	Toe ulceration at distal tip of 1 or more toes	None	None
Schepers et al. [25]	2010	Peer-reviewed journal	4	3	16	13	9	2	43	11 (1–27)	66.8 (38.9–85.8)	Toe ulceration at distal tip (6.8 months [1–24])	1 [2.3%]	Iatrogenic volar plate injury → amputation (1 [2.3%])
Tamir et al. [6]	2013	Peer-reviewed journal	4	16	31	37	16	3	103	22 (16–29)	65 (48–89)	Toe ulceration at distal tip (33 weeks [1–156])	None	Transfer ulceration to adjacent toe (9); plantar skin rupture (3); minor infection (1); pain (1). Total (14 [13.6%])
Rasmussen et al. [26]	2013	Peer-reviewed journal	4	24	25	9	5	2	65	31 (2–48)	62.8 (37–91)	Toe ulceration at distal tip in 27 toes and impending ulceration in 38 toes	3 [3.6%], no ulceration in preventative tenotomy group	Transfer ulceration (2 [3.1%])
van Netten et al. [27]	2013	Peer-reviewed journal	4	15	16	15	1	0	47	23 (11–60)	69 (41–93)	Toe ulceration at distal tip in 38 toes (96 day [9–525]); grade 0 ulceration in 9 toes	7 [14.9%], no ulceration in preventative tenotomy group	Amputation (3 [6.4%])

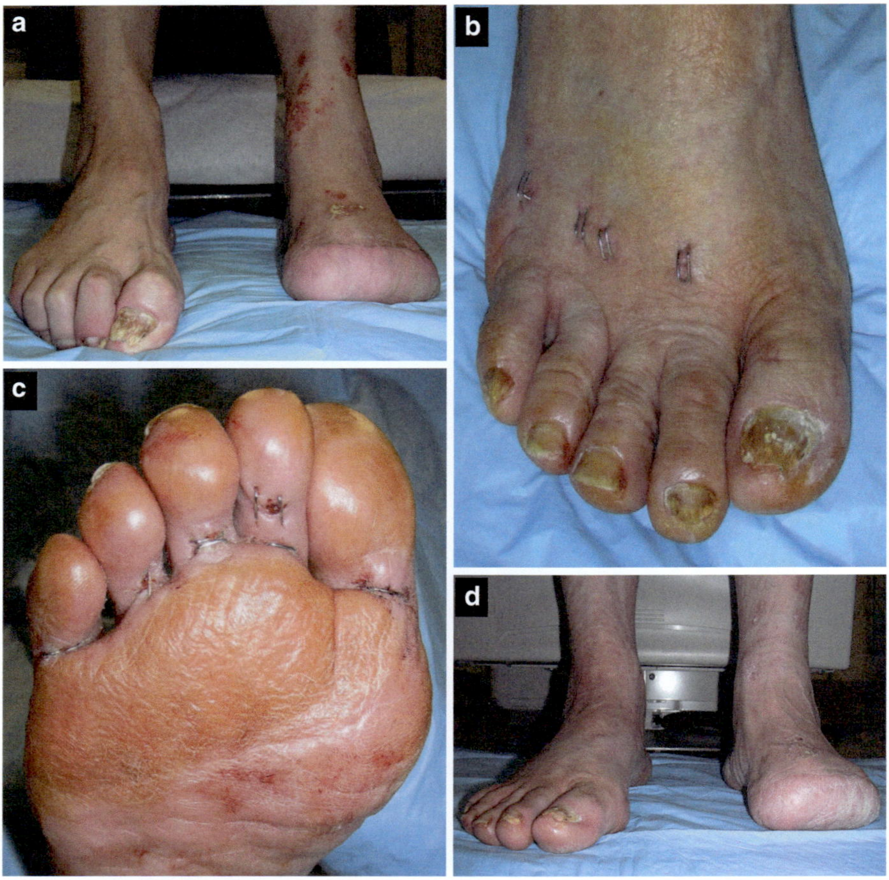

Fig. 25.4 Clinical photograph of a patient who underwent a transmetatarsal amputation after a series of toe amputations (left foot) and developed severe claw toes of all toes and intermittent distal tuft ulcerations to the second and third toes (right foot) (**a**). Clinical photograph of the dorsal (**b**) and plantar (**c**) forefoot following prophylactic percutaneous flexor digitorum longus and flexor digitorum brevis tenotomy, as well as percutaneous extensor digitorum longus tenotomy and capsulotomy to all the lesser toes. Note that the extensor hallucis longus and flexor hallucis longus tendons were also transected in the same setting. Clinical photograph demonstrating rectus albeit nonfunctional toes free of ulceration to the right forefoot following the above procedures (**d**)

References

1. Viswanathan V, Kumpatla S. Pattern and causes of amputation in diabetic patients: a multicentric study from India. J Assoc Physicians India. 2011;59:148–51.
2. Singh N, Armstrong D, Lipsky B. Preventing foot ulcers in patients with diabetes. JAMA. 2005;293(2):217–28.
3. Boyko EJ, Ahroni JH, Stensel V, Forsberg RC, Davignon DR, Smith DG. A prospective study of risk factors for diabetic foot ulcer. The Seattle diabetic foot study. Diabetes Care. 1999;22(7):1036–42.

4. Thomas R, Brenton K, Harris B, Ham R, Rees G, Gorvett T, et al. Foot ulceration in a secondary care diabetic clinic population: a 4-year prospective study. Diabetes Res Clin Pract. 2010;90(2):e37–9.
5. Myerson MS, Shereff MJ. The pathological anatomy of claw and hammertoes. J Bone Joint Surg Am. 1989;71(1):45–9.
6. Tamir E, Vigler M, Avisar E, Finestone AS. Percutaneous tenotomy for the treatment of diabetic toe ulcers. Foot Ankle Int. 2014;35(1):38–43.
7. Guyton GP, Saltzman CL. The diabetic foot: basic mechanisms of disease. J Bone Joint Surg Am. 2001;83(7):1084–96.
8. Lipsky BA. A report from the international consensus on diagnosing and treating the infected diabetic foot. Diabet Metab Res Rev. 2004;20(Suppl 1):S68–77.
9. Lipsky BA, Berendt AR, Embil J, De Lalla F. Diagnosing and treating diabetic foot infections. Diabetes Metab Res Rev. 2004;20(Suppl):S56–64.
10. Zgonis T, Roukis TS. A systematic approach to diabetic foot infections. Adv Ther. 2005;22(3):244–62.
11. Frykberg RG, Zgonis T, Armstrong DG, Driver VR, Giurini JM, Kravitz SR, et al. Diabetic foot disorders: a clinical practice guideline. J Foot Ankle Surg. 2006;45(Suppl):S2–66.
12. Andersen CA, Roukis TS. The diabetic foot. Surg Clin N Am. 2007;87(5):1149–77.
13. Thomas JL, Blitch EL 4th, Chaney DM, Dinucci KA, Eickmeier K, Rubin LG, et al. Diagnosis and treatment of forefoot disorders. Section 1: digital deformities. J Foot Ankle Surg. 2009;48(2):230–8.
14. Roukis TS, Markewych B. Minimal incision surgery: can it have an impact in diabetic limb salvage? Podiatry Today. 2009;22(3):37–49.
15. Roven MD. Phalangeal set. Clin Podiatr. 1985;2(3):483–9.
16. Landsman AS, Cook E, Cook J. Tenotomy and tendon transfer about the forefoot, midfoot, and hindfoot. Clin Podiatr Med Surg. 2008;25(4):547–69.
17. Roven MD. Tenotomy, tenectomy and capsulotomy for the lesser toes. Clin Podiatr. 1985;2(3):471–5.
18. Roukis TS, Schade VL. Percutaneous flexor tenotomy for treatment of neuropathic toe ulceration secondary to toe contracture in persons with diabetes: a systematic review. J Foot Ankle Surg. 2009;48(6):684–9.
19. Laborde JM. Treatment of forefoot ulcers with tendon lengthenings. J South Orthop Assoc. 2003;12(2):60–5.
20. Laborde JM. Tendon lengthenings for forefoot ulcers. Wounds. 2005;17(5):122–30.
21. Laborde JM. Neuropathic toe ulcers treated with toe flexor tenotomies. Foot Ankle Int. 2007;28(11):1160–4.
22. Laborde JM. Neuropathic plantar forefoot ulcers treated with tendon lengthenings. Foot Ankle Int. 2008;29(4):378–84.
23. Laborde JM. Tendon lengthening: is it a viable option for forefoot ulcers? Podiatry Today. 2005;18(7):24–34.
24. Tamir E, McLaren AM, Gadgil A, Daniels TR. Outpatient percutaneous flexor tenotomies for management of diabetic claw toe deformities with ulcers: a preliminary report. Can J Surg. 2008;51(1):41–4.
25. Schepers T, Berendsen HA, Oei IH, Koning J. Functional outcome and patient satisfaction after flexor tenotomy for plantar ulcers of the toes. J Foot Ankle Surg. 2010;49(2):119–22.
26. Rasmussen A, Bjerre-Christensen U, Almdal TP, Holstein P. Percutaneous flexor tenotomy for preventing and treating toe ulcers in people with diabetes mellitus. J Tissue Viability. 2013;22(3):68–73.
27. van Netten JJ, Bril A, van Baal JG. The effect of flexor tenotomy on healing and prevention of neuropathic diabetic foot ulcers on the distal end of the toe. J Foot Ankle Res. 2013;6(1):3. https://doi.org/10.1186/1757-1146-6-3.

Chapter 26
Lesser Metatarsal-Phalangeal Joint Fusion as an Adjunctive Procedure for the Treatment of the Complex Hammer Digit

Robert Joseph

Presentation and History

Lesser metatarsal-phalangeal joint fusion is a less common but highly effective adjunct procedure for the treatment of the complex hammer digit. The complex hammer digit is a multi-planar deformity that presents as a flexion contracture of the digit with subluxation or dislocation of the metatarsal-phalangeal joint (Fig. 26.1 *complex hammer digit*). This is distinguished from the simple hammer digit that presents as a flexion contracture of the digit without metatarsal-phalangeal joint instability (Fig. 26.2 *simple hammer digit*). Metatarsal-phalangeal joint pathology is not only the hallmark difference between the complex and simple hammer digits but the critical indication for adjunct procedures that stabilize the metatarsal-phalangeal joint when performing hammer digit correction surgery. Neglect of metatarsal-phalangeal joint instability when surgically correcting the complex hammer digit may result in a higher incidence of floating toe syndrome or recurrence of deformity. Hence joint fusion and techniques such as plantar plate repair and flexor tendon transfer procedures are essential for the treatment of the complex hammer digit [1–9].

Lesser metatarsal-phalangeal joint fusion has historically been a less favored technique for stabilizing the lesser metatarsal-phalangeal joints as these joints were once considered "essential joints" for foot function. The inherent challenge of achieving adequate fixation across such small joints combined with the small cubic content of bone for fusion had promulgated misperceptions and aversion toward fusions because of the risk of nonunion with this procedure in comparison with fusion of the first metatarsal-phalangeal joint. Advances in instrumentation, technique, and appreciation of foot biomechanics have mitigated some of these concerns, while recent reports demonstrate nonunion rates that are similar to those of

R. Joseph (✉)
Department of Podiatric Medicine and Radiology, Scholl College of Podiatric Medicine at Rosalind Franklin University of Medicine and Health Sciences, North Chicago, IL, USA

E. A. Cook, J. J. Cook (eds.), *Hammertoes*,
https://doi.org/10.1007/978-3-319-16552-3_26

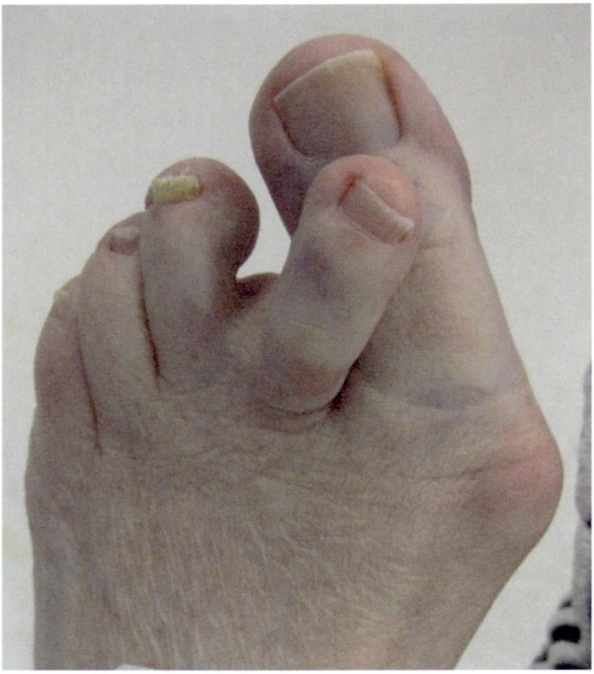

Fig. 26.1 Complex hammer digit: clinical presentation of a complex hammer digit that presents as an overlapping hammertoe

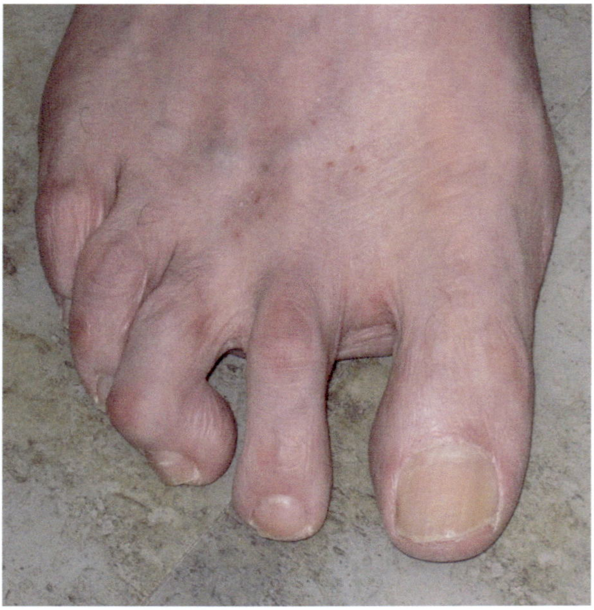

Fig. 26.2 Simple hammer digit: clinical presentation of the simple hammer digit. The simple hammer digit appears as a flexion contracture of the digit without gross instability of the metatarsal-phalangeal joint

first metatarsal-phalangeal fusion. Consequently, first metatarsal-phalangeal joint fusion is becoming a more attractive procedure for stabilizing the proximal phalanx when surgically correcting the complex hammer digit [10–15].

Diagnosis and Assessment of the Complex Hammer Digit and Metatarsal-Phalangeal Joint Instability

The primary indication for lesser metatarsal-phalangeal joint fusion is joint instability caused by disruption of the plantar plate complex. The plantar plate complex consists of the plantar plate and its associated ligaments. Avascular necrosis of a metatarsal is also a less common indication for fusion.

Clinical evaluation of the complex hammer digit includes static and dynamic evaluation of metatarsal-phalangeal joint function. Pre-dislocation syndrome (PDS) is the first stage of joint dysfunction that often presents concomitantly with hammer digits. PDS is a result of injury, attenuation, and inflammation of the capsular structures of the metatarsal-phalangeal joint that include the plantar plate. Pre-dislocation syndrome is *not* an indication in itself for metatarsal-phalangeal joint fusion. Often times, PDS resolves with conservative care or secondarily following surgical correction of the simple hammer digit once the retrograde forces created by the contracted proximal phalanx are reduced with surgery. Evaluation of PDS typically demonstrates pain with palpation of the plantar aspect of the metatarsal-phalangeal joint and a negative Lachman test.

Worsening of PDS to the point of joint subluxation may warrant consideration of joint fusion with hammer digit surgery. Joint subluxation can be noted with a positive Lachman test. A decision to fuse a subluxable joint is controversial however, and the ultimate decision for fusion should depend on the severity of joint instability and extent of plantar plate injury. As the severity of cartilage and ligament injury worsens, the likelihood of incomplete cartilage healing of the plantar plate increases since cartilage has a poor metabolic capacity for healing. Joint stabilization by fusion may be warranted under circumstances where the overall capacity and durability of bone healing is deemed more predictable than the severity of cartilage injury, and healing is therefore unlikely to provide a favorable long-term outcome. Severe attenuation and disruption of the plantar plate or a combination of collateral ligament and plantar plate injuries are compelling situations that support a rationale that the severity of joint injury may not be favorable for healing despite surgical repair and joint fusion may be a more predictable joint stabilizing procedure. Advanced imaging such as ultrasound (Fig. 26.3a–d *ultrasound of normal and abnormal plantar plate*) or MRI (Fig. 26.4 *MRI of plantar plate and collateral ligament tear*) may be useful in assessing the severity and magnitude of plantar plate injury and substantiating a decision for fusion in these circumstances. It is unclear whether there is a specific grade of plantar plate injury or threshold of degeneration that suggests the plantar plate complex may be beyond the physiologic limits of healing.

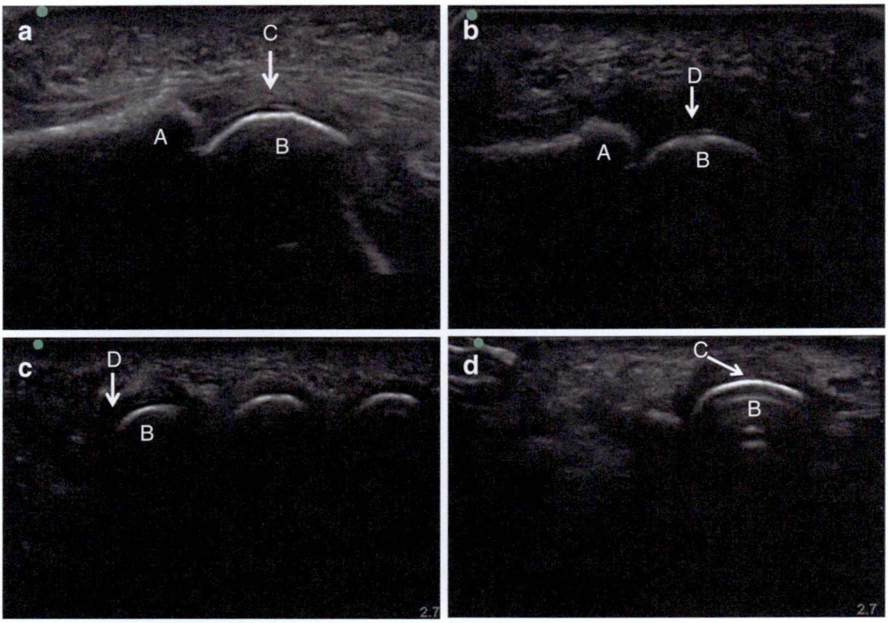

Fig. 26.3 (**a**) longitudinal image of an intact plantar plate: (**a**) proximal phalanx, (**b**) metatarsal head, (**c**) intact plantar plate, (**d**) plantar plate tear (Images courtesy of the Weil Foot and Ankle Institute). (**b**) Longitudinal ultrasound image of a plantar plate tear. (**c**) Transverse ultrasound image of a plantar plate tear. (**d**) Transverse ultrasound image of an intact plantar plate

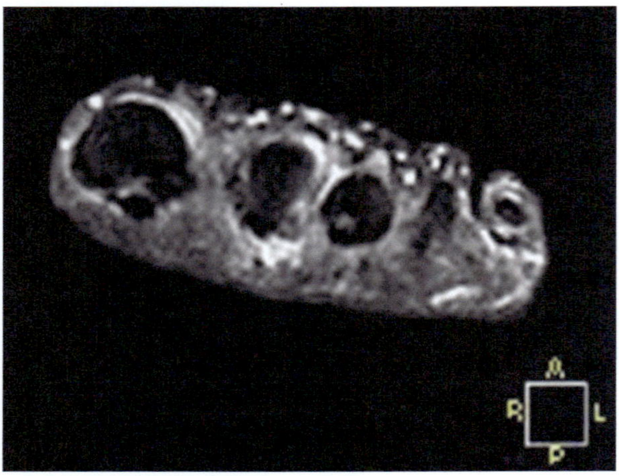

Fig. 26.4 T2-weighted MRI of a plantar plate and collateral ligament tear of the second digit. (Images courtesy of the Weil Foot and Ankle Institute)

The end stage of metatarsal-phalangeal joint dysfunction manifests as dislocation of the proximal phalanx. This often presents with diffuse attenuation or obliteration of the plantar plate and rupture of collateral ligaments. This is truly a complex condition with translational, rotational, and angular elements of deformity. This most commonly appears as an “overlapping” or “underlapping” hammer digit deformity. Neither MRI nor ultrasound is necessary to identify this stage of disease or substantiate an indication for fusion, as it is unlikely that the supportive structures of the metatarsal-phalangeal joint can be repaired or have the capacity for healing such severe injury [16–23].

Technique

Fusion Site Preparation

A dorsal linear incision is made approximately 3 cm proximal to the metatarsal-phalangeal joint. The incision is extended distally to the level of the proximal interphalangeal joint. All contracture of the extensor hood is released during dissection. The joint capsule of the metatarsal-phalangeal joint and proximal interphalangeal joint is then transected, and the collateral ligamentous structures are released. Full release of collateral ligaments of the metatarsal-phalangeal joint enables adequate exposure of the metatarsal head for visualization and placement of internal fixation (Fig. 26.5 *surgical exposure of joint*).

The joint surfaces of the metatarsal-phalangeal joint are then denuded of articular cartilage with a curette, small cup and cone reamer, or transverse osteotomy technique. Osteotomy is preferred if shortening of a congenitally long metatarsal is required. When performing an osteotomy, between 25 and 40% of the distal metatarsal head is resected. This maximizes the cross-sectional surface area for fusion while preserving adequate width across the metatarsal head to allow placement of staple fixation. The osteotomy should be performed such that the proximal phalanx will be aligned in a final position of 5–10° of dorsiflexion from the weight-bearing

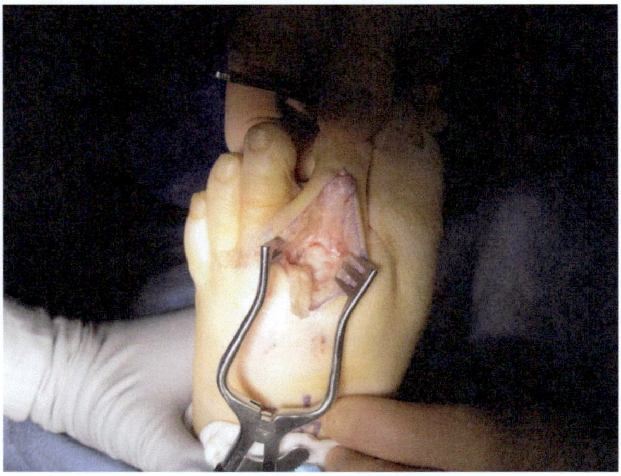

Fig. 26.5 Surgical exposure of the metatarsal-phalangeal joint through a dorsal incision. (Images courtesy of Marc Greenberg, DPM)

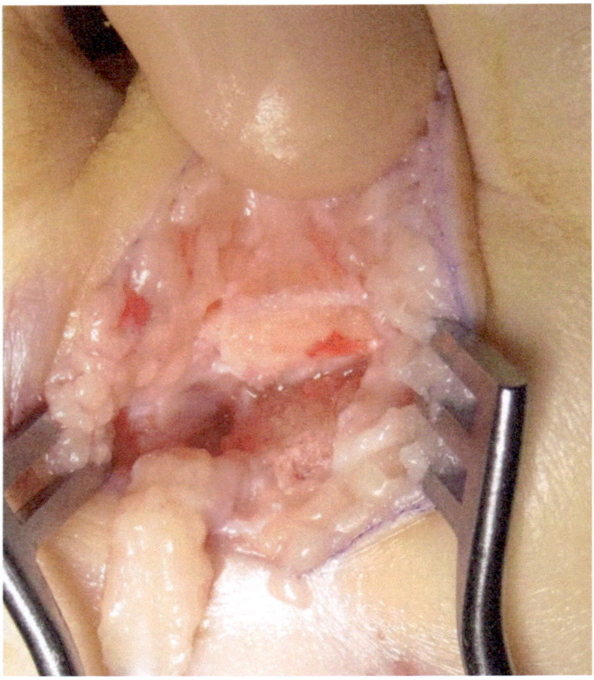

Fig. 26.6 Metatarsal-phalangeal joint resection by osteotomy technique in preparation for fusion. (Images courtesy of Marc Greenberg, DPM)

surface. This position facilitates toe off with gait and shoe gear accommodation (Fig. 26.6 *joint resection*).

The base of the proximal phalanx should also be conservatively resected to the level of subchondral bone when preparing the metatarsal-phalangeal joint for fusion. Aggressive resection of the base of the proximal phalanx critically reduces the surface area and cubic bone mass for fusion as well as the ability to place internal fixation. The flared curvature and round base of the proximal phalanx creates a disproportionately greater decrease in the surface area of fusion with each millimeter of bone resected from the phalanx. Hence caution should be taken to resect as little bone as possible from the proximal phalanx (Fig. 26.6 *joint resection*).

Fixation Construct

Following joint preparation, the fusion site is stabilized with the phalanx aligned at 5–10° of dorsiflexion using a retrograde 0.62 Kirschner wire. Two compression staples are then positioned parallel with the Kirschner wire across the dorsal medial and lateral aspects of the fusion site. Each staple is positioned obliquely with the

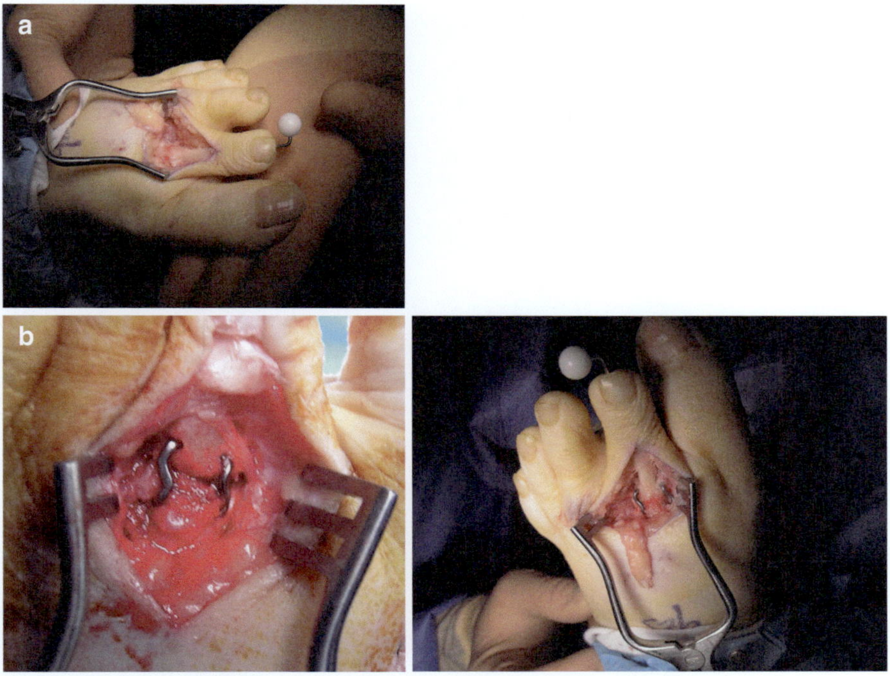

Fig. 26.7 (**a**) Stabilization of the metatarsal-phalangeal joint fusion in a position of 5° dorsiflexion using a retrograde 0.62 Kirschner wire. (Images courtesy of Marc Greenberg, DPM). (**b**) Symmetric placement of two parallel compression staples across the fusion site to achieve uniform compression across the fusion site and along the axis of the Kirschner wire. (Images courtesy of Marc Greenberg, DPM)

legs of each staple pointed centrally toward with Kirschner wire. The Kirschner wire aligns compression forces created by the staples equally across the fusion site and along the axis of the wire (Fig. 26.7a, b *K-wire stabilization of digit*). Symmetric alignment of the staples about the Kirschner wire is essential. Proper orientation of the Kirschner wire and staples forms a "butterfly" sign that can be observed on an anterior-posterior radiographic projection of the foot whereby the staples resemble the symmetrical wings of a butterfly and the Kirschner wire resembles the body of the butterfly (Fig. 26.8 *butterfly sign*). This sign suggests that the staples are symmetrically oriented along the axis of the Kirschner wire and will more likely to distribute even compression across the fusion site. The function of this construct may be likened to that of an intramedullary compression rod. The nonunion rate of this construct is reported to be 12.9%. This is similar to the nonunion rate of 9% reported in Karlock et al. in his series of 11 patients using a conventional staple and Kirschner wire fixation construct. The Kirschner wires remain in place for approximately 4–6 weeks before being removed.

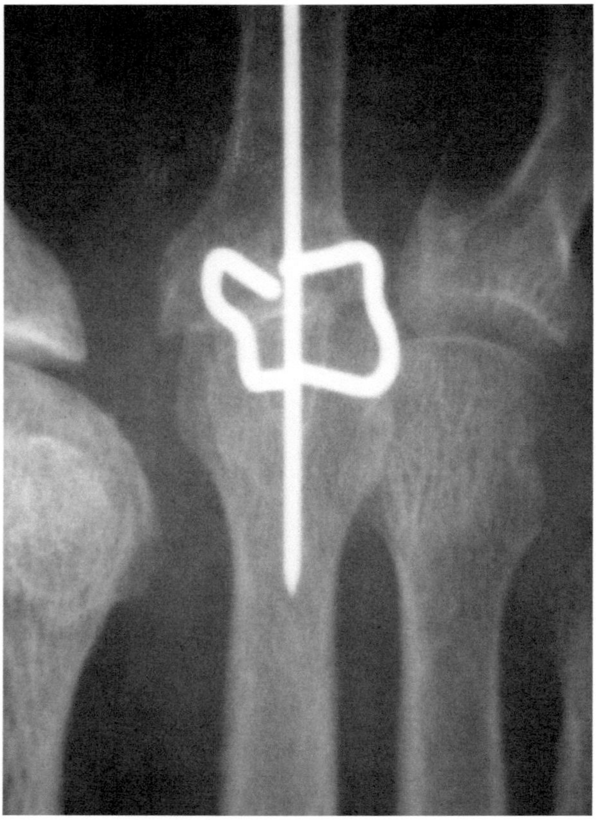

Fig. 26.8 Radiographic appearance of the "Butterfly" sign that demonstrates symmetric placement of two compression staples around a central Kirschner wire. The "Butterfly" sign suggests symmetric compression across the fusion site and along the axis of the Kirschner wire

Postoperative Care

Patients remain non-weight-bearing with a short leg cast or CAM boot for 5 weeks postoperatively followed by partial weight-bearing with a CAM boot that is advanced to full weight-bearing over a period of 4 weeks. Kirschner wire fixation is removed with the onset of partial weight-bearing. Patients may return to unrestricted shoe gear at 10 weeks postoperatively.

Outcome

There are several unique considerations when comparing lesser metatarsal-phalangeal joint fusions with fusion of the first metatarsal-phalangeal joint. The primary consideration is that the first metatarsal-phalangeal joint has greater cubic bone content than a lesser metatarsal-phalangeal joint and is thereby able to accommodate more robust fixation that allows immediate postoperative weight-bearing. The author's experience and research suggest that 75% of nonunions associated with this procedure involve hardware failure and have occurred when patients begin weight-bearing prior to the mean duration of non-weight-bearing (4.7 weeks) in his original study. Hence immediate weight-bearing is not recommended with this procedure due to concern that the fixation construct cannot compensate for the inherent weakness of bone during the early phases of bone healing. It is therefore recommended that patients remain non-weight-bearing for a period of 5 weeks after surgery followed by an additional 4–5 weeks of guarded weight-bearing with use of a CAM boot. Radiographic union is most commonly observed by postoperative week 8. Patients are transitioned to regular shoe gear at postoperative week 10. Clinical union is observed most commonly between 8 and 10 weeks postoperatively. This procedure has been shown to significantly reduce pain associated with the complex hammer digit and improve patient function while allowing the patient to return to regular shoe gear.

Lesser metatarsal-phalangeal joint fusion has several distinct advantages over alternate procedures commonly used to stabilize the lesser metatarsal-phalangeal joints. Most procedures stabilize joint function by attempting direct repair of structures such as the plantar plate or indirectly stabilizing the joint by splinting the digit with a combination of tendon transfers and fusion of the interphalangeal joint. It is difficult to assess how these procedures affect dynamic function of the foot when they are performed in a static context with the patient under anesthesia. This assessment is unreliable considering that tendon transfer procedures predominantly stabilize digit function through active tendon contraction that cannot truly be evaluated in the operating room. This leaves the surgeon to passively evaluate digit stabilization by evaluation of the resting tension of transferred tendons. The plantar plate also stabilizes the digit during dynamic function so is likewise difficult to evaluate in the operating room. These intraoperative assessments may be less predictive of the true functional stabilization of the joint and the ultimate resting position of the digit.

The advantage of metatarsal-phalangeal joint fusion is that the function and position of the joint remain constant during static and dynamic function of the foot when it is fused and is therefore predictable. There is no ambiguity in the resting position of the phalanx as that is determined intraoperatively. This reduces the risk of floating toe syndrome due to an unpredictable intraoperative assessment.

In the authors' opinions, this technique is not without pitfalls that make fusion of this joint challenging in comparison with fusion of the first metatarsal-phalangeal joint. The fused position of the phalanx is of critical importance to prevent digit impingement in the toe box of shoe gear but must allow sufficient sagittal plane angulation of the digit to accommodate toe-off pressures during ambulation. The author's standard technique is to place the digit in 5–10° of dorsal angulation from the weight-bearing plane of the foot to accommodate these needs. This angulation can result in transfer of retrograde force through the metatarsal that can result in several complications however.

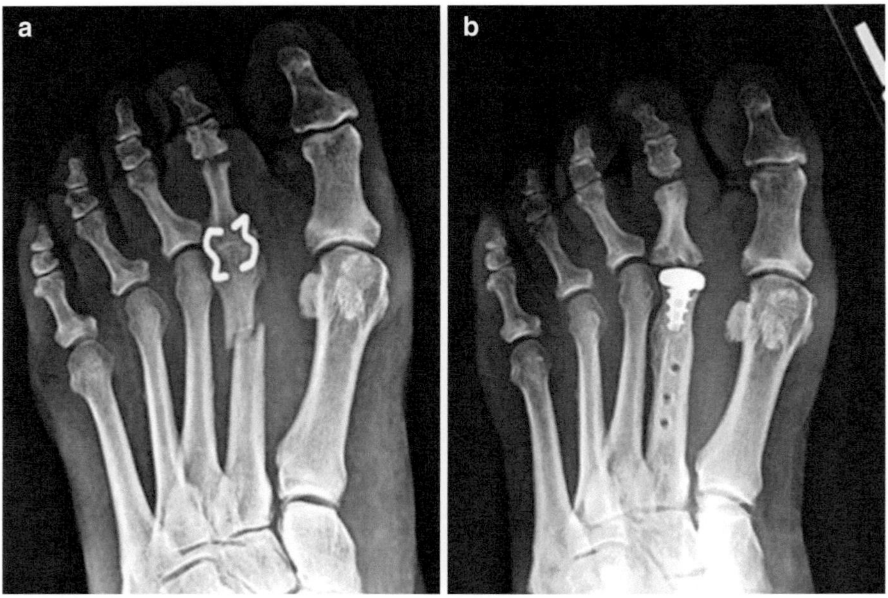

Fig. 26.9 (**a**) Metatarsal shaft fracture caused by increased retrograde forces created by fusion of the metatarsal-phalangeal joint in a cavus foot type with a congenitally long second metatarsal. (**b**) Revision takedown of a second metarsal-phalangeal joint fusion and replacement with hemi-metallic implant. Hemi-joint was placed following ORIF plating and healing of a second metatarsal fracture that was precipitated by fusion of the metatarsal-phalangeal joint. (Images courtesy of Marc Greenberg, DPM)

Fusion of the metatarsal-phalangeal joint increases the lever-arm axis of the metatarsal that potentially increases stress on the metatarsal and pressure on the plantar foot. Dorsal angulation of the phalanx can increase this stress by creating a retrograde force. This can result in fracture of the metatarsal shaft with weight-bearing (Fig. 26.9a *metatarsal fracture secondary to fusion*). In circumstances where a congenitally long digit, long lesser metatarsal, short first metatarsal, cavus foot type, or hypermobile first ray further contributes to a potential overloading syndrome, the author will concomitantly perform a proximal interphalangeal joint arthroplasty in combination with transverse osteotomy technique to maximize shortening of the metatarsal rather than utilizing a curettage technique for removal of articular cartilage. The combination of arthroplasty and transverse osteotomy techniques naturally provides the greatest effective reduction of the metatarsal lever arm; however care must be taken to avoid over shortening of the digit which may result in a flail toe (Fig. 26.10 *flail toe*). Aggressive removal of bone from the metatarsal head and proximal phalanx may also limit options for placement of internal fixation in a region already noted to have significantly less cubic bone content than the first metatarsal-phalangeal joint, a factor that potentially limits fusion healing and durability.

Salvage considerations for these complications include conversion of the fusion to implant arthroplasty or amputation (Fig. 26.9b *Stress fracture of metatarsal following fusion that required take down*).

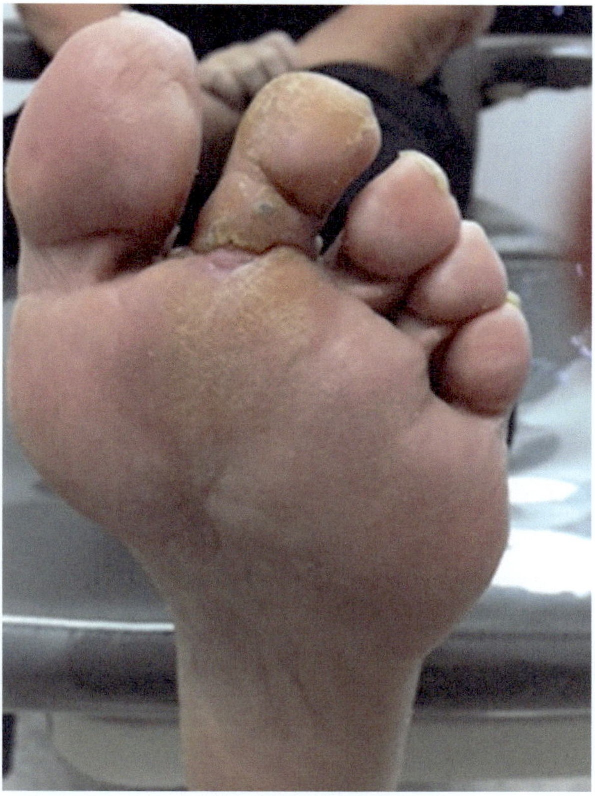

Fig. 26.10 Preulcerative hyperkeratosis caused by excessive retrograde pressure from a metatarsal-phalangeal joint fusion in a patient with a congenitally long second metatarsal and mild cavus foot type. (Images courtesy of Marc Greenberg, DPM)

References

1. Myerson MS, Jung HG. The role of toe flexor-to-extensor transfer in correcting metatarsophalangeal joint instability of the second toe. Foot Ankle Int. 2005;26:675–9.
2. Umans HR, Elsinger E. The plantar plate of the lesser metatarsophalangeal joints: potential for injury and role of MR imaging. Magn Reson Imaging Clin N Am. 2001;9:659–69. xii
3. Deland JT, Sung IH. The medial crosssover toe: a cadaveric dissection. Foot Ankle Int. 2000;21:375–8.
4. Goldner JL, Ward WG. Traumatic horizontal deviation of the second toe: mechanism of deformity, diagnosis, and treatment. Bull Hosp Jt Dis Orthop Inst. 1987;47:123–35.
5. Mendicino RW, Statler TK, Saltrick KR, Catanzariti AR. Predislocation syndrome: a review and retrospective analysis of eight patients. J Foot Ankle Surg. 2001;40:214–24.
6. Deland JT, Lee KT, Sobel M, DiCarlo EF. Anatomy of the plantar plate and its attachments in the lesser metatarsal phalangeal joint. Foot Ankle Int. 1995;16:480–6.
7. Fortin PT, Myerson MS. Second metatarsophalangeal joint instability. Foot Ankle Int. 1995;16:306–13.
8. Bhatia D, Myerson MS, Curtis MJ, Cunningham BW, Jinnah RH. Anatomical restraints to dislocation of the second metatarsophalangeal joint and assessment of a repair technique. J Bone Joint Surg Am. 1994;76:1371–5.
9. Baravarian B, Thompson J, Nazarian D. Plantar plate tears: a review of the modified flexor tendon transfer repair for stabilization. Clin Podiatr Med Surg. 2011;28:57–68.

10. Lehman DE, Smith RW. Treatment of symptomatic hammertoe with a proximal interphalangeal joint arthrodesis. Foot Ankle Int. 1995;16:535–41.
11. Mesiha M, Zurakowski D, Soriano J, Nielson JH, Zarins B, Murray MM. Pathologic characteristics of the torn human meniscus. Am J Sports Med. 2007;35:103–12.
12. Gregg J, Marks P, Silberstein M, Schneider T, Kerr J. Histologic anatomy of the lesser metatarsophalangeal joint plantar plate. Surg Radiol Anat. 2007;29:141–7.
13. Ellington JK, Jones CP, Cohen BE, Davis WH, Nickisch F, Anderson RB. Review of 107 hallux MTP joint arthrodesis using dome-shaped reamers and a stainless-steel dorsal plate. Foot Ankle Int. 2010;31:385–90.
14. Karlock LG. Second metatarsophalangeal joint fusion: a new technique for crossover hammertoe deformity. A preliminary report. J Foot Ankle Surg. 2003;42:178–82.
15. Hamilton GA, Ford LA, Patel S. First metatarsophalangeal joint arthrodesis and revision arthrodesis. Clin Podiatr Med Surg. 2009;26:459–73. Table of Contents
16. Stainsby GD. Pathological anatomy and dynamic effect of the displaced plantar plate and the importance of the integrity of the plantar plate-deep transverse metatarsal ligament tie-bar. Ann R Coll Surg Engl. 1997;79:58–68.
17. Johnston RB 3rd, Smith J, Daniels T. The plantar plate of the lesser toes: an anatomical study in human cadavers. Foot Ankle Int. 1994;15:276–82.
18. Bouche RT, Heit EJ. Combined plantar plate and hammertoe repair with flexor digitorum longus tendon transfer for chronic, severe sagittal plane instability of the lesser metatarsophalangeal joints: preliminary observations. J Foot Ankle Surg. 2008;47:125–37.
19. Hansen ST. Functional reconstruction of the foot and ankle in. Philadelphia: Lippincott Williams and Wilkins; 2000. p. 31.
20. Heinegard D, Saxne T. The role of the cartilage matrix in osteoarthritis. Nat Rev Rheumatol. 2011;7:50–6.
21. Joseph RM. Osteoarthritis of the ankle: bridging concepts in basic science with clinical care. Clin Podiatr Med Surg. 2009;26:169–84.
22. Amalinei C, Caruntu ID, Giusca SE, Balan RA. Matrix metalloproteinases involvement in pathologic conditions. Romanian J Morphol Embryol. 2010;51:215–28.
23. Jeffries LC, Rodriguez RH, Stapleton JJ, Zgonis T. Pan-metatarsophalangeal joint arthrodesis for the severe rheumatoid forefoot deformity. Clin Podiatr Med Surg. 2009;26:149–57.

Chapter 27
Flail Toe Correction: Interpositional Bone Graft and Syndactylization Approaches

Michael S. Downey

Presentation/History

The flail toe or floppy toe deformity is a condition in which one or more toes of a foot lack stability and structural integrity as the result of excessive bone loss (from surgery, infection, trauma, or tumor) and/or gross motor instability from resection or overlengthening of the tendinous structures to the toe. Excessive resection of bone during the performance of a proximal interphalangeal joint arthroplasty is the most common etiology, but the actual rate of flail or floppy toe following the arthroplasty procedure has not been reported in the literature [1]. The flail or floppy toe deformity should be differentiated from a floating toe deformity or syndrome. McGlamry [2] defined "floating toe syndrome" as a condition in which one or more toes on a foot fail to purchase the weight-bearing surface of the ground during stance or gait. The floating toe deformity is typically at the level of the metatarsophalangeal joint and results from insufficient loading of the plantar plate during stance and gait. Floating toe deformity is commonly seen following shortening or elevating metatarsal osteotomies; following a plantar plate tear, with congenital brachymetatarsia; or following any condition that causes the flexor mechanism and plantar plate of a toe to function inadequately and improperly load during weight-bearing.

M. S. Downey (✉)
Division of Podiatric Surgery, Penn Presbyterian Medical Center, Philadelphia, PA, USA

Department of Surgery, Temple University School of Podiatric Medicine, Philadelphia, PA, USA

The Podiatry Institute, Decatur, GA, USA

Private Practice, Philadelphia, PA/Southern NJ, USA
e-mail: Michael.Downey@uphs.upenn.edu

E. A. Cook, J. J. Cook (eds.), *Hammertoes*,
https://doi.org/10.1007/978-3-319-16552-3_27

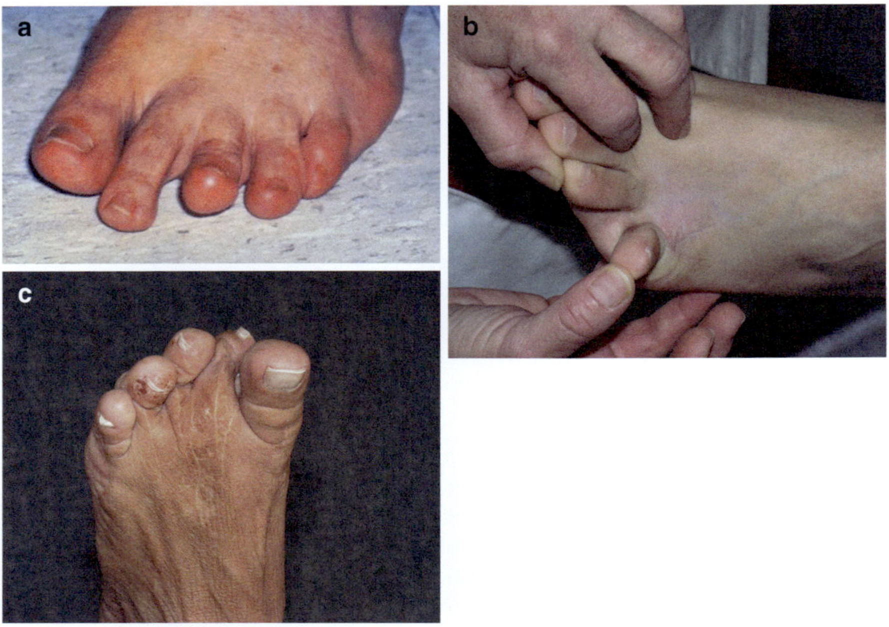

Fig. 27.1 (**a**) Flail third toe. Note the toe has no inherent stability and is shortened due to previous surgical bone removal from the toe. (**b**) Floppy fifth toe after excessive removal of bone from proximal interphalangeal joint (PIPJ) arthroplasty. (**c**) Multiple flail and floppy toes following lesser digital PIPJ arthroplasties with excessive bone resection

The patient with a flail or floppy toe deformity typically presents with a toe that is short, often deformed, and usually lacking functional motor control (Fig. 27.1a–c). The patient will often complain of instability and pain in the toe when trying to apply hosiery or shoes, when the toe bends back upon itself. Patients also frequently complain of burning pain, instability of the toe when standing or walking, metatarsalgia, and cosmetic concerns [3].

Conservative measures for the flail or floppy toe deformity are primarily palliative and include strappings, taping, splints, pads, extra-depth shoes, insoles or orthotics, and pain management modalities such as nonsteroidal anti-inflammatory drugs (NSAIDs) and corticosteroid injections. Surgical procedures for the correction of the flail and floppy toe generally attempt to stabilize and/or lengthen the involved toe. Numerous surgical procedures have been described in the literature, including syndactylization to an adjacent toe [4, 5], implant arthroplasty [6], free autogenous or allogenous bone graft arthrodesis of the proximal interphalangeal joint [1, 3, 7], and gradual bone graft lengthening with autologous bone graft and external fixation [8]. Amputation of the involved toe has also been described when the pain in the toe is intractable and other methods have failed or are contraindicated [9].

Diagnosis/Assessment

Assessment of the flail or floppy toe deformity involves both a clinical examination and weight-bearing radiographs of the involved foot. The clinical examination should include assessments of the digital parabola, passive and active range of motion of the toes including the involved toe, and an evaluation of the neurovascular status of the involved toe. Weight-bearing radiographs of the foot will assist in this assessment and also allow an inspection of the bone stock within the involved toe and surrounding toes. If the contralateral foot is normal and uninvolved, radiographs of that foot be may be desirable to allow comparisons between normal and abnormal. The attitude of the affected toe in all three cardinal body planes should be determined along with the status of the metatarsophalangeal joint.

Once a flail or floppy toe is diagnosed, and after conservative measures have failed or proven insufficient, surgery can be considered. The surgical options include the following:

- Soft tissue rebalancing and reconstruction
- Implant arthroplasty
- PIPJ arthrodesis
- Bone graft lengthening
- Syndactylization
- Amputation

The patient's age, health, neurovascular status, activity level, desired shoe gear, and severity of deformity will all be factors in the choice of the optimal surgical approach. If the deformity is primarily soft tissue in nature, then soft tissue rebalancing and reconstruction (as discussed elsewhere in this text) would be the preferred approach. If the toe has sufficient remaining bone stock, a proximal interphalangeal joint (PIPJ) implant arthroplasty and PIPJ end-to-end arthrodesis without a bone graft are the favored approaches. Quite often with the flail or floppy toe, the toe is short and has a loss of bone stock. In this situation, a bone graft lengthening of the toe should be considered. Syndactylization of the unstable toe to a contiguous toe is a salvage approach that can be considered when the patient is not a good candidate for a soft tissue and/or bone reconstructive procedure or has failed other surgical reconstructive attempts. Finally, amputation is always an alternative when other approaches have failed or if the patient's age, health, and neurovascular status combine to make reconstructive approaches contraindicated. With any of the surgical approaches, the long-term biomechanical effect of the foot and function should always be considered.

Surgical Techniques

In this chapter, bone graft lengthening and syndactylization procedures will be discussed.

Bone Graft Lengthening Approach/Outcomes

The bone graft lengthening procedure typically involves an interpositional, autogenous bone graft utilized to span the void created by previous bone loss (Fig. 27.2a, b). Most commonly, the bone loss in a flail or floppy toe is at the PIPJ level, and the bone graft will be used to bridge the gap between the distal aspect of the remaining stump of the proximal phalanx and the proximal aspect of the base of the middle phalanx. The bone graft when healed will be creating a consolidated bone of the proximal and middle phalanges, mimicking the result obtained with a PIPJ arthrodesis procedure. Due to the small, coronal cross section of a phalangeal bone, and the likely impaired vascularity of the previously resected bone, an interpositional autogenous bone graft is preferred to allogenous bone grafts.

The surgery is done with the patient in the supine position and most commonly with the use of an ankle tourniquet for hemostasis (Fig. 27.3a, b). Ideally, the toe should be addressed first as intraoperative measurements are preferred for determining how much autogenous bone will be needed. The area of previous bone loss is

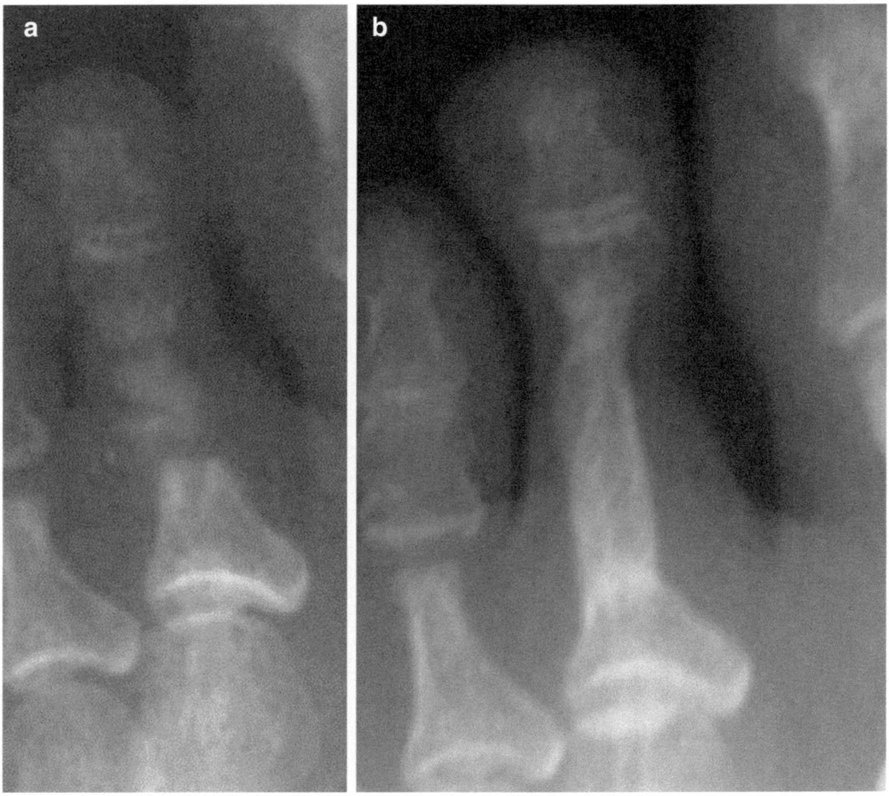

Fig. 27.2 (**a–b**) Preoperative and postoperative radiographs of patient having undergone an interpositional bone graft reconstruction of a flail toe

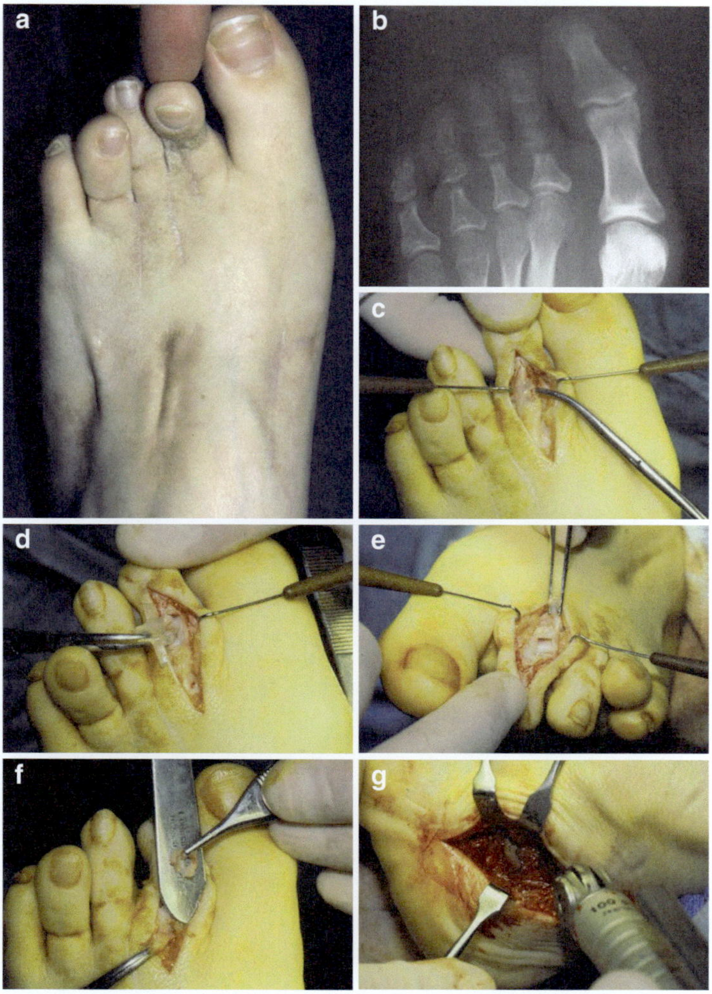

Fig. 27.3 – Interpositional bone graft reconstruction of flail second toe. (**a**, **b**) Preoperative and radiographic appearance of flail second toe. Note excessive bone removal at PIPJ level and interposed Swanson-type silicone implant. (**c**, **d**). Initial surgical exposure of second toe with removal of the implant. (**e**, **f**) Removal of all fibrous tissue present and freshening of bone ends of distal aspect of proximal phalanx and proximal aspect of base of middle phalanx. Measurements are then taken for the amount of bone graft required. (**g**, **h**) Corticocancellous, autogenous bone graft harvested from the ipsilateral, lateral calcaneal wall. Note the retained fixation staple from a previous Dwyer calcaneal osteotomy. Bone graft removal done with a combination of power saw and osteotomes. (**i**, **j**) Resulting donor defect in lateral calcaneus is backfilled with osteoconductive bone graft material. (**k**) The bone graft is carefully contoured into its final shape for insertion into the toe. (**l**) The bone graft is sequentially, longitudinally skewered with a K-wire. (**m**) K-wire with skewered bone graft driven centrally through the middle phalanx and distal toe. (**n**) K-wire then retrograded into the proximal phalanx and in this case across the second metatarsophalangeal joint. (**o**, **p**). Final clinical and radiographic appearance of the foot on the day of surgery. (**q**, **r**). Three-year follow-up clinical and radiographic appearance. Note the graft has fully incorporated and healed to both the proximal and middle phalanges and a stable, functional toe has resulted with a good digital parabola

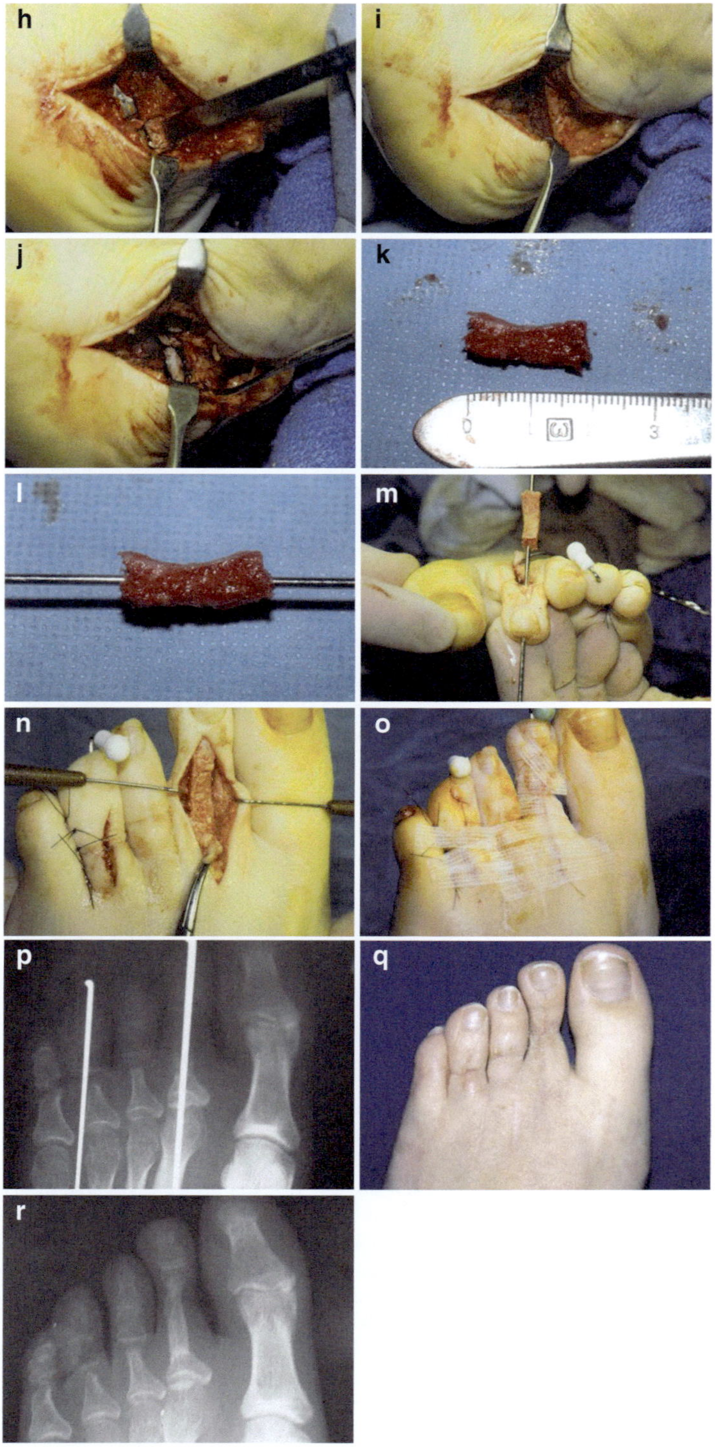

Fig. 27.3 (continued)

opened and explored, and all intervening fibrous tissue is excised (Fig. 27.3c–f). The bone ends that will oppose the bone graft are then resected and/or freshened utilizing a combination of bone cutting forceps, bone rongeur, or small power burr (2 mm ball type) until good, bleeding bone is achieved. In the case of a PIPJ bone graft procedure, the base of the middle phalanx may not have been previously resected, and in such cases the cartilage and subchondral bone plate must be fully resected. All resections should be done in tabletop fashion to achieve good postoperative alignment of the toe. Once the interpositional bone graft bed site has been prepared, measurements are taken to determine the amount of bone graft needed. A smooth lamina spreader, or similar instrument, may be helpful in distracting the site and assessing the optimal length to be achieved. The goal of the bone graft lengthening is not always to achieve the maximal length possible but a length that ideally restores a more normal digital parabola and restores weight-bearing function and propulsion to the toe.

Once appropriate measurements have been taken, the donor site for the autogenous bone graft can be opened. There are many potential sites for obtaining an autogenous bone graft for this technique, but the lateral calcaneus is the consensus preferred location. Most commonly, an incision will be made over the posterior-lateral calcaneal body, just posterior to the peroneal tendons and sural nerve, and the graft will be harvested from the superior-central shoulder of the posterior calcaneal body or the lateral wall of the calcaneus (Fig. 27.3g–j). Harvesting of autogenous calcaneal bone grafts has been well described in the literature with a low rate of complications [10]. The harvested, autogenous bone graft should be a rectangular-shaped, corticocancellous graft, with one or two sides of cortical bone. The graft donor site can be backfilled with any osteoconductive bone graft substitute material, although materials that harden in situ are preferred.

Next, the harvested graft is carefully fashioned into its final shape using a combination of power saw, bone cutting forceps, and bone rongeur (Fig. 27.3k). The graft is then carefully stabilized and a 0.035″ (0.9 mm) Kirschner wire (i.e., K-wire) is passed longitudinally through the graft in essence skewering the graft. The 0.035″ (0.9 mm) K-wire is then removed, and sequentially a 0.045″ (1.1 mm) K-wire and then a 0.062″ (1.6 mm) K-wire are passed through the channel created previously by the 0.035″ (0.9 mm) K-wire. A 0.062″ (1.6 mm) K-wire is preferred for final fixation, and once inserted through the graft, that K-wire is not removed (Fig. 27.3l). The K-wire is then passed centrally through the base of the middle phalanx and driven distally until it exits the distal pulp of the toe (Fig. 27.3m). Again, using the 0.035″ (0.9 mm) K-wire and the 0.045″ (1.1 mm) K-wire, a channel is created in the distal aspect of the proximal phalangeal stump. The 0.062″ (1.6 mm) K-wire is then driven into the channel created by these K-wires in the proximal phalanx (Fig. 27.3n). If the metatarsophalangeal joint necessitated concomitant release and realignment, the 0.062″ (1.6 mm) K-wire may be driven across the metatarsophalangeal joint maintaining it in the desired alignment (Fig. 27.3o, p). If no correction of the metatarsophalangeal joint is needed, the K-wire may be maintained in the subchondral area of the proximal phalangeal base. If a tourniquet was utilized, it may be released prior to closure to ensure that good capillary refill returns to the surgically lengthened toe. Standard wound closure is then performed.

Postoperatively, the patient is maintained in a non-weight bearing cast or alternatively a CAM walker boot or padded surgical shoe that off-loads the toe and decreases any potential for K-wire fatigue and breakage. The K-wire is typically maintained in place for a minimum of 6 weeks and preferably for 8 weeks. Serial radiographs are performed to assess osseous consolidation and the optimal time for K-wire removal. If the K-wire crossed the metatarsophalangeal joint, a short course of physical therapy for the joint may be needed. Once healed, the patient is permitted to return to all activities and shoes to tolerance (Fig. 27.3q, r).

Since first being described in 1992 [7], the reported outcomes of the interpositional, autogenous, bone graft reconstruction for the flail and floppy toe have been very good. In a retrospective analysis, Mahan, Downey, and Weinfeld [3] reported on 22 procedures in 13 patients. Their mean patient age was 49.6 years old (range: 22–68 years old), and their mean follow-up time was 27 months (range: 4–48 months). In their study, all of the patients had autogenous bone grafts – 18 from the ipsilateral calcaneus, 1 from the medial aspect of the first metatarsal head, 1 from the head of the fifth metatarsal, 1 from the third metatarsal neck, and 1 from the fourth metatarsal neck. They described a successful result as reduction of pain, correction of toe length, correction of deformity, improvement in toe stability, and consolidation of the bone graft with at least one graft-host junction union at either the proximal or distal site. Using this criteria, 18/22 (82%) of the procedures were successful initially, and 20/22 (91%) were successful after one additional surgery. The mean consolidation time at the proximal bone graft-host junction was 15.9 weeks (range: 8.5–37.0 weeks) and for the distal bone graft-host junction was 14.5 weeks (range: 8.5 –24.0 weeks). The mean consolidation time for both junctional sites in the same toe was 15.56 weeks. At the proximal bone graft-host junction, 2/22 (9%) had a nonunion, and in one case (5%) the bone graft resorbed. At the distal bone graft-host junction, 1/22 (5%) resulted in a nonunion, and in one case (5%) the bone graft resorbed. Thus, 3 nonunions occurred (2 proximal and 1 distal) at the 44 graft-host sites (7%), and 1 graft (5%) showed complete resorption. Upon clinical examination, the authors noted that the successfully repaired toes remained stable, had an improved digital parabola, had restored flexor power, and had reduced pain. No digital ischemia or vascular complications were found in this series.

In 2010, Myerson and Filippi found similarly successful results in their series of flail and floppy toes [1, 11]. They reported on 13 cases of the bone graft reconstructive technique used for flail toes. Their mean patient age was 43 years old (range: 23–72 years old), and they followed 12 of the 13 patients (one was lost to follow-up) for a mean time of 31 months (range: 6–70 months). In the 12 patients available for follow-up, 3 had a calcaneal autograft, and 9 had an iliac crest autograft. Consolidation of the bone grafts occurred in 9/12 (75%) of their patients. At final follow-up, these authors concluded that 7/12 (58%) of their patients were asymptomatic, 3/12 (25%) patients had persistent metatarsalgia, and 2/12 (17%) patients had stiffness at the corresponding metatarsophalangeal joint. Eleven of the 12 patients (92%) stated they would undergo the procedure again. In these authors' series, 2/12 (17%) patients had ischemic complications in the distal toe tip, with one (8%) of the patients having a resultant 2 mm loss of tissue at the toe tip.

In 2009, Lamm and Ades [8] described a case report where a 2-stage surgical reconstructive procedure was done to lengthen a flail toe. Stage one involved excision of the scar tissue at the proposed graft site with the application of an external fixation device to distract the toe out to an appropriate length. Stage 2 involved the insertion of an autogenous calcaneal bone graft into the void created by the distraction. The second stage was done approximately 5 weeks after the first stage, and the external fixator was removed after 10 weeks. No neurovascular compromise was noted, and complete consolidation of the bone graft was noted at 3 months follow-up. The authors noted that at 5 months postoperative, the patient was pleased with both the cosmetic and functional results of the surgery.

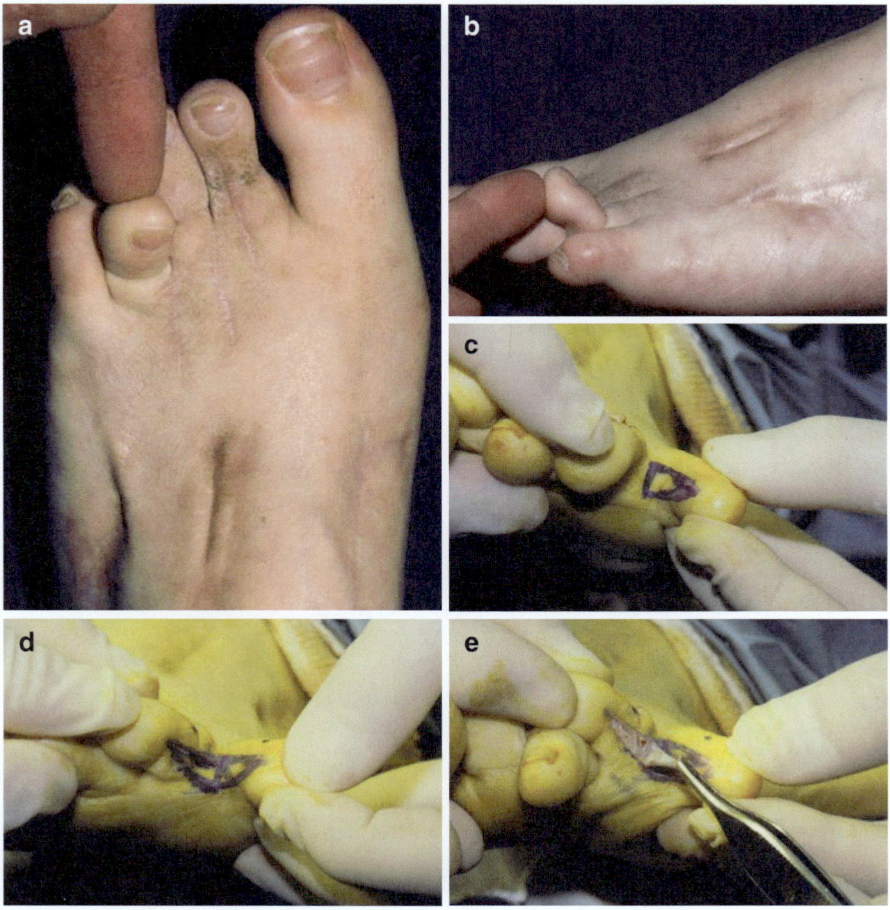

Fig. 27.4 – Syndactyly of floppy fourth toe to stable fifth toe. (**a**, **b**) Preoperative clinical appearance of floppy fourth toe. (**c**) Drawing of skin wedge to be excised. (**d**) Transfer of mirror image of skin wedge to corresponding toe. (**e**) Excision of skin wedge. (**f**) Loose placement of sutures prior to tightening and final closure. (**g**, **h**) Three-year clinical appearance of syndactylized fourth and fifth toes. The toes have remained stable and in good alignment

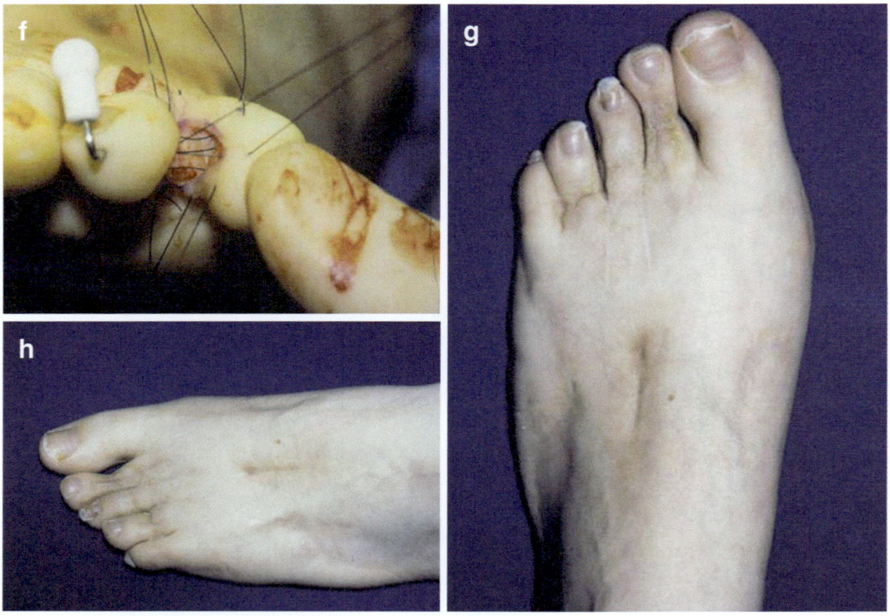

Fig. 27.4 (continued)

Syndactylization Approach/Outcomes

The syndactylization approach typically involves the anastomosis of the affected flail or floppy toe to a neighboring more stable toe (Fig. 27.4a, b). The procedure is often considered a "webbing" of two toes together, although describing it in this fashion to a patient will almost assuredly be met with a negative response due to the stigma associated with the thought of a toe "webbing" procedure. The procedure does eliminate the web space between the two involved toes and relies on a more stable toe to maintain correction of an unstable, flail, or floppy toe [12, 13]. The syndactylization of two adjacent toes can also be performed to eliminate a recalcitrant, interdigital heloma molle or other interdigital skin pathology [14]. The use of syndactylization has also been described as an adjunctive procedure in the salvage reconstruction of a subluxated, dislocated, and/or degenerative lesser metatarsophalangeal joint [15]. It should be noted that syndactyly has limited ability to correct and maintain length of a shortened toe and the potential exists for the unstable toe to "pull" the more stable toe into a position of deformity, resulting in continued instability of the toes and a poor cosmetic result.

The surgery is done with the patient in the supine position and most commonly with the use of an ankle tourniquet for hemostasis. A surgical skin marker, preferably one with gentian violet ink, is used to carefully mark out the skin wedge to be removed on one of the toes (Fig. 27.4c). Carefully placing the most dorsal aspect of the proposed incision slightly down the side of the toe and just short of the end of the toe will allow the appearance of a cleft or space between the webbed toes, improving the cosmetic outcome. Once the planned skin wedge has been marked on a toe, the deformed toe can be pulled to its desired position on the corresponding stable toe. The two toes are then pressed together transferring the mirror image of the previous ink impression on from one toe to the other (Fig. 27.4d). Once this has been accomplished, the resulting skin ellipse between the two toes is excised (Fig. 27.4e). It should be remembered that this is only a skin ellipse, and there is no need to make the incisions into the subcutaneous tissue. By so doing, there should be no violation of the subcutaneous neurovascular structures when the procedure is done optimally. In the case of a recalcitrant heloma molle or interdigital lesion, the skin ellipse will include the excrescence. Again, if desired, the tourniquet can be released and good hemostasis achieved as needed prior to closure. Closure of the syndactylization is then performed with nonabsorbable skin sutures only. Placement of all of the skin sutures loosely and untied first allows easier visibility during their insertion, and optimal cosmetic closure (Fig. 27.4f).

Postoperatively, the patient is allowed to heel weight bear immediately in a surgical shoe. Light walking is permitted until suture removal at 2–3 weeks. Postoperative splinting for an additional 2–3 weeks is sometimes desirable to aid in the maintenance of the correction (Fig. 27.4g, h).

The recent literature is sparse regarding the outcomes following surgical syndactylization of the lesser toes for a flail or floppy toe deformity, as most of the reports center on desyndactylization techniques and results. Bartel [12] provided a literature review of the results of syndactylization of the lesser toes and concluded that syndactylization "is an excellent salvage technique for flail toes." Reported complications included infection, hematoma, and wound dehiscence. Instability and recurrent deformity were noted to occur more frequently if the webbing is not carried distally enough, if it is too small in its size, or if the deforming musculotendinous and contracture of the flail or floppy toe are not adequately addressed. A patient's preoperative concerns regarding the cosmetic result of toe webbing can usually be allayed through preoperative counseling, including a discussion of appropriate patient expectations.

References

1. Myerson MS, Filippi J. Interphalangeal joint lengthening arthrodesis for the treatment of the flail toe. Foot ankle Int [Internet]. 2010 [cited 2016 Jan 11];31(10):851–6. Available from: http://www.ncbi.nlm.nih.gov/pubmed/20964962.
2. McGlamry ED. Floating toe syndrome. J Am Podiatry Assoc [Internet]. 1982 [cited 2016 Jan 11];72(11):561–8. Available from: http://www.ncbi.nlm.nih.gov/pubmed/7142651.
3. Mahan KT, Downey MS, Weinfeld GD. Autogenous bone graft interpositional arthrodesis for the correction of flail toe. A retrospective analysis of 22 procedures. J Am Podiatr Med Assoc

[Internet]. 2016 [cited 2016 Jan 11];93(3):167–73. Available from: http://www.ncbi.nlm.nih.gov/pubmed/12756306.
4. Marek L, Giacopelli J, Granoff D. Syndactylization for the treatment of fifth toe deformities. J Am Podiatr Med Assoc [Internet]. 1991 [cited 2016 Jan 11];81(5):248–52. Available from: http://www.ncbi.nlm.nih.gov/pubmed/2061821.
5. Stewart WP. Syndactylism in podiatric surgery. Clin Podiatr Med Surg [Internet]. 1986 [cited 2016 Jan 11];3(1):65–76. Available from: http://www.ncbi.nlm.nih.gov/pubmed/2937524.
6. Sgarlato TE, Tafuri SA. Digital implant arthroplasty. Clin Podiatr Med Surg [Internet]. 1996 [cited 2016 Jan 11];13(2):255–62. Available from: http://www.ncbi.nlm.nih.gov/pubmed/9118016.
7. Mahan KT. Bone graft reconstruction of a flail digit. J Am Podiatr Med Assoc [Internet]. 1992 [cited 2016 Jan 11];82(5):264–8. Available from: http://www.ncbi.nlm.nih.gov/pubmed/1640375.
8. Lamm BM, Ades JK. Gradual digital lengthening with autologous bone graft and external fixation for correction of flail toe in a patient with Raynaud's disease. J Foot Ankle Surg [Internet]. 2009 [cited 2016 Jan 11];48(4):488–94. Available from: http://www.ncbi.nlm.nih.gov/pubmed/19577729.
9. Field LM. An "ultimate solution" for a painful toe. J Dermatol Surg Oncol [Internet]. 1979 [cited 2016 Jan 11];5(5):402–3. Available from: http://www.ncbi.nlm.nih.gov/pubmed/458008
10. Mahan KT, Hillstrom HJ. Bone grafting in foot and ankle surgery. A review of 300 cases. J Am Podiatr Med Assoc [Internet]. 1998;88(3):109–18. Available from: http://www.ncbi.nlm.nih.gov/pubmed/9542352.
11. Myerson MS, Filippi J. Bone block lengthening of the proximal interphalangeal joint for managing the floppy toe deformity. Foot Ankle Clin [Internet]. 2010 [cited 2016 Jan 11];15(4):663–8. Available from: http://www.ncbi.nlm.nih.gov/pubmed/21056864.
12. Bartel E. Syndactylization of the lesser toes. Oper Tech Orthop. 1999;9(1):51–4.
13. Jahss MH. Chronic and recurrent dislocations of the fifth toe. Foot Ankle Int. 1981;1(5):275–8.
14. Kurtz CM, Guthrie JD Jr. Syndactylization: a surgical approach to heloma molle. J Foot Surg [Internet]. 1984;23(5):407–9. Available from: http://www.ncbi.nlm.nih.gov/htbin-post/Entrez/query?db=m&form=6&dopt=r&uid=0006094645.
15. Feeney S, Rees S, Tagoe M. Hemiphalengectomy and syndactylization for treatment of osteoarthritis and dislocation of the second metatarsal phalangeal joint: An outcome study. J Foot Ankle Surg. 2006;45(2):82–90.

Chapter 28
Recurrent Hammertoe Deformity

Elena Manning and Michael L. Sganga

Presentation/History

Hammertoe is a very common lesser toe deformity and accounts for 34% of all foot and ankle conditions in older adults [1]. Classically hammertoe surgery includes resection of the proximal interphalangeal joint [2]. Coughlin and others have shown that either a rigid or fibrous union does not have an effect on clinical outcome [2]. Many different fixation techniques are available ranging from a simple Kirschner wire to a wide variety of implants.

The most common complication of hammertoe surgery is floating toe, which is a continued hyperextension at the level of the MTPJ after arthroplasty. Other complications are distal IP joint plantar contracture after PIPJ fusion, non-unions or malunions, fibrous unions, pin-tract infection, and internal fixation displacement [3].

There are many reasons that patients are dissatisfied with the outcome of their surgeries. This is frequently due to unequal or unrealistic expectations, persistent pain, stiffness, and recurrent or residual deformity. A component of stiffness will almost always occur with hammertoe correction as the interphalangeal joint is being resected. We recommend that this should be discussed with the patient prior to surgery to ensure realistic expectations.

Recurrence can result from inadequate initial correction. Inadequate initial correction can occur due to improper fixation, malposition, or incorrect procedure selection.

E. Manning
Department of Surgery, Division of Podiatry, Mount Auburn Hospital, Cambridge, MA, USA

M. L. Sganga (✉)
Orthopedics New England, Natick, MA, USA

E. A. Cook, J. J. Cook (eds.), *Hammertoes*,
https://doi.org/10.1007/978-3-319-16552-3_28

Diagnosis/Assessment

As with all conditions, a detailed history of the problem and full examination are needed. One must fully examine the foot in comparison to the other foot and fully examine old scars. In addition any malalignment of the hallux must be appreciated and addressed. Examination of the hammertoe deformity should also include localizing the point of maximum tenderness and areas of subluxation or dislocation and assessing the flexibility of the deformity [4].

Conservative treatment options for recurrent issues are similar to treatment options of hammertoes at initial presentation. These options include but are not limited to footwear modifications, orthotics, physical therapy, strappings, medications, and the option to do nothing [4].

One of the most common deformities causing patient dissatisfaction after hammertoe surgery is recurrent flexion at the PIP joint and MTP joint extension. A common cause of recurrence after PIP joint fusion is DIP joint flexion contracture. This can present either rigid or flexible in nature. A percutaneous flexor tenotomy is easier to perform and has decreased risk of stiffness, but another option is a flexor to extensor tendon transfer although this can result in further stiffness. If it is rigid deformity at the DIP joint, then surgical options are to convert the PIP joint fusion to an excision arthroplasty with or without a flexor tenotomy [4].

Over-shortening should be avoided during the initial surgery and can lead to a flail toe. It is difficult to treat a recurrence due to over-shortening as length is difficult to reestablish. There are reports in the literature of regaining length with the use of a bone graft and transfixation wire [4]. Flail toes are extremely difficult to repair. In the literature revisional surgery for a flail toe includes amputation and syndactylization. However, these are often when all other treatment has failed. Syndactylization is preferred by this author in these cases as it preserves digital structure and if done properly can have a cosmetically pleasing result. Patients often find amputations difficult to accept and cosmetically displeasing.

Persistent swelling such as a “sausage toe” is another common complication, and edema can take 6–12 months to dissipate. Further surgery is not indicated for post-op edema in these cases. Compression using Coban or compression socks has shown improvement with time [4].

Recurrent hammertoe deformities in the coronal plane should be assessed at the level of the deformity. If there is coronal deformity of the toe at the level of the arthroplasty or arthrodesis, the bone cuts should be examined for inadequate or angled bone cuts. Surgical correction of these deformities would include revision surgery with repeat bone resection at the PIP joint with plantarflexory osteotomies. Other options could include wedge resections within the phalanx, but due to the size of the bone and limited fixation, it is very difficult to execute.

Treatment/ Surgical Technique

Surgical treatment of a recurrent hammertoe should be done on a case-by-case basis focusing on the etiology. Multiple factors need to be accounted for, and usually patient satisfaction is the key. There are many situations that can present: a revision of another surgeon's work, a late complication ranging from many months to several years out, or your own complication.

If it is your patient that has returned to you for revision, then they trust you, and all you have to do is focus on their concerns and the aspects of the surgery that did not turn out satisfactorily. This could mean bony regrowth at the fusion or arthroplasty site, extensor contracture, or even recurrence. In any case, have an open and honest discussion with your patient what is painful, what is displeasing, and what the patient wishes to accomplish in further treating the offending toe or toes. This does not always mean surgery, but when it does do not repeat the same mistake or pitfall. If there are extensor tendon contracture or scarring and a floating toe, address that with a skin plasty and tendon lengthening, and be aggressive to get the result you and the patient want.

The authors have found success when revision is undertaken following a very clear conversation about what will be addressed and when expectations are managed properly. We find it very helpful to add a plantar sulcus skin wedge excision or plasty to platarflex at the MTP joint and allow for some transverse plane correction by widening the wedge on the side needing tightening. This is often not visible to the patient and will require a few weeks of limited weight bearing, but typically we do not keep these patients non-weight bearing.

The authors prefer to start with an algorithm that takes on a stepwise approach. First, one should look at the toe clinically and then assess the MTP joint. Special attention must be paid to digital alignment overall, the PIPJ and DIPJ as well as the prior incision line. The motion and position of the toe as well as function of the flexors and extensors in both seated and full weight bearing should be evaluated. Finally, we progress to evaluate the foot as a whole to ensure there is no metatarsus adductus, first ray or great toe pathology, adjacent digits, or soft tissue pathology driving the recurrence. Careful assessment is key, and these authors then make notes of each alignment issue seen and ask the patient what aspects are bothersome and causing pain or issue.

A flexor tenotomy in office is a great procedure to address recurrence, tight flexors, or a stiff rigid digit. The authors utilize a technique with local anesthesia and an 18-gauge needle at the MTP joint sulcus from a lateral or medial approach. From this we can attain a release of the flexor tendons and even MTPJ or PIPJ capsule release if indicated. A pearl with this technique is to have the patient flex the digit against the bevel of the needle to resect the tendon and then apply a Steri-Strip to the area after the procedure. Patients are in a postoperative shoe for 7–10 days and can remove all dressings and shower at 3–5 days postoperative.

The key to success overall is to address the patients' concerns and be realistic with them regarding possible revision and outcomes.

Case: Failed Hammertoe

This is the case of a 68-year-old male with Parkinson's disease and shuffling gait. He has a history of rigid hammertoe deformities causing distal ulcerations *as well as a history of mallet toe on the right third toe. He had a flexor tenotomy done on*

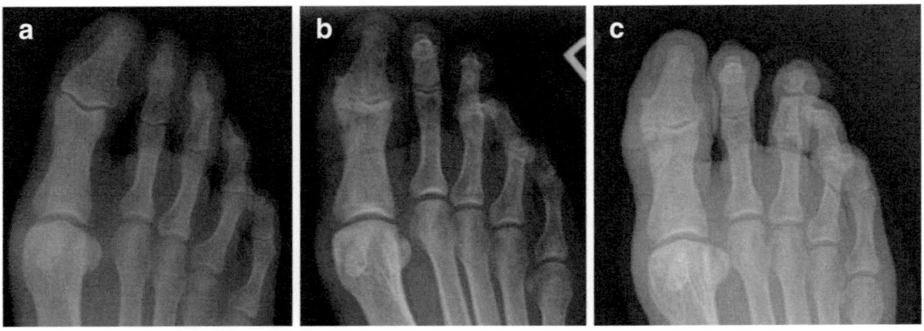

Fig. 28.1 Anterior-posterior weight-bearing radiographs. (**a**) Right third mallet toe presents with pre-ulcerative lesion. (**b**) Status post right third flexor tenotomy developing a rigid hammertoe deformity. (**c**) Status post DIPJ arthroplasty

the right third toe at the level of the MTPJ. This was done in an effort to correct his hammertoe deformity as he was having continued ulceration at the distal tuft of the toe secondary to his gait. He tried multiple forms of conservative treatment including gel toe caps but continued to have ulcerations which were at high risk for recurrent cellulitis. The flexor tenotomy allowed more flexibility at the deformity, yet over time the deformity reoccurred. Patient then developed a rigid hammertoe deformity needing a DIPJ arthroplasty which in this case resolved the issue (Fig. 28.1).

Clinical pearls/pitfalls

- Hammertoe deformities are very common, and recurrent deformity after surgery is unfortunately fairly common as well.
- It is important to assess for any other deformities driving the recurrence including first ray pathology and metatarsal phalangeal joint pathology. This is especially true with the hallux valgus and a great indication for a stand-alone akin procedure.
- It is most important to find the cause of the recurrence, and most importantly if it is due to incorrect procedure, initially do not repeat the same mistake. Thus initial examination, patient expectations, and procedure selection are key to success.

References

1. Jay RM, Malay SD, Landsman AS, Nathan J, Huish J, Younger M. Dual-component intramedullary implant versus Kirschner wire for proximal interphalangeal joint fusion: a randomized controlled clinical trial. J Foot Ankle Surg. 2016;55(4):697.
2. Klammer G, Baumann G, Moor BK, Farshad M, Espinosa N. Early complications and recurrence rates after Kirschner wire transfixion in lesser toe surgery: a prospective randomized study. Foot Ankle Int. 2012;33(2):105–12.
3. Kramer WC, Parman M, Marks RM. Hammertoe correction with k-wire fixation. Foot Ankle Int. 2015;36(5):494–502.
4. Solan MC, Davies MS. Revision surgery of the lesser toes. Foot Ankle Clin. 2011;16(4):621–45.

Chapter 29
Lesser Metatarsal Head with Avascular Necrosis and Revision PIPJ Distraction Arthrodesis

Jacob Wynes

Presentation/History

A 53-year-old female presents with a pertinent past medical history notable for prior right knee arthroscopy with meniscectomy, high tibial osteotomy, and notable prior left hallux valgus correction. Her presenting complaint was for left second digit medial drift and pain to the ball of her foot in keeping with collateral ligamentous disruption and elongated second metatarsal relative to the adjacent metatarsals (Fig. 29.1).

Initially, the patient underwent a Weil metatarsal osteotomy (WMO) in a dorsal distal to plantar proximal orientation, proximal interphalangeal joint (PIPJ) arthrodesis with intramedullary polyetheretherketone (PEEK) intramedullary implant, and collateral ligament repair. Restoration of the sagittal, frontal, and transverse plane was achieved (Fig. 29.2).

Nine months later, recurrence of the digital medial deviation and sub-metatarsal two pain was noted, and revision was performed including implant/hardware removal and Girdlestone flexor digitorum longus (FDL) tendon transfer in conjunction with insertion of a 0.062 inch Kirschner wire to maintain tri-planar position across the metatarsophalangeal joint (MTPJ) (Fig. 29.3).

Following this intervention, the patient's wire partially extruded, and subtle recurrence of the deformity developed in the transverse and sagittal plane. Thereafter, the patient was lost to follow up and did not return again until months later (Fig. 29.4).

J. Wynes, DPM, MS, FACFAS (✉)
Department of Orthopaedics, University of Maryland School of Medicine, Baltimore, MD, USA
e-mail: jwynes@som.umaryland.edu

E. A. Cook, J. J. Cook (eds.), *Hammertoes*,
https://doi.org/10.1007/978-3-319-16552-3_29

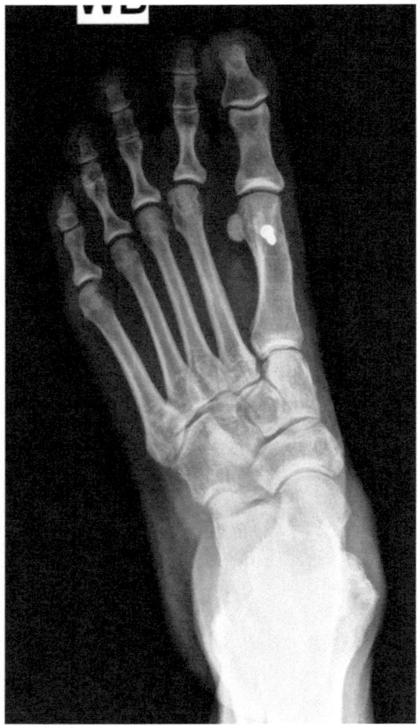

Fig. 29.1 Anterior-posterior (AP) plain film radiograph of the patient's initial presentation, with first metatarsal shortening, second metatarsal elongation, and complete lateral collateral ligamentous disruption of the second metatarsophalangeal joint

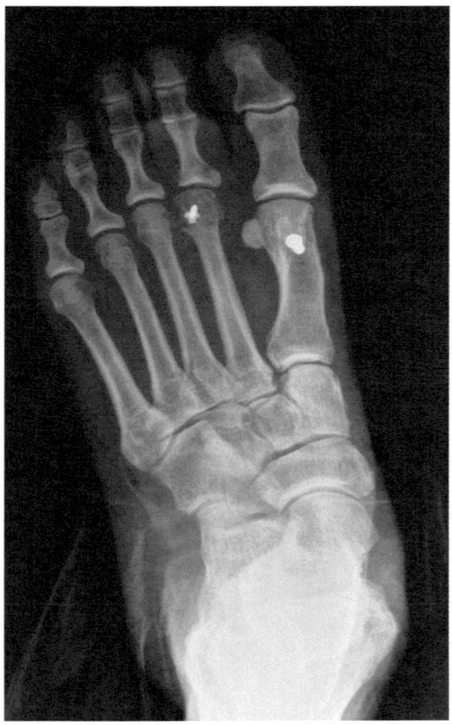

Fig. 29.2 AP radiograph demonstrating improvement in the anatomic parabola and improved transverse plane alignment

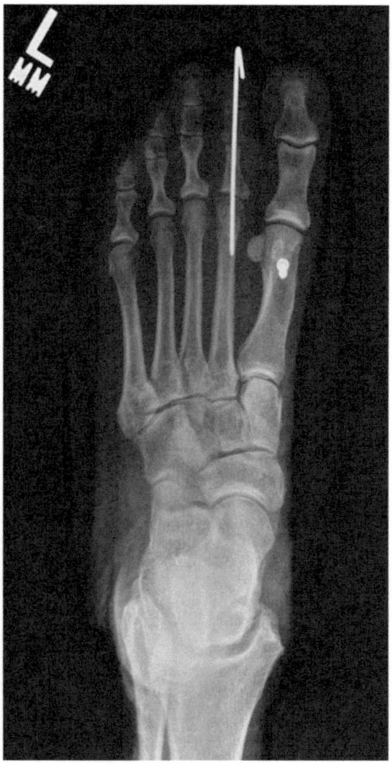

Fig. 29.3 AP radiograph illustrating removal of symptomatic intramedullary and second metatarsal implant with flexor digitorum longus (FDL) transfer and 0.062 inch Kirschner wire (K-wire) fixation

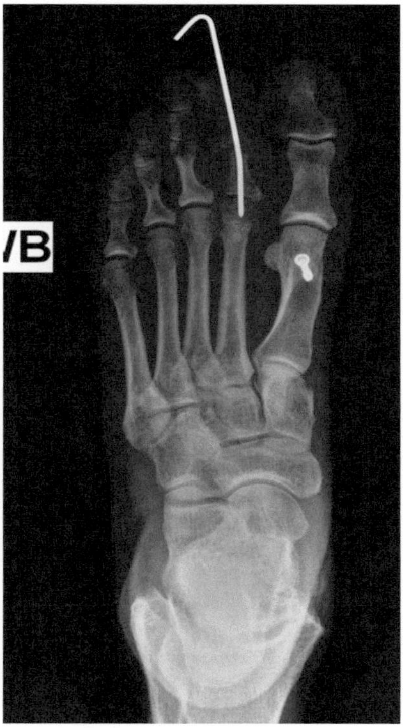

Fig. 29.4 AP radiograph depicting partial extrusion of the K-wire

Diagnosis/Assessment

Diagnosis at the time of definitive surgical intervention was hypertrophic nonunion of the second proximal interphalangeal joint and avascular necrosis of the second metatarsal with plantar plate/collateral ligament attenuation (Fig. 29.5a, b).

Treatment/Surgical Technique (Figs. 29.6 and 29.7)

Arthrodiastasis was achieved using a monolateral external fixator (Orthofix M100®, Lewisville, Tx) and distracting 2 mm acutely in association with core decompression of the metatarsal head using bone marrow aspirate concentrate (Arthrex® Angel system, Naples, Fl) harvested from the ipsilateral calcaneus. Deep bone culture and pathology were sent of the proximal phalanx and second metatarsal in addition which was negative (Figs. 29.8 and 29.9).

Outcomes/Case Resolution

The patient was allowed to weight bear in a controlled ankle motion (CAM) walker boot perioperatively. At 3 weeks, the patient developed a fracture of the proximal second metatarsal metaphysis, which ended up healing uneventfully (Fig. 29.10).

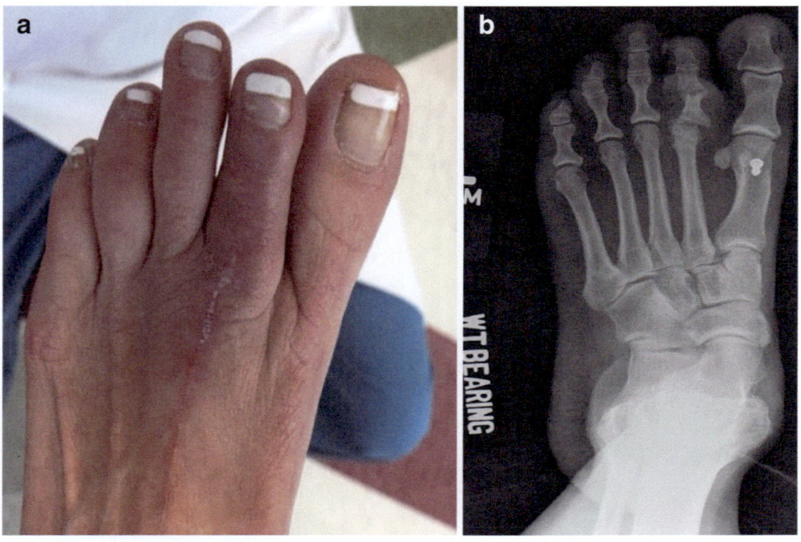

Fig. 29.5 (**a**, **b**) Clinical and radiographic presentation after loss to follow up with second MTPJ subluxation noted and recurrent transverse plane deformity. Patient reported symptomatic submetatarsal two pain and cosmetic concerns with respect to digital length

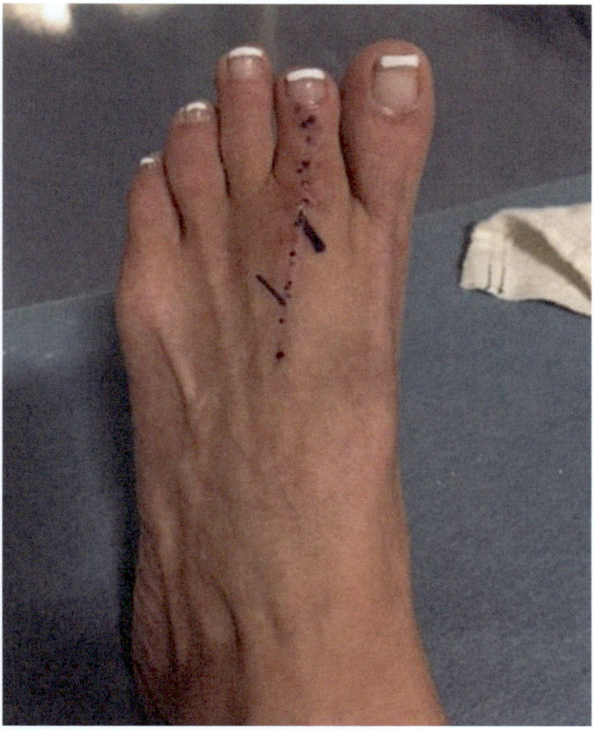

Fig. 29.6 Preoperative planning of skin incisions for lengthening skin Z-plasty and incisional approach for extensor digitorum longus lengthening, plantar plate reconstruction, metatarsophalangeal joint (MTPJ) lateral collateral ligament reconstruction, and interpositional PIPJ arthrodesis using calcaneal bone graft

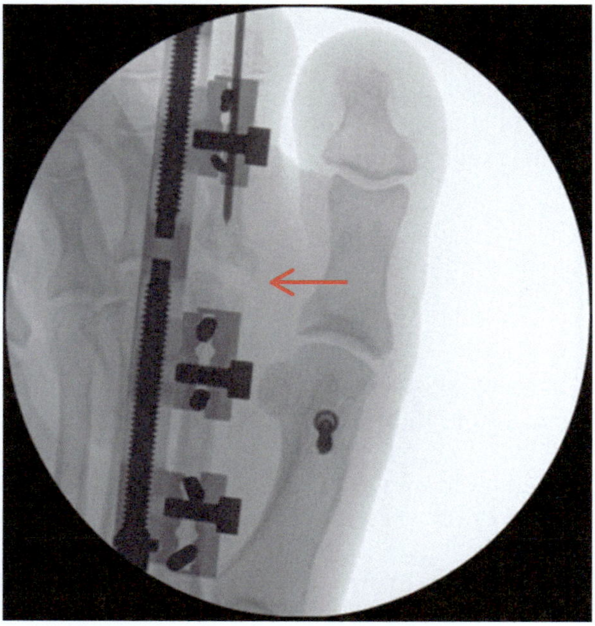

Fig. 29.7 Intraoperative fluoroscopy illustrating placement of monolateral fixator and acute 2 mm distraction (red arrow) and status post core decompression with bone marrow aspirate concentrate

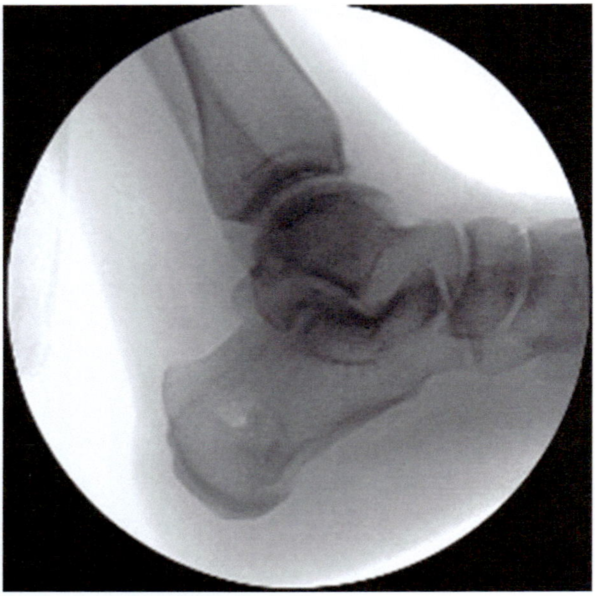

Fig. 29.8 Intraoperative fluoroscopy demonstrating site of unicortical autogenous bone graft harvested from the ipsilateral calcaneus

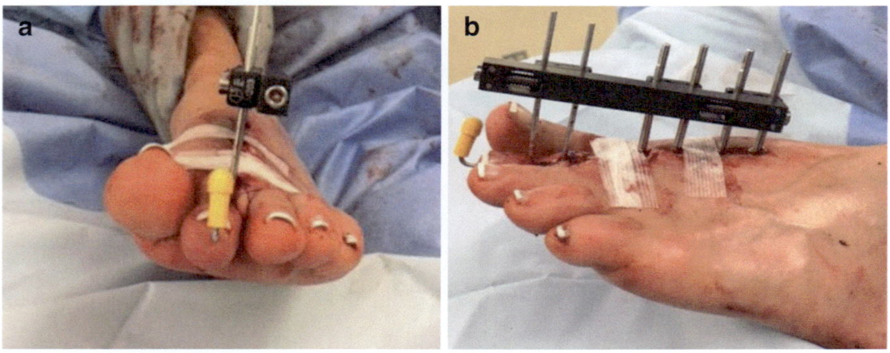

Fig. 29.9 (**a**, **b**) Intraoperative monolateral fixator construct depicting orthogonal pin placement and K-wire placement for the autogenous interpositional bone graft. Note, slight overcorrection with plantarflexion of the second MTPJ

Three-week status post definitive procedure with intact monolateral external fixator and 0.062 inch Kirschner wire within the PIPJ interpositional arthrodesis site (Fig. 29.11).

Once healing was confirmed at the proximal aspect of the second metatarsal, the patient's external fixator was removed in the office without issue under aseptic conditions (Fig. 29.12).

Months after external fixator removal, the patient remained active and able to perform all activities without pain or discomfort. Radiographic parameters show

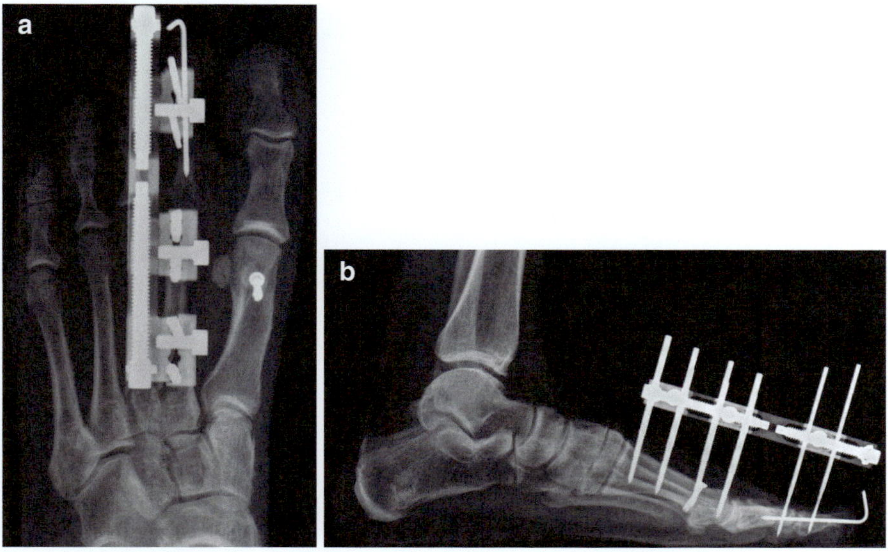

Fig. 29.10 (**a**, **b**) AP and lateral radiographs at 3-week follow-up with intact fixation and tri-planar correction achieved at the second MTPJ

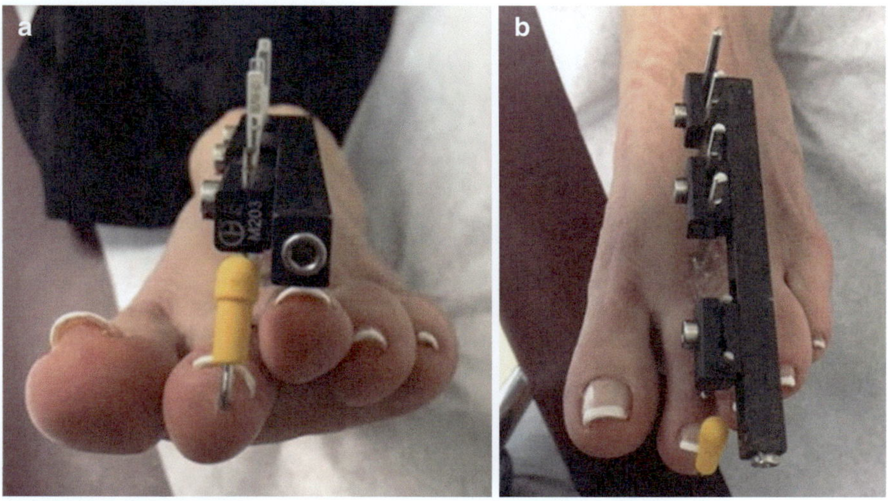

Fig. 29.11 (**a**, **b**) Clinical pictures 6 weeks postoperative demonstrating skin flap healing with restoration of length as well as sagittal and transverse plane alignment

restoration of the anatomic parabola and maintenance of trabeculation within the metatarsal head without further articular collapse. Clinically, the patient's active/passive dorsiflexion is to 35° at the second MTPJ and active/passive plantarflexion to 15°. There was a negative digital Lachman/dorsal drawer test in addition (Figs. 29.13, 29.14, and 29.15).

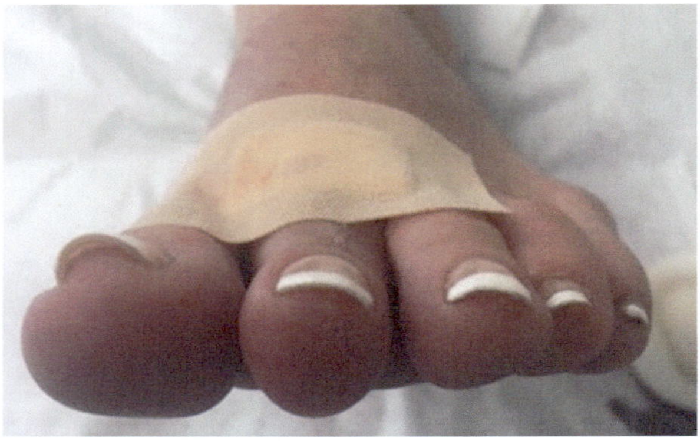

Fig. 29.12 Clinical picture of uneventful hardware removal of K-wire and monolateral external fixator

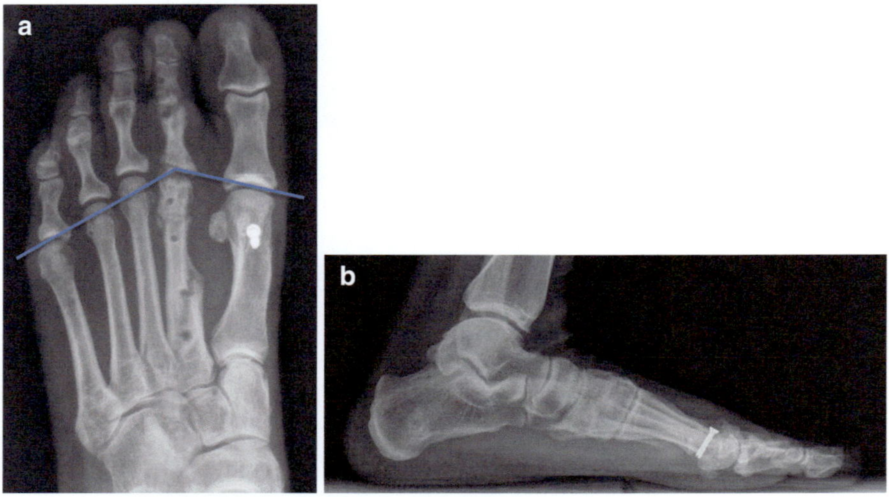

Fig. 29.13 (**a**, **b**) AP and lateral radiograph status post definitive reconstruction and lucency consistent with placement of monolateral external fixator. Normal anatomic parabola achieved of 140°

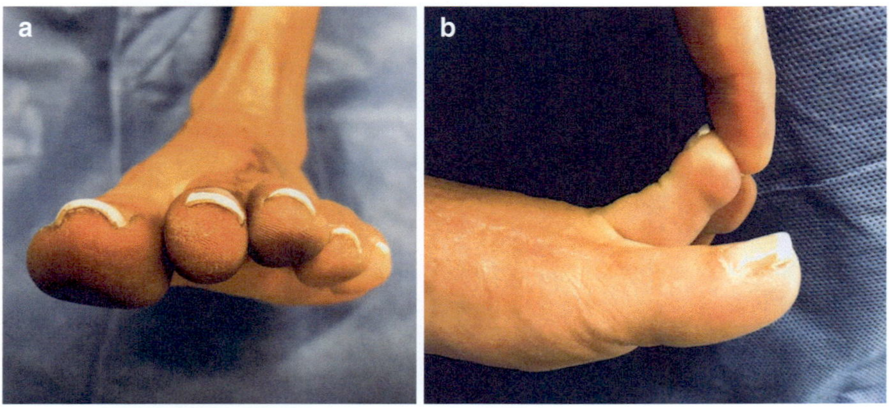

Fig. 29.14 (**a**, **b**) Coronal and sagittal clinical pictures demonstrating anatomic tri-planar alignment and passive range of motion equivalent to adjacent digits

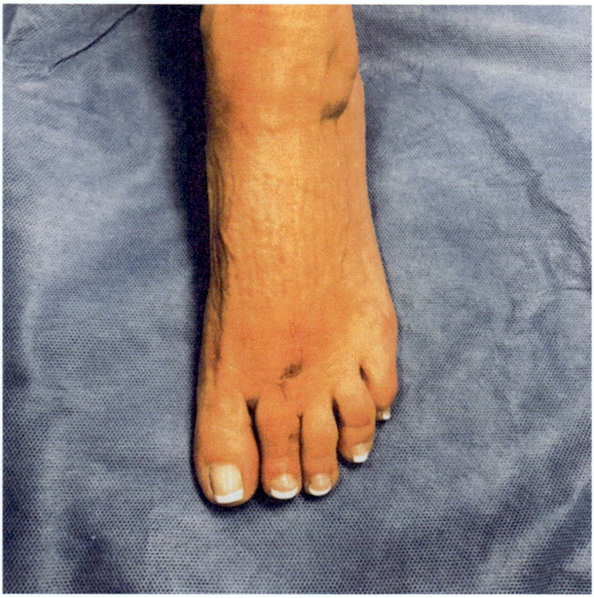

Fig. 29.15 AP clinical view of the foot at the patient's most recent clinical follow-up

Clinical Pearls

- A dorsal approach to foot reconstruction is a viable utilitarian approach to correct triplanar instability of the second MTPJ.
- Surgeon should be cognizant of the relative elongation of the second metatarsal relative to the first metatarsal as this could precipitate second MTPJ instability, lateral collateral ligament attenuation, and metatarsalgia.
- Incorporation of arthrodiastasis in combination with bone marrow aspirate concentrate allows for maintenance/restoration of length to the second ray complex while promoting revascularization to the bone and prevention of recurrent shortening.
- Careful colinear placement of the monolateral fixator with orthogonal fixation allows for stability of the construct during weight bearing.
- Using a Z-plasty incision allows for excellent exposure, and one should maintain acuity to no less than 60° to avoid apical necrosis. The monolateral external fixator allows an excellent means of minimizing edema and allows the skin envelope to heal uneventfully.
- Pin site care should include cleansing the area of the skin peripheral to the pins to mitigate colonization leading to pin site infection. Use of gauze peripheral to the pin sites further enables the mechanical management of pistoning which further decreases the risk of pin site irritation.
- Distraction of the leser MTPJ should not exceed 2–3 mm acutely as this could predispose to vasospasm and digital dysvascularity. This is accomplished with a third clamp integrated to the fixator using smaller 1.6 mm half pins.

This case illustrates the complex nature of managing second MTPJ pathology, particularly with pre-existing transverse plane instability. This patient presented with second metatarsal elongation that has been shown to be a driving force for collateral ligamentous disruption secondary to biomechnical overload [1, 2]. The literature is replete with success of dorsal foot reconstruction for lateral collateral ligamentous pathology [3, 4]. Iatrogenic shortening of the first metatarsal should always be considered as a nidus for this pathology as was evident prior to the patient's initial presentation [5].

Avascular necrosis of the second metatarsal may be treated with dorsal angulation metatarsal osteotomies, marrow stimulation, and interpositional arthroplasty; yet options may be limited when second ray length is an issue. In keeping with the technique utilized, Dr. Freiberg was the first to advocate for core decompression of the second metatarsal [6]. The goal of bone marrow aspirate concentrate is to stimulate mesenchymal stem cells to differentiate to functional osteoblasts [7]. Additionally, control of the catabolic environment and regulation of the cytokine cascade create regenerative effects to osteochondral damage [8].

Arthrodiastasis is a surgical technique used to promote morphoangiogenesis and serves to decrease subchondral sclerosis adjacent to joint surfaces through stress shielding. Studies have also shown an increase in intra-articular proteoglycan synthesis. Nociceptive fibers are located within the joint capsule, ligaments, periosteum, and subchondral bone. By distracting this allows for decreasing intra-articular pressure and thereby diminishes the nociceptive influence. Numerous reports have demonstrated efficacy with hip avascular necrosis in pathology such as Legg-Calvé-Perthes [9]. In the foot and ankle, it has been commonly employed for end-stage osteoarthritis of the first MTPJ and ankle joints [10–14]. It also has had utility in the management of osteochondral lesions within the tarsal bones [15].

References

1. Fleischer AE, Klein EE, Ahmad M, Shah S, Catena F, Weil LS Sr, Weil L Jr. Association of abnormal metatarsal parabola with second metatarsophalangeal joint plantar plate pathology. Foot Ankle Int. 2017;38(3):289–97.
2. Weber JR, Aubin PM, Ledoux WR, Sangeorzan BJ. Second metatarsal length is positively correlated with increased pressure and medial deviation of the second toe in a robotic cadaveric simulation of gait. Foot Ankle Int. 2012;33(4):312–9.
3. Phisitkul P, Hosuru Siddappa V, Sittapairoj T, Goetz JE, Den Hartog BD, Femino JE. Cadaveric evaluation of dorsal intermetatarsal approach for plantar plate and lateral collateral ligament repair of the lesser metatarsophalangeal joints. Foot Ankle Int. 2017;38(7):791–6.
4. Co AY, Ruch JA, Malay DS. Radiographic analysis of transverse plane digital alignment after surgical repair of the second metatarsophalangeal joint. J Foot Ankle Surg. 2006;45(6):380–99.
5. Ahn J, Lee HS, Seo JH, Kim JY. Second metatarsal transfer lesions due to first metatarsal shortening after distal chevron metatarsal osteotomy for hallux valgus. Foot Ankle Int. 2016;37(6):589–95.
6. Freiberg AA, Freiberg RA. Core decompression as a novel treatment for early Freiberg's infraction of the second metatarsal head. Orthopedics. 1995;18(12):1177–8.

7. Makihara T, Yoshioka T, Sugaya H, Aoto K, Wada H, Uemura K, Tanaka K, Akaogi H, Yamazaki M, Mishima H. Feasibility and efficacy of autologous bone marrow aspirate transplantation combined with human parathyroid hormone 1–34 administration to treat osteonecrosis in a rabbit model. Bone Marrow Res. 2017;2017:2484689.
8. Castagnini F, Pellegrini C, Perazzo L, Vannini F, Buda R. Joint sparing treatments in early ankle osteoarthritis: current procedures and future perspectives. J Exp Orthop. 2016;3(1):3.
9. Laklouk MA, Hosny GA. Hinged distraction of the hip joint in the treatment of Perthes disease: evaluation at skeletal maturity. J Pediatr Orthop B. 2012;21(5):386–93.
10. Van Valburg AA, van Roermund PM, Marijnissen AC, et al. Joint distraction in treatment of osteoarthritis: a 2 year follow-up of the ankle. Osteoarthr Cartil. 1999;7:474–9.
11. Marijnissen AC, van Roermund PM, van Melkebeek J, et al. Clinical benefit of joint distraction in the treatment of severe osteoarthritis of the ankle: proof of concept in an open prospective study and in a randomized controlled study. Arthritis Rheum. 2002;46:2893–902.
12. Paley D, Lamm BM. Ankle joint distraction. Foot Ankle Clin. 2005;10(4):685–98.
13. Ploegmakers JJW, van Roermund PM, van Melkebeek J, et al. Prolonged clinical benefit from joint distraction in the treatment of ankle osteoarthritis. Osteoarthr Cartil. 2005;13(7):582–8.
14. Ramanujam CL, Kissel S, Stewart A, Zgonis T. First metatarsophalangeal joint arthrodiastasis and biologic resurfacing with external fixation: a case report. Clin Podiatr Med Surg. 2012;29(1):137–41.
15. Saxena A, Fullem BW. A unique procedure for treatment of osteochondral lesions of the tarsal navicular: three cases in athletes. J Foot Ankle Surg. 2013;52(2):249–53.

Index

E. A. Cook, J. J. Cook (eds.), *Hammertoes*,
https://doi.org/10.1007/978-3-319-16552-3

Q

R

MIX
Papier aus verantwortungsvollen Quellen
Paper from responsible sources
FSC® C105338

If you have any concerns about our products,
you can contact us on
ProductSafety@springernature.com

In case Publisher is established outside the EU,
the EU authorized representative is:
Springer Nature Customer Service Center GmbH
Europaplatz 3, 69115 Heidelberg, Germany

Printed by Libri Plureos GmbH
in Hamburg, Germany